B Palmer
9/93 $40—

EVALUATING RADIOGRAPHS

EVALUATING RADIOGRAPHS

By

QUINN B. CARROLL, M.Ed., R.T.

Director
Radiography Department
Midland College
Midland, Texas

Photography by

William S. Heathman, B.S., R.T.

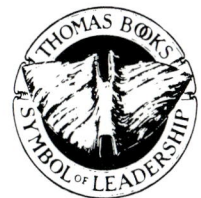

CHARLES C THOMAS • PUBLISHER
Springfield • Illinois • U.S.A.

Published and Distributed Throughout the World by

CHARLES C THOMAS • PUBLISHER
2600 South First Street
Springfield, Illinois 62794-9265

© *1993 by* CHARLES C THOMAS • PUBLISHER

ISBN 0-398-05878-4

Library of Congress Catalog Card Number: 93-8350

With THOMAS BOOKS *careful attention is given to all details of manufacturing
and design. It is the Publisher's desire to present books that are satisfactory as to
their physical qualities and artistic possibilities and appropriate for their particular
use.* THOMAS BOOKS *will be true to those laws of quality that assure a good
name and good will.*

Printed in the United States of America
SC-R-3

Library of Congress Cataloging-in-Publication Data

Carroll, Quinn B.
    Evaluating radiographs / by Quinn B. Carroll ; photography by
William S. Heathman.
        p.   cm.
    Includes index.
    ISBN 0-398-05878-4 (cloth)
    1. Radiography, Medical—Evaluation.   I. Title.
    [DNLM: 1. Radiography—methods.   WN 200 C319e   1993]
RC78.C349   1993
616.07'572—dc20
DNLM/DLC   93-8350
for Library of Congress   CIP

To
Margaret Nielsen Carroll
Jason
Melissa
Chad
Tiffani
Brandon
Tyson

PREFACE

This textbook does not contain very many good radiographs! And for a good reason: Positioning textbooks generally present ideal radiographs to illustrate the products of correct positioning. These are of little help, however, in determining the corrective actions needed to ensure that *repeated* radiographs are done right.

Because of the great number of variables with which they must cope, all radiographers have to repeat exposures occasionally in daily practice. Yet, no radiograph should have to be repeated more than one time. On observing the original image, the radiographer should be able to assess all of the needed adjustments in both technique and positioning in order to produce an optimum view when the exposure is repeated. For example, on a single view the density may need to be darker, certain artifacts removed, rotation of the body part corrected and perhaps a little less angulation of the x-ray beam employed.

An incomplete education has produced many technologists with an ability to recognize when a spine position (for example) is rotated, but not *which way* it is rotated and *how much,* or with the ability to see when the x-ray beam angle for a sunrise view of the knee is off, but not whether it is angled *too much* or *not enough.* What value is there in recognizing that something is wrong about a radiographic image if one cannot accurately determine the type and amount of adjustment needed to correct it?

Don Q. Paris published a wonderful book in 1983, *Craniographic Positioning with Comparison Studies,* the first to address this issue, but limited the scope of the text to skull positions only. It is a daunting task to attempt to address fully the evaluation of all aspects of the radiographic image, including not only all anatomical areas of interest but also the technical quality of the image. To make the amount of information manageable for both the student and the author, this text (1) excludes nonroutine or rare procedures and views, (2) only demonstrates *incorrect* positions for most procedures, using correct positions only on those very challenging and rare cases such as mastoid series or SI joints, and (3) focuses primarily upon reliable skeletal criteria and combines procedures which share criteria where ever possible. For example, the amount of rotation in the pelvis can be determined by the bony structures whether it is for a cystogram, IVP, sacrum, pelvis, or barium enema. Therefore, the appearance of soft tissue organs in contrast studies (which is highly variable) is covered only briefly.

Section II of this book may be best used by laying it alongside your positioning manual for comparison with correctly positioned views. The author has made every effort to keep the text clear, concise, and to the point, and would appreciate any suggestions for future editions.

The capability to evaluate radiographs is fundamental to each technologist's performance and to keeping patient dose from unnecessary retakes at a minimum. It is hoped that this text will contribute substantially to that goal.

QBC

ACKNOWLEDGMENTS

I would like to extend grateful acknowledgment to William S. Heathman, R.T., for his photography and help in producing this textbook, as well as for his personal friendship.

Special thanks to Shawna Loyd for the massive amount of hand development of photographs and special darkroom techniques required for a work of this nature, and for the assistance of Vanessa Gunn and Lori Fuson in the photographic darkroom.

I am grateful for the professional support of Eileen F. Piwetz and Charles J. Engbretson throughout my educational career, and for my earliest role model of professionalism in health care, Sherri Uzelac, R.T.

CONTENTS

PART II—POSITIONING QUALITY

EVALUATING RADIOGRAPHS

PART I
GENERAL CONSIDERATIONS

Chapter 1

IDENTIFICATION, ASSESSMENT AND LABELLING

Careful identification of the patient and labelling of the radiograph seem to be such simple tasks that they may not be taken seriously by many students and radiographers. Yet the consequences of an error in this regard can be among the most profound in the practice of radiography. Consider the following: Approximately 500 radiology patients die each year due to allergic reactions to contrast agents used for intravenous urography and other procedures. Suppose the wrong patient was brought into the radiographic room for such a procedure, and this patient was highly allergic? Such mistakes can and do happen. One radiographer called for a "Mr. Johnson" and performed a complete IVP series. Afterward it was discovered that there had been two patients in the waiting area with the surname "Johnson." The IVP patient was still waiting, and the wrong patient, who had endured the injection and procedure, had not been assertive enough to fully question the radiographer's proceeding.

This is only one of many examples of improper identification which could lead to serious injury and malpractice lawsuits. Further, when any medical case with a radiologic component goes to court, radiographs may be required as evidence, at which time any stickers or writing made on a radiograph after exposure will be called into question, especially if they contradict original information "flashed" or radiographically exposed onto the film. The same emphasis must be placed on proper "right" and "left" marker placement and other labelling on the radiograph pertinent to diagnosis.

As radiologists are in less direct contact with patients, they rely increasingly upon the technologist to acquire pertinent clinical histories which are essential to proper diagnosis. It is natural that the technologist should obtain and note this information, because the condition of the patient directly bears upon the projections that the radiographer may decide to take, and upon anticipated adjustments in radiographic technique that may prevent repeated exposures.

As an integral member of the radiological health care team, the radiographer must assume professional responsibility for careful identification and assessment of each patient and for proper identification and labelling of each radiograph.

ASSESSING THE REQUISITION AND THE PATIENT

The requisition received by the radiographer should state the exact anatomical area to be radiographed, and the suspected diagnosis or purpose of the procedure. If there is any question regarding the views desired, the radiographer or a supervisor should contact the referring department or office for clarification. For example, a requisition for "AP and Lateral Hips," without *right* and *left* hips specifically noted, should be clarified: Are two views of one hip desired, or is this a bilateral examination? Frequently the suspected diagnosis or purpose of the procedure may be absent on the written requisition, and this information must be obtained by questioning the patient.

In any case, the patient should always be briefly questioned about his or her history and condition, both as a confirmation of data on the requisition and for information that might be germane to how the procedure should be performed. Common changes made in radiographic procedures due to historical information include:

1. Any optional views that might be indicated beside the routine views normally taken
2. Any modifications in positioning that might be indicated or positioning aids that might be needed
3. Any modifications in technical factors that might be anticipated to produce the proper image density, contrast, and sharpness

One patient, for example, demonstrated the entrance wound of a sliver just behind the medial malleolus of the ankle. The radiographer elected to take an additional, nonroutine view—an external oblique which projected this sliver free of superimposition of any bones that would interfere with a confident diagnosis. Tangential views are often indicated for superficial foreign bodies such as slivers, Figure 1.

The condition of the patient is the greatest variable which the radiographer faces in producing quality radiographs. In addition to being aware of the normal variations in body habitus, tissue composition, age, bony structure, stage of respiration, presence of contrast agents, and thickness of body parts, one must also be conscious of abnormal changes

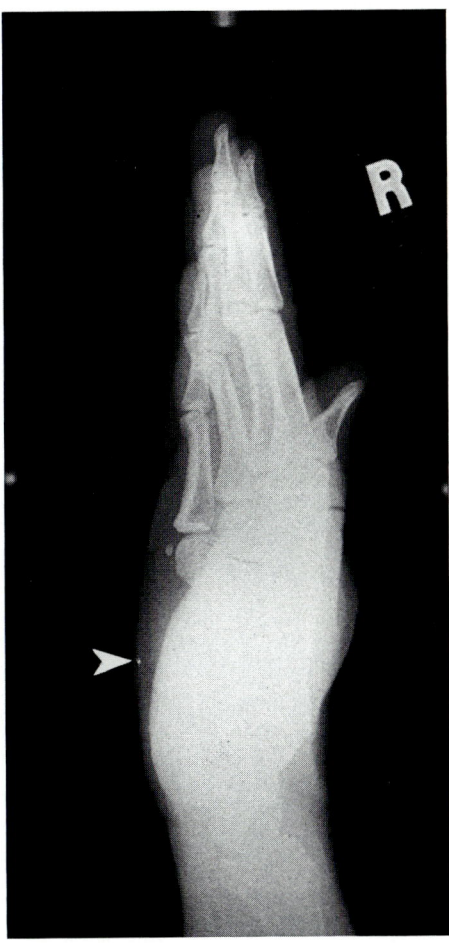

Figure 1. A nonroutine *tangential* projection (lateral oblique) of the hand demonstrating a small metal sliver (arrow) superficially lodged in the palm. A soft tissue technique of 46 kVp at the usual mAs was employed.

due to pathology or medical intervention. An example of medical intervention which alters the course of a radiologic examination is hip surgery. If a total hip prosthesis or a surgical pin has been implanted, the centering for the AP view of the bilateral hips would be modified: Instead of centering as usual to the pelvis, the AP view must be centered four to six inches lower in order to include the entire length of the hip prosthesis or surgical pin, Figure 2. Failure to gather historical information such as previous surgery before initiating the radiologic examination results in unnecessary repeats and expense, as well as increased patient exposure to radiation.

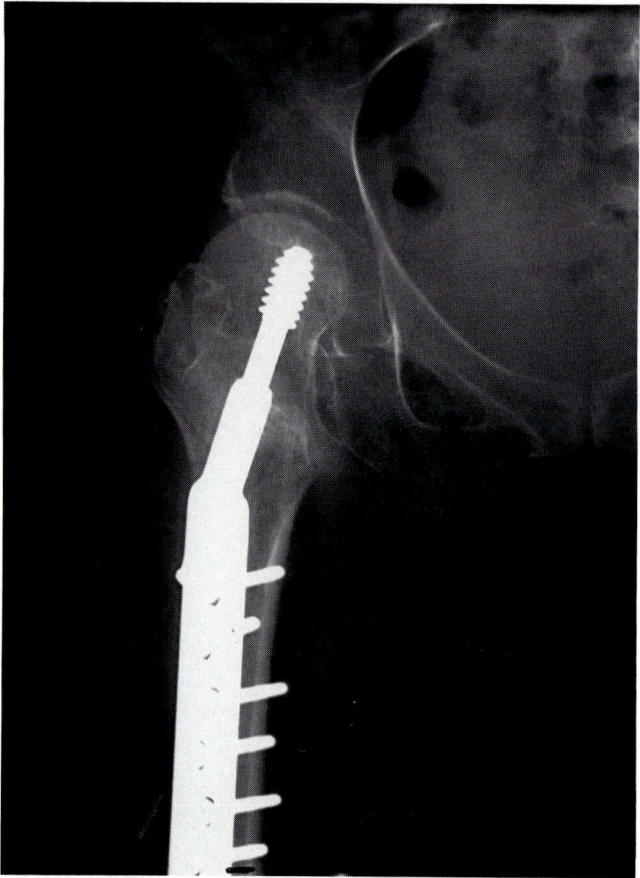

Figure 2. An AP projection of the unilateral hip clipping off the bottom of the surgical hip pin. This centering would have been acceptable for a normal hip, but a history of hip pinning indicates a modification in centering, four inches lower.

Such information can be obtained from:

1. The requisition
2. The patient when possible
3. The patient's chart

Radiographers should have at least a rudimentary ability to interpret patients' charts. Careful observation of the patient frequently provides readily apparent signs of conditions that bear on technique selection. It should be emphasized that obtaining pertinent patient history and assessing conditions that affect radiographic technique are the responsibility of the *radiographer,* not the referring physician or the radiologist.

Not all diseases are radiographically visible. Many do not appreciably affect the densities present in the image, and are therefore of no concern in determining techniques. For a pathological condition to require a technique adjustment, it must substantially alter the presence and amount of the five radiographically demonstrable materials. These five types of substances, in order of increasing x-ray attentuation, are:

1. Gas, such as air
2. Fat
3. Fluid (or more properly, liquid)
4. Bone
5. Metals

Generally, soft tissues such as connective tissues, muscles and visceral organs are of "fluid" density, equal to water radiographically. Barium and iodine compounds are, chemically, metals. Using soft tissue or fluid as a background, gas (air) and fat are demonstrated against the soft tissue because of extreme differences in their physical density. On the other hand, bone and metals including contrast agents are demonstrated because of their atomic numbers (large atoms).

Additive Conditions

Abnormal conditions which lead to an increase in *fluid, bone,* or *metal* are, for radiographic purposes, generally considered as *additive conditions.* They require added exposure, or increased technique factors, in order to be properly demonstrated. In the case of excessive bone tissue or metals, the increase in technique is necessitated mostly because of their high average atomic numbers (large atoms). For fluid accumulation in the lungs, an increase in factors is required because the fluid is nearly a thousand times more dense than the air which is normally present (there are one-thousand molecules of fluid for every molecule of air). Fluid distention of the abdomen, on the other hand, does not substantially change atomic numbers nor tissue density, but results in an increase in part thickness, and requires a doubling of the technique for every four centimeters of added thickness. In each of these cases, more x-ray photons are absorbed by the body tissues, and if an increase in technical

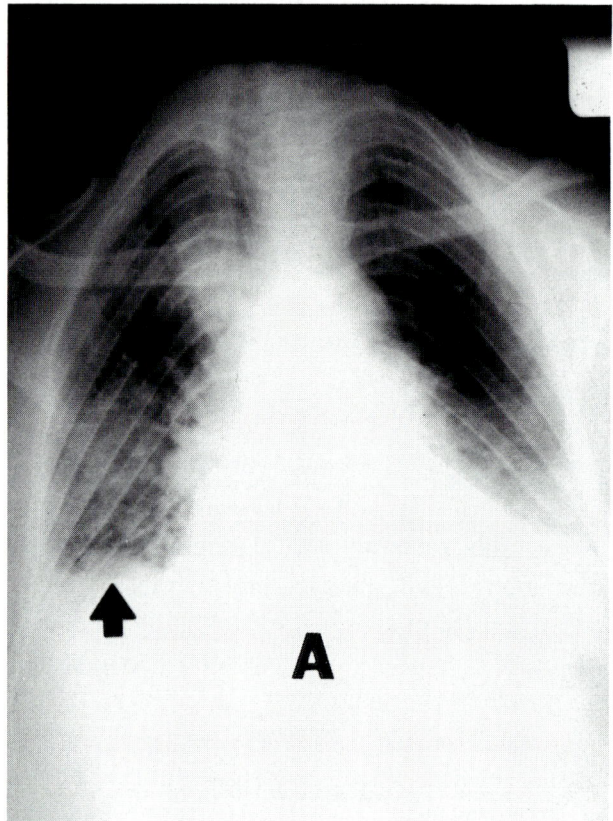

Figure 3-A. The pulmonary edema (arrow) is radiographically additive and requires an increase in technique.

factors is not effected, an underexposed, light radiograph will result, Figure 3-A.

For additive diseases, technique may need to be increased from 35 percent (⅓) to over 100 percent (doubling) if the disease is in an advanced stage. *As a rule of thumb, additive diseases require a 50 percent increase in overall technique.* Some examples of additive diseases which are commonly encountered in radiography include acromegaly, osteoarthritis, osteochondroma, osteopetrosis, osteomyelitis, Pagets disease, advanced syphilis, osteoarthritis, actinomycosis, fibrous carcinomas, cardiomegaly, cirrhosis, pneumoconiosis, pulmonary tuberculosis, ascites, pulmonary edema, hydrocephalus, hydropneumothorax, pleural effusion, and pneumonia.

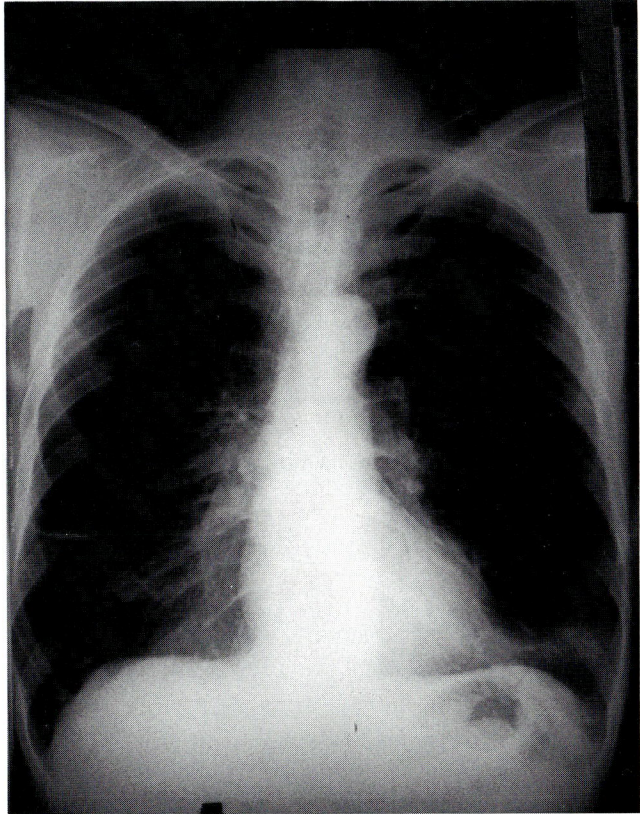

Figure 3-B. Emphysema is radiographically destructive and requires a decrease in technique.

It is well to reiterate the difference between fluid distention of the abdomen and obesity. When the abdomen is truly distended due to ascites or severe infection, the skin is tight and rather hard to the touch. The obese patient, on the other hand, presents very loose, flaccid skin that is soft to the touch. For two patients measuring the same thickness, the technique increase required for the fluid-distended patient will be considerably *more* than that for the obese patient.

Destructive Conditions

Abnormal conditions which lead to an increase in *air* or *fat*, or to a *decrease* in normal body fluid or bone, are radiographically considered as *destructive conditions*. These require a reduction from typical exposure techniques in order to be properly demonstrated. Both air and fat are significantly less dense than fluid, and absorb fewer x-ray photons.

For destructive diseases, overall technique may need to be reduced by 30 to 50 percent, Figure 3-B. *As a rule of thumb, destructive diseases require a 30 percent decrease in technique.* Examples of destructive diseases commonly encountered in radiography include aseptic necrosis, various bone carcinomas, Ewing's tumor, exostosis, gout, Hodgkin's disease, hyperparathyroidism, osteitis fibrosa cystica, osteoporosis, osteomalacia, rheumatoid arthritis, blastomycosis, bowel obstructions, emphysema and pneumothorax. Dark radiographs result when these diseases are advanced unless technique is reduced.

Trauma

The challenges in determining optimum radiographic techniques for most trauma patients relate to the above discussion of disease conditions, particularly in regard to presence of excess fluids or gasses within the tissues. For example, pneumothoraces are common in trauma patients and, due to excessive aeration, require a reduced technique. Internal bleeding in the abdomen or hematomas in the brain may require a 30 percent increase in mAs, while blood pooling in the lungs can necessitate increases from 30 to 100 percent more than normal.

Casts and splints also require an increase in technique, from 50 to 100 percent, or the resulting radiograph will be too light. These are further discussed in Chapter 3.

Postmortem Radiography

Experienced radiographers learn to expect considerable pooling of blood and fluids in dead bodies, particularly in the head, thorax, and abdomen. An increase in technique, typically about 35 percent increase in mAs, may be anticipated. Even shortly after death, blood and fluids will begin to pool in the lungs, and since postmortem radiographs are taken with the body recumbent, the fluids will pool across the entire lung field. In addition, bear in mind that postmortem radiography is by definition an *expiration* chest technique. Without the normal air insufflation of the lungs, an increase in technique is indicated. *Postmortem chest techniques must be increased by at least 30 percent (one-third),* and may require a 50 percent increase, depending on the amount of time since death. This 30 percent rule should be applied on the *first* exposure attempted, or a repeated exposure will very likely be needed.

Soft-Tissue Technique

Frequently trauma patients will present with suspected small foreign bodies such as slivers of wood, glass, or metal, or swallowed bones. These are better visualized by using a reduced *soft tissue technique.*

Metal and most types of glass are actually highly radiopaque, but very small slivers of the same can be difficult to detect. Chicken bones or similar objects which may become lodged in the laryngopharynx are often not very dense in cortical bone and have only slight radiographic contrast. Wood splinters are especially troublesome: Because of the air pockets they contain, they may show up early on as a slightly *darker* density, radiolucent against a soft tissue background. But in a brief period of time wood splinters will absorb fluid from the surrounding tissues and become very difficult indeed to distinguish from tissue. The technique employed must be tailored to demonstrate soft tissue, rather than the usual bone tissue.

To maximize the visualization of these small foreign objects, image contrast must be enhanced and overall density must be lightened up. A reduction in kVp will accomplish both of these objectives, as demonstrated in Figure 1. There should be no attempt to "compensate" for the drop in kVp by adjusting mAs. As a rule of thumb, *for soft tissue techniques, subtract ten to twelve kVp from the average technique without changing mAs.* In addition to demonstrating small foreign bodies, such techniques show any damage to soft tissues. Soft tissue visualization is most frequently called for in radiography of the hands and of the neck.

Body Habitus

Perhaps the first characteristic the radiographer takes note of in assessing the condition of patients is their overall body habitus and the thickness of the part of interest. Many radiographs turn out too light simply because the radiographer was negligent in making a careful assessment of *both* the thickness and the type of body habitus that the patient presents.

Generally, *radiographic technique must be doubled for every four centimeters of additional part thickness beyond the average.* Likewise, technique should be reduced by one-half for every four centimeters less than average thickness. Failure to assess the part thickness and adjust technique by this "four-centimeter" rule will result in radiographs that are too light or too dark.

The radiographer must also assess the body habitus and the tissue composition of the part to be radiographed. As mentioned earlier, fluid-equivalent tissues require more technique than fatty tissues to produce optimum image density. This means that a large muscular patient will require much more technique than an obese patient of similar size. Age and sex have a bearing on body habitus. Generally, females and young children have more body fat than males. The bones of young children are cartilagenous and not fully calcified, requiring less penetrating power (kVp) of the x-ray beam. Very old patients lose calcium and other minerals from their bones and also require reduced technique. Of course, there are exceptions to these general statements, and the radiographer must assess the condition of each patient in terms of overall habitus.

Body habitus may be categorized into four general types: Sthenic, hypersthenic, hyposthenic and asthenic. The *sthenic* patient is healthy and active, with a physique relatively heavy in bone and muscle. Average techniques are based upon the sthenic body habitus.

The *hypersthenic* patient is characterized by a soft and rounded physique with an excess of subcutaneous fat, and tends to become obese. Generally, technique must be increased according to the "four-centimeter rule" for such patients due to their larger thickness.

Note that a very large patient is not necessarily hypersthenic in habitus. Some patients are unusually tall, big-boned, and muscle-bound. This is a sthenic habitus, yet it requires a much *greater* increase in technique than the "four-centimeter rule" calls for.

The *hyposthenic* patient is healthy, but much thinner than average. Technique should be reduced by the "four-centimeter rule."

The *asthenic* patient is physically weak and emaciated from pathological conditions or advanced age. This patient appears linear and delicate with stringy muscles. Beside reducing technique for the smaller size of the body, a further reduction in x-ray beam penetration (kVp) is often required for asthenic patients because of the extreme loss of bony minerals and dehydration of tissues.

There are physical differences in the mass, density, and shape of various bones for different human races, which are often substantial enough to require adjustments in radiographic technique. This is particularly true for skull radiography. A workable rule of thumb cannot be stated for any particular anthropological group, for at least two reasons: First, there is too much variation within a racial group, and second, racial groups have become widely intermixed. However, an observant radiographer will recognize those patients whose skull appears to be *brachicephalic,* that is, relatively round and broad in shape rather than oval. Brachicephalic skulls typically have a greater bony mass than average, and require about one-third more technique than average for all views.

In addition to assessing the patient's age, habitus and condition, the radiographer must beware of any clothing items, jewelry, prostheses such as false eyes, or orthopedic devices which might be safely removed to prevent artifacts from obscuring important diagnostic information on the resulting radiograph. Artifacts are further discussed in Chapter 3.

RADIOGRAPH IDENTIFICATION AND LABELLING

Patient identification must be "flashed" or photographically exposed onto the film in the blocker area whenever possible. If the wrong identification is flashed onto a film, it is often possible to correct it prior to development by "triple-flashing," flashing the correct ID three times. This will almost obliterate the original information and is usually legible. If the error is not corrected prior to processing, stickers with the correct information must be placed so as to completely cover the original data.

The *minimum* information that should be included in identifying each radiograph is:

1. Patient name or ID number
2. Date of the procedure
3. Institution performing the procedure

In addition, many departments require the patient's date of birth or age, time of day the procedure was performed, or other data.

"Right" and "left" markers must be used strictly to label the anatomy, and not the position. For example, they should never be used to indicate which side is down on decubitus or oblique positions. Such practices greatly increase the probability of errors. The only function of the marker is to indicate which side of the anatomy is right or left.

On radiographs of the extremities, markers should be placed lateral to the anatomy. On a typical radiograph there are several acceptable locations where a marker may be placed. Common sense must be employed to assure that the marker location is not likely to superimpose the *anatomy of interest.* For example, on a PA chest radiograph it is acceptable for the marker to be placed over the shoulder bones because they are not of interest, Figure 4. The lungs, which are of interest, are narrower at the top and leave plenty of room in the upper corners of the film for marker placement. The lungs are broadest near the bottom, and markers should never be placed in this region of the cassette. The same rules apply to placement of the film identification blocker.

One might ask why the radiologist wouldn't know right from left

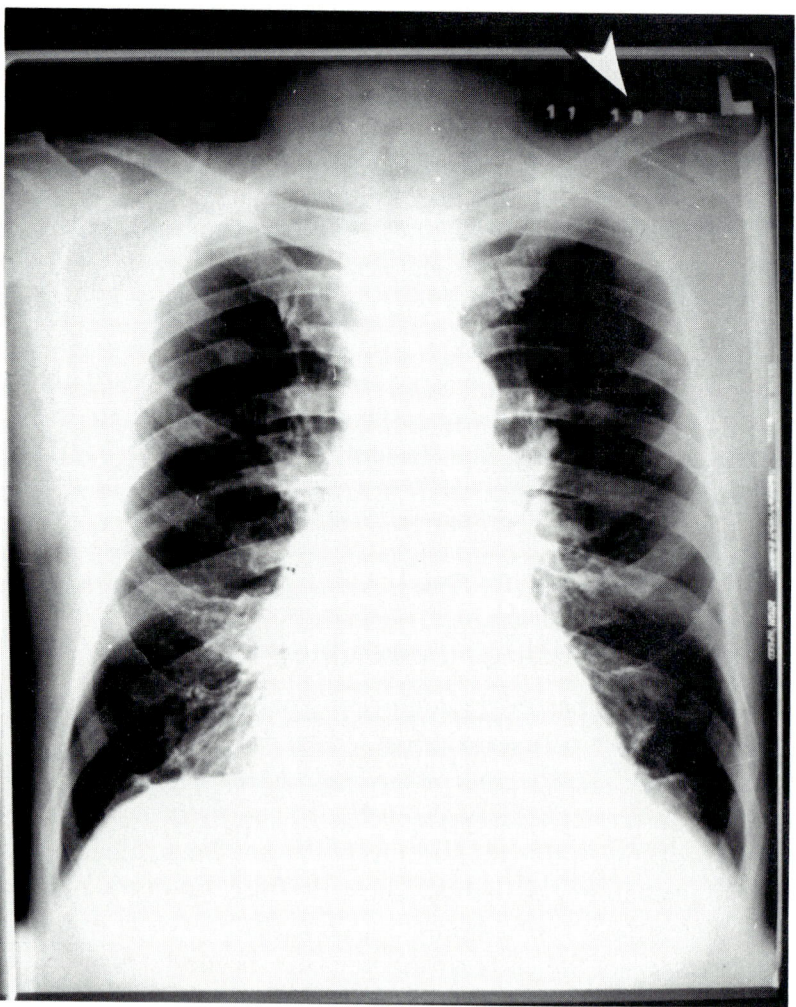

Figure 4. Placement of the blocker over the shoulder bones (arrow) is acceptable since the shoulder anatomy is not of direct interest on a chest series.

without markers on the radiograph. Patients may present with partial or complete situs inversus. In partial situs inversus, the patient's heart is reversed in position with the apex to the right, but the abdominal organs such as the stomach are in their usual location. This condition is obvious. However, in complete situs inversus *all* organs, both thoracic and abdominal, are reversed in position. Repeat radiographs may be requested to confirm the diagnosis, but it is essential that the right or left marker be placed correctly.

Special markers are available and should be used to indicate when the radiograph is taken in upright, decubitus, or other special positions, to indicate postevacuation, postvoiding, scout views or timed radiographs. The above guidelines should be followed in placing these markers as well. This type of information should never be written on a processed radiograph when lead markers are available. Legally, the lead markers are more reliable as evidence. On many mobile procedures, and occasionally on routine radiographs, other special information must be written on the radiograph with permanent ink or placed on special labels.

Chapter 2

RADIATION PROTECTION

The general topic of radiation protection can fill an entire course, but this discussion shall be limited to those radiation protection practices that are visible on a finished radiograph and therefore become part of the criteria in critiquing the image. These include the size and type of film cassette used, proper collimation of the x-ray field size, and lead shielding used on the patient. Since the quality of positioning and technique used in producing the radiograph (discussed in Parts II and III of this book) determine whether repeat exposures are needed, it might be said that anything which assures good radiographic quality on the first exposure is a preventative form of good radiation protection practice.

CASSETTE AND FILM TYPE

Modern radiology departments frequently use two or more types of image receptor systems (screen/film combinations) in their cassettes. For general radiography, most departments use cassettes variously labelled as "medium," "regular," or "high" speed. For distal extremity radiographs, *extremity cassettes* or *detail cassettes* are often preferred in order to maximize sharpness. These cassettes are much "slower" than the regular cassettes, and require from three to seven times greater exposure to produce adequate image density. Astute radiologists require chest radiographs to be taken with special high latitude "chest cassettes" and "chest film." These cassettes and film are designed to produce a longer scale of grays in the image (with lower contrast), in order to visualize more details in the lungs and heart. Used correctly, exposures for these systems are about the same as those for the regular cassettes.

However, if film and screens are mismatched, or if the wrong type of screen cassette is used for the anatomy, the resulting image quality will be poor and a repeated exposure will be needed, causing excess radiation to the patient. If special extremity film is loaded into a regular cassette, or if regular film is loaded into an extremity cassette, the image will usually turn out light. Some types of extremity film have emulsion on only one side. This emulsion side holds the image. It appears duller than the nonemulsion side. The side of the film without emulsion has a very glossy sheen, appears shiny and feels slick by comparison.

If high latitude "chest" film is mistakenly loaded into a regular cassette, the resulting radiograph will appear unusually gray and "washed out" as shown in Figure 5. If regular film is misloaded into a "chest" cassette, the chest radiograph will appear unusually contrasty, too black and white. Either case will require a repeated exposure to the patient, because the radiologist must have consistent image quality for proper diagnoses.

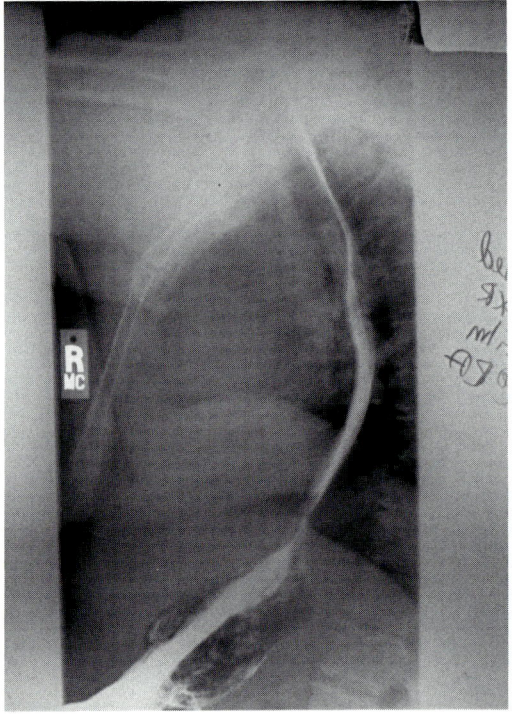

Figure 5. High latitude chest film mistakenly loaded into a regular speed cassette for an esophagram. Note the washed out light gray appearance.

COLLIMATION AND CASSETTE SIZE

The minimizing of patient exposure should be of paramount concern to every radiographer, and limiting the size of the x-ray beam is one of the most effective ways to minimize exposure. By controlling field size, organs with critical sensitivity to radiation such as the gonads, thyroid gland, and lenses of the eyes can be kept outside of the primary beam. The difference between including a particular organ of the body within the direct x-ray beam and placing it just outside the edge of the x-ray beam is a ratio of 1/100. That is, the organ will receive approximately one hundred times more radiation inside the beam than it does just outside the edge of the beam.

Several devices are available for collimating the field size and shape. Modern radiographic units are required to have rectangular collimators. Cones and cylinders provide a smaller, round field which is more fitting for anatomy such as the gall bladder or the sinuses. The field size should generally not be more than 20 percent larger than the anatomy of interest. On the other hand, overcollimating (collimating too tight) to the point of clipping off any anatomy of interest, as shown in Figure 6 will result in a repeated exposure, which doubles the necessary amount of radiation to the patient. A key point in avoiding this error is to remember that the edges of the collimated light field can be, and often are, as much as one-half inch inaccurate. The edges of the actual x-ray beam may be one-half inch *inside* or one-half inch *outside* of the light field. Therefore, on extremity procedures such as a hand series, *always allow at least one-half inch of light field around each edge of the anatomy.*

Selection of an appropriate cassette size as an issue in radiation protection bears emphasis. When an oversized cassette is used, the technologist will be less likely to collimate properly and critical organs such as the eye lens may be unnecessarily exposed, as shown in Figure 7. The cassette size should be just large enough to be sure the anatomy of interest is completely depicted with a reasonable margin for error. What, then, is reasonable? An additional 10 to 20 percent of the anatomy size will usually suffice—an extra inch to two inches around each side of a ten-inch anatomical part. Of course, for pediatric radiography, a bit more margin for error is needed to account for possible movement.

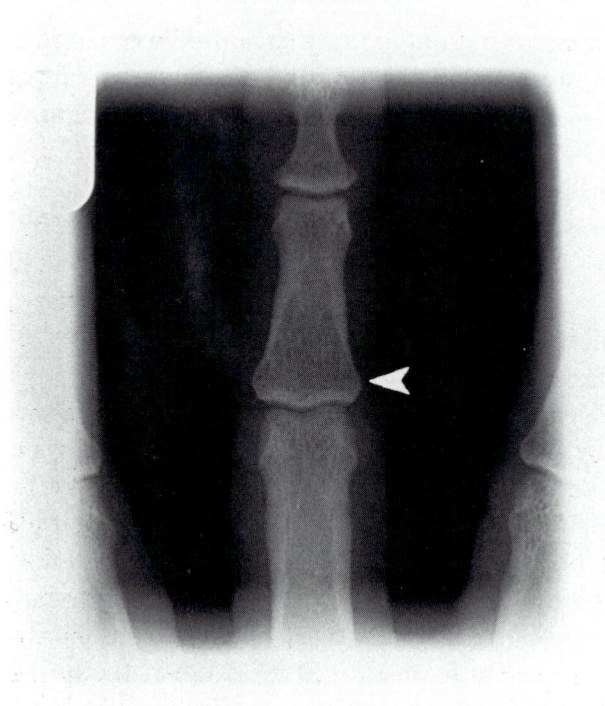

Figure 6. This PA finger was correctly centered to the PIP joint (arrow), but overcollimation resulted in clipping the anatomy.

SHIELDING

It is important to use lead shielding of the gonads on any procedure in their vicinity *if the shielding will not obscure the anatomy of interest.* Whenever there is a substantial risk of getting the lead shield over any anatomy of interest, it should not be used. Often, the use of tape or other methods to hold a small shield in place will allow the best compromise for both a good radiograph and good protection. A common mistake is to use too large a gonad shield on a premature infant for a hip radiograph, where even slight off-centering of slippage of the shield will obscure the right or left acetabulum or femoral head. Most often, shields can be used if they are properly placed, Figure 8. Placing a lead waist apron too high for a chest radiograph risks obscuring the costophrenic angles of the

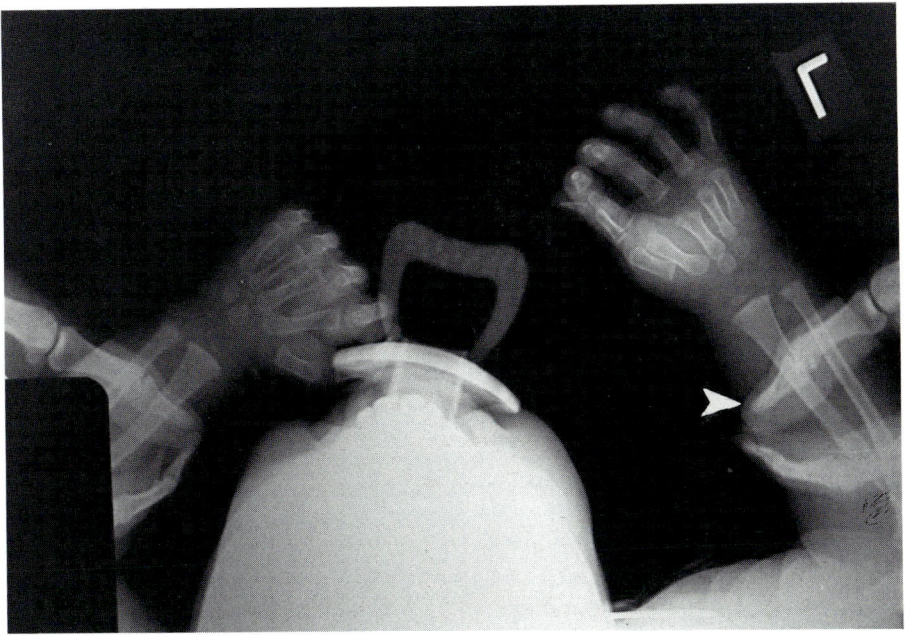

Figure 7. A misguided attempt to perform a bilateral hand view on a child, using excessive film and field size. The child's eyes, highly sensitive to radiation, are in the primary beam, and the parents hands (arrow) are being exposed.

lungs. Placing the top of the apron at the level of the iliac crest reliably covers the gonads for either sex, Figure 9.

MINIMIZING REPEATED EXPOSURES

It cannot be overstated that the single greatest contributor to unnecessary radiation dose to patients is the repeating of exposures due to poor positioning or poor technical quality. A repeat doubles the dose to the patient. High repeat rates can be reduced by:

1. Proper education and training in both positioning and selection of technique
2. Continuing education
3. Repeat analysis for departments and individuals
4. Quality control programs for processors and radiographic units
5. The proper use of technique charts

These topics are fully covered in good radiographic imaging textbooks.

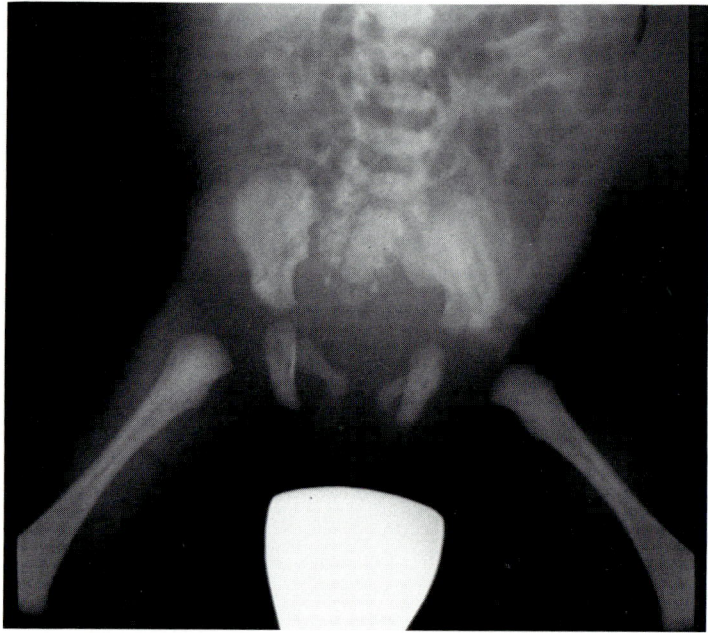

Figure 8. Proper placement of a lead gonad shield on a male infant for an AP pelvis view, avoiding superimposition of bony anatomy.

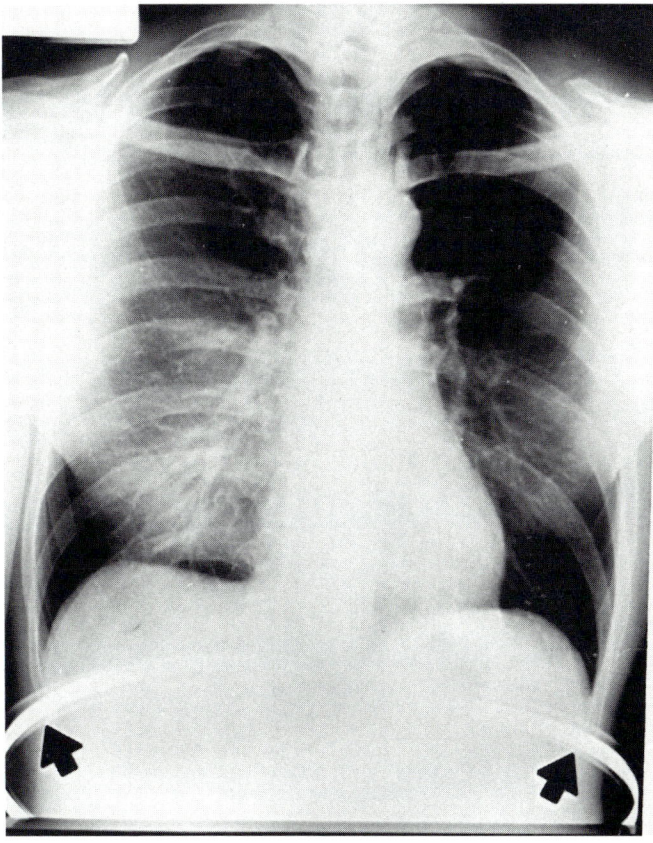

Figure 9. The ring from a lead waist apron (arrows) almost superimposes the costophrenic angles of the lungs on this PA chest view. Any higher placement of the apron may have resulted in a repeat.

Chapter 3

EXPOSURE-RELATED ARTIFACTS

In assessing the patient prior to a radiographic procedure, the radiographer must be aware of any removable prosthetic or orthopedic devices, casts, parts of clothing or items in the hair which may impede full visualization of the anatomy of interest. Carelessness during the procedure can also result in parts of equipment, such as electrical cables or intravenous lines, getting in the way of the exposure and causing artifacts on the radiograph. When patients must be held, carelessness can result in the radiographer's own hands or the hands of a parent being superimposed over the anatomy of interest, as shown in Figure 7 in the last chapter. The patient's own head, arms, or hands sometimes get in the way, as on the mammogram in Figure 10.

An *artifact* may be defined in a dictionary as "a product of artificial character due to an extraneous agency." That is, it is not natural, and it is caused or created by something outside itself, such as a human. On a radiograph, an artifact is an image which does not represent the real anatomy of the patient, and that is either created by the process of producing the radiograph or caused by a man-made object.

Understanding the geometry of the x-ray beam helps to eliminate and diagnose the specific causes of many artifacts: As an object is placed farther and farther from the film cassette (or nearer to the x-ray tube), its projected "shadow" on the radiograph will become more magnified in size and more blurry at the edges, Figure 18. A sharp, clear artifact which appears to have a realistic size was probably caused by an object near, on or *in* cassette. A slightly blurred artifact was most likely caused by an object on or near the surface of the patient. A grossly magnified and blurred artifact was most likely caused by an object suspended over the patient or attached to the x-ray tube itself.

Prior to beginning a radiographic procedure, the technologist also makes an estimation of the probability that the patient motion might occur during the exposure, knowing that small children, retarded patients, inebriated patients, trauma patients who are suffering much pain, and

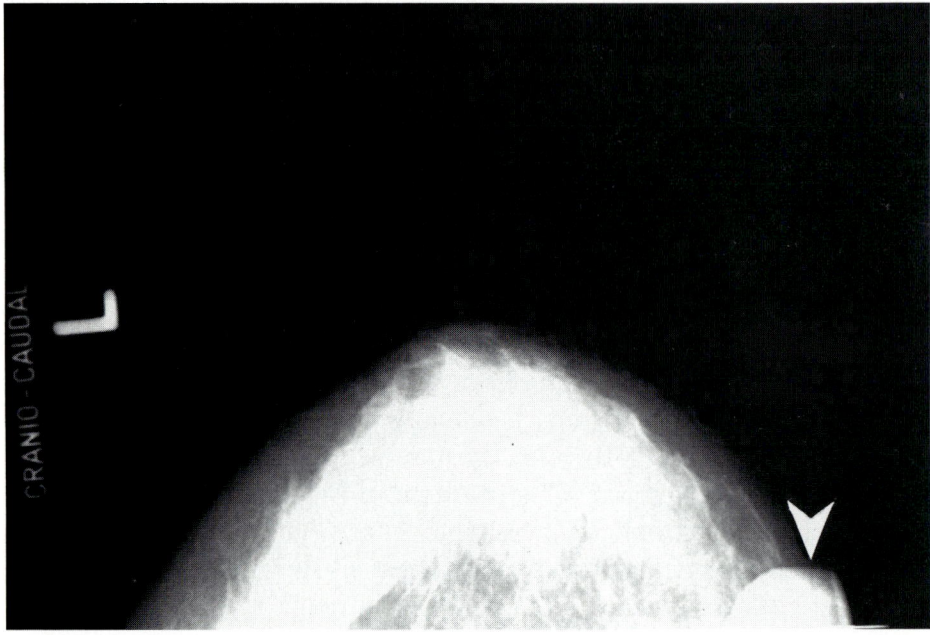

Figure 10. A cranio-caudal projection for a mammogram in which the patient's nose (arrow) was caught in the beam and projected over the anatomy of interest.

senile patients are more likely to move. In such cases when the probability of motion is high, extra immobilization methods and modified techniques must be anticipated and used on the first attempts at producing quality radiographs.

PATIENT–RELATED ARTIFACTS

Below is a partial listing of the types of items which might be inadvertently left on the patient's person during a radiographic exposure. Most of these objects are radiopaque and show up "white" or lighter than soft tissue on the image.

> Necklaces, rings, and other jewelry
> Hairpins, barrettes, wigs, and other hair ornaments
> Keys, cigarette lighters and other items left in pockets
> Glasses, hearing aids, dentures, false eyes, and other prosthetic or cosmetic devices
> Snaps, buttons, thick seams, and ornaments on clothing
> Blood-soaked hair or braided hair

Folded, matted or blood-soaked clothing, gowns, sheets, blankets, or
  gauze

Figures 11 and 12 demonstrate two examples of negligence on the part of
the radiographer in assessing the patient prior to exposure. Remember,
proper assessment includes talking to the patient and *asking if he/she has
any hairpins, prostheses, false eyes, removable orthodontic devices, etc.* in addition to careful observation. For chest radiographs, braided hair, pony-
tails or pig-tails must be set on top of the shoulders, sometimes with tape,
to keep them out of the lung fields.

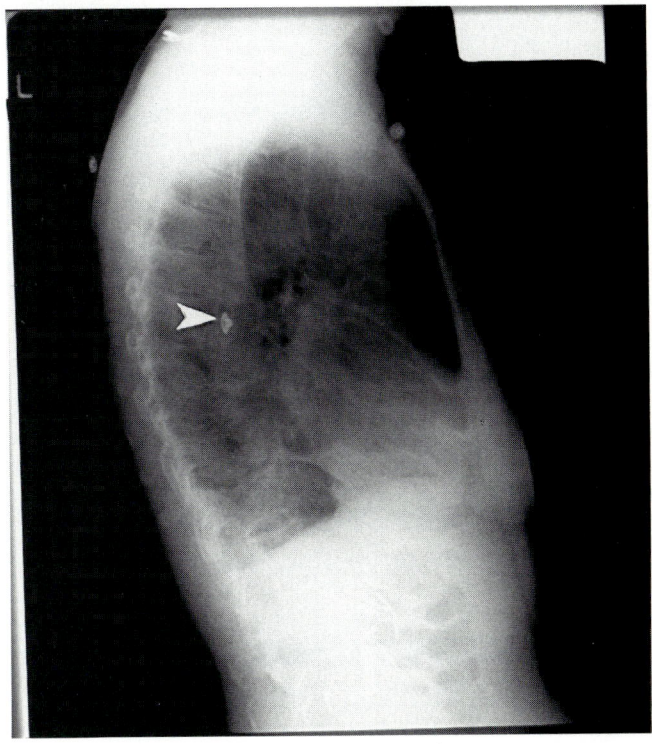

Figure 11. Patient gown snap (arrow) projected into lung field, a common hindrance for
radiographers.

Intravenous lines, catheters, electrical leads, or other equipment attached
to the patient must be moved aside whenever possible. If they cannot be
completely removed from the projected image area, an attempt should
be made to at least minimize their superimposition over the *anatomy of
interest.* For example, never leave coils of electrical leads over the lung

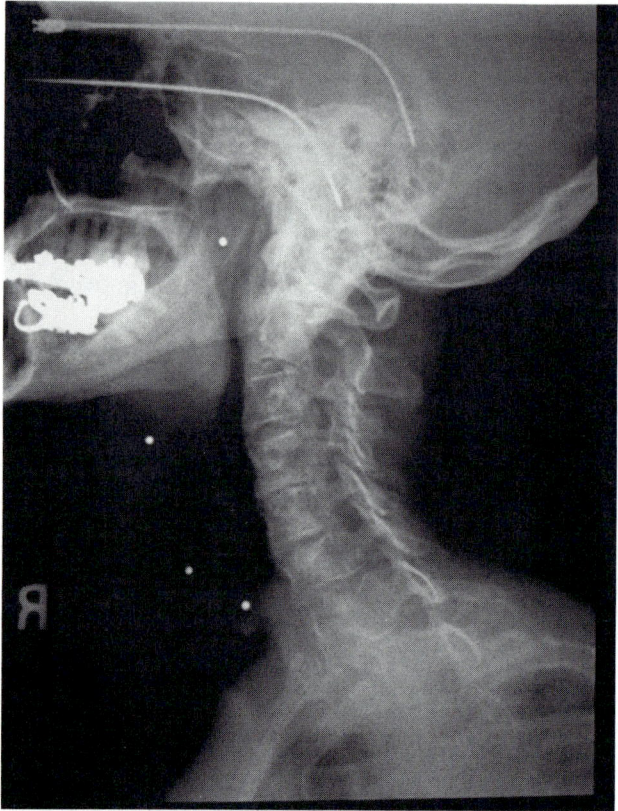

Figure 12. The patient's eye glasses were not removed for this oblique cervical spine view, and one temple nearly superimposes the atlanto-occipital joint area.

fields when they might be unwound and pulled to the side so that only a single lead wire to each lead is in the anatomy, Figure 13.

Also beware of folds in sheets and gowns as the patient is placed on the radiographic table. Radiographers often assume that folds or seams in clothing, gowns, sheets or pillows will not show up on the radiograph. Figure 14, a fold in a pillow, illustrates the error in such thinking. Especially at lower kilovoltage techniques, care must be taken to smooth out sheets under the patient, remove undershirts, take off packed gauze, etc., or these cloth materials may indeed show up.

Complete preparation of the patient for fluoroscopic procedures is essential. Generally, patients should be kept NPO (allowed nothing by mouth) for at least 8 hours prior to a fluoroscopic procedure, and cleansing enemas must be effectively performed for colon studies. Figure 15

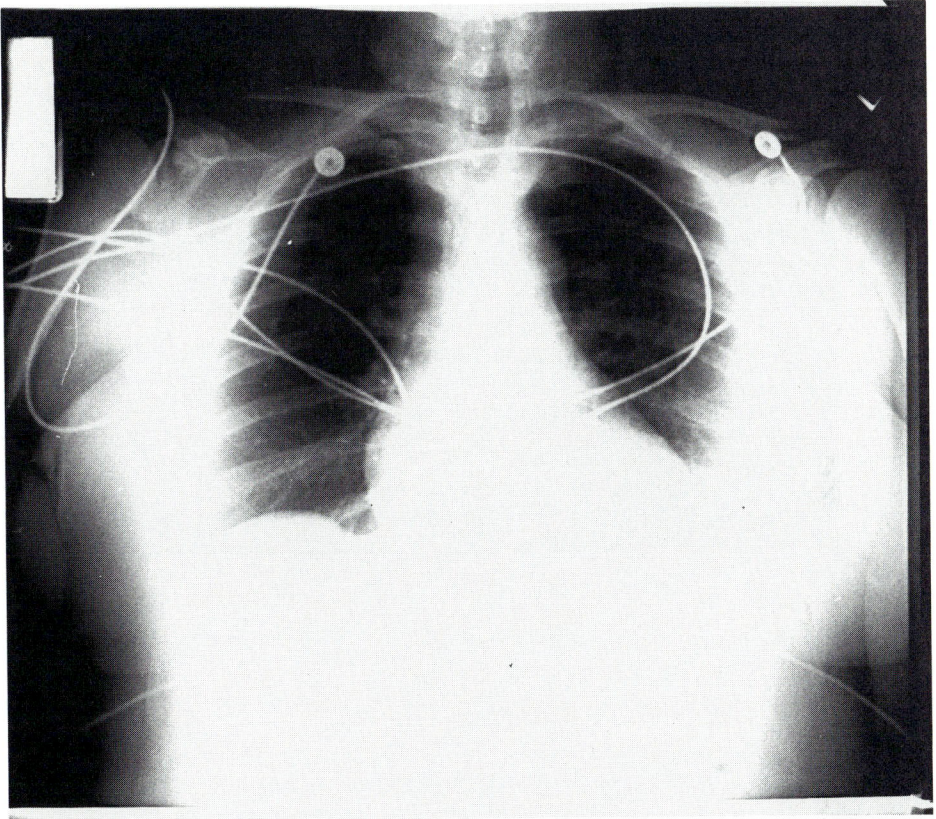

Figure 13. Electrical leads unnecessarily coiled over the lung fields on a portable chest view.

illustrates the mottled appearance of food in the stomach during an unprepared Upper GI series. The food causes dark artifacts breaking up the barium bolus and rendering any useful diagnosis hopeless. Such studies must be repeated after the patient is successfully prepared.

There are many kinds of foreign bodies, such as bullet fragments, slivers, swallowed objects or objects inserted into the skin, nose, ears, penis, vagina, or rectum that might be considered as "artifacts," particularly if they superimpose anatomy of interest, Figure 16. More often, however, foreign bodies *are* the "anatomy" or pathology of interest and will not be further discussed here.

Some radiopaque items such as casts cannot be removed. These may require technique adjustments or positioning modifications in order to minimize the deleterious effect of the artifacts.

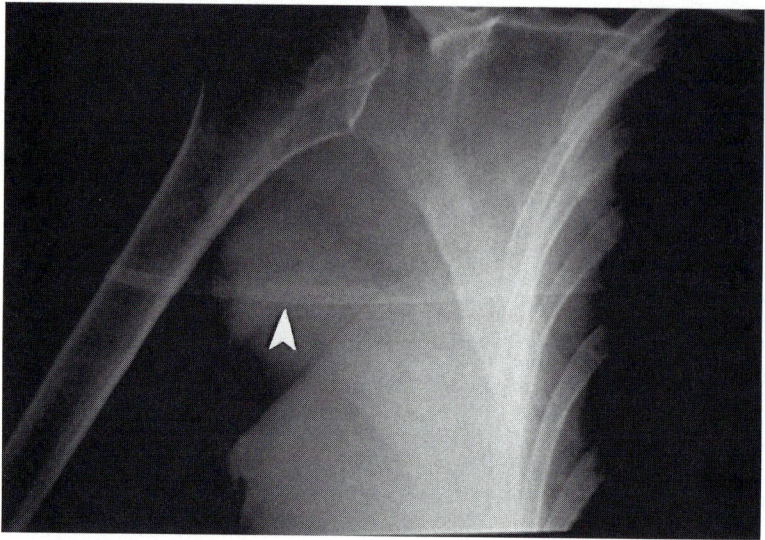

Figure 14. A fold in a pillow (arrow) shows up on this shoulder view.

Casts and Splints

For proper demonstration of anatomy superimposed by casts or splints, radiographic techniques must certainly be adjusted upward. But to determine the extent of this increase, one must take into consideration the composition of the materials used, their thickness and configuration, and whether they are wet or dry. Radiographs taken *after* a limb of the body has been set and casted are called *post-reduction radiographs.*

Full plaster casts require a minimum doubling of overall exposure factors from the usual technique for that body part. This doubling can be achieved either by doubling the mAs or by increasing the kVp by 15 percent. Full plaster casts which are still wet, having just been applied, require *three* times the overall technique. Unusually thick plaster may be applied around the femur or the torso. A full cast of this type which is dry will require a *tripling* of the usual technique. A plaster cast of this thickness which is still wet can require as much as *four times* the original technique.

Often, "half-casts" are secured to a limb by wrapping a partial cast with an Ace™ bandage. For this situation, use a *50 percent* increase in technique. That is, half again as much mAs, or approximately 8 percent more kVp. Remember to employ the increase only when the projection of the part of interest passes through the cast material. For example, on a lateral

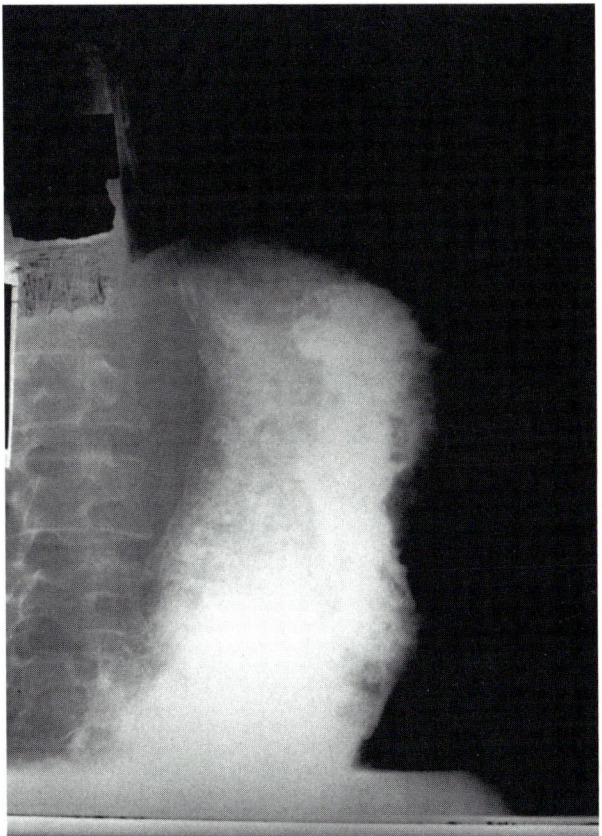

Figure 15. An "unprepped" patient reports to radiology for an UGI series after a full breakfast. Note the darker mottle within the barium bolus of the stomach.

view of a forearm in a half-cast, the bones may not be covered by the cast, and a normal technique should be used.

Fiberglass mesh has become popular as a casting medium. Fiberglass is very radiolucent, allowing the x-ray beam to pass through it virtually unaffected. Normal techniques may be used in most cases when *pure* fiberglass is used. However, fiberglass is often mixed in roughly equal proportions with plaster. For casts made of mixed fiberglass and plaster, a general rule of thumb is to increase mAs by *50 percent,* or kVp by 8 percent, as in Figure 17.

Projections must sometimes be made through splints of wood or aluminum, or through plastic devices. These materials may require from 35 to 65 percent increases in overall technique. Whether the splint is applied to one side or to both sides of the limb, the radiographer must

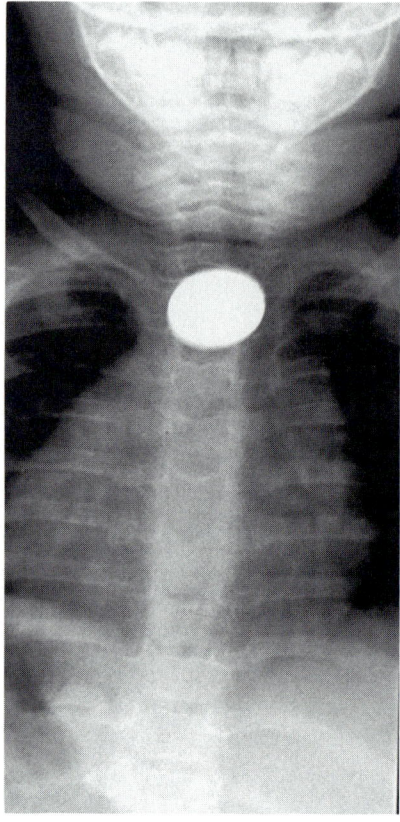

Figure 16. A swallowed foreign body in a child. This coin is lodged in the esophagus and is positioned broadside as it is squeezed between the spine and the trachea. If it were in the trachea, it would appear on end for an AP projection.

assess the *total thickness* of material to be traversed by the x-ray beam. For example, the mAs should be increased by 35 percent ($1/3$) for one-half inch of wood, or by 50 percent ($1/2$) for one inch. As a rule of thumb, *increase mAs by 50 percent for wood or aluminum splints.*

It is not possible to completely eliminate the artifacts caused by casts or splints, but a proper increase in technique will darken the image density to enhance the visibility of the anatomy through the obstructing material.

RADIOGRAPHIC OR PATIENT CARE EQUIPMENT

The radiographer must always be aware of any type of equipment which lies between the x-ray tube and the film cassette. Anything which

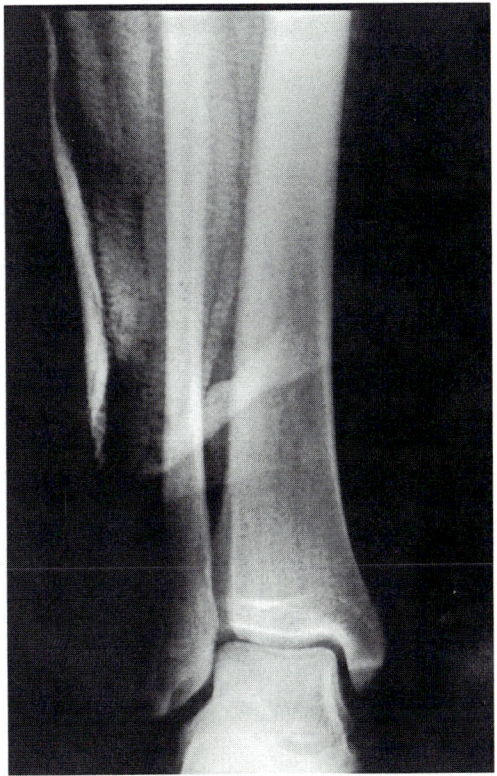

Figure 17. A distal leg in a mixed fiberglass/plaster cast. A technique of 66 kVp and 10 mAs, 50 per cent more mAs than the 6.8 listed on the technique chart for a leg, was used.

falls within the collimated light field, whether it is near the x-ray tube, over the patient, on the patient or behind the patient, will be imaged as an artifact and may obscure essential diagnostic information.

A common example of troublesome radiographic equipment would be the electrical cables which connect to the x-ray tube, especially on older machines. Sometimes these cables are not properly secured to the ceiling crane or tube armature, and it is possible when turning the tube and collimator into certain positions to get the cables in front of the tube. Note in Figure 18 how the magnification and blurriness of the artifact indicate that it is far from the film, i.e., near the x-ray tube.

Troublesome patient care equipment includes air hoses and attachments for ventilators and other respiratory care equipment, intravenous lines, and electrical leads for electrocardiographs. Again, the amount of magnification and blur indicate the relative distance from the film,

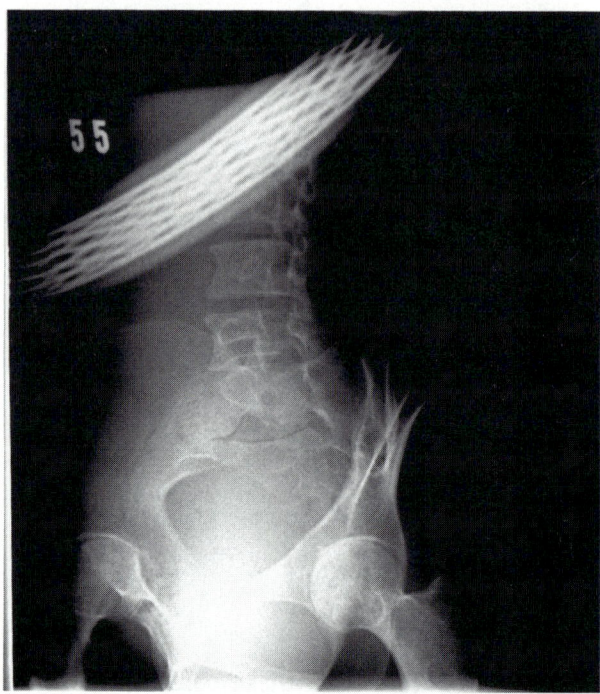

Figure 18. An electrical cable dangling in front of the x-ray tube during this exposure appears extremely blurred and magnified due to its distance from the film.

which is helpful in diagnosing the cause of the artifact. The ventilation hose and plastic attachments in Figure 19 are subtle artifacts, first, because they were hanging in the air over the patient and at that distance were blurred and magnified, and second, because they are made of thin plastic which has low x-ray absorption characteristics. The IV line in Figure 20 also has low absorption characteristics, but was caught between the patient and the cassette so that it is not magnified and shows sharp edges. The electrical leads in Figure 13 illustrate slight but detectable blurring, indicating that they lay atop the patient.

ACCIDENTAL EXPOSURE

Accidental exposures to the film can take on a number of appearances and have a variety of causes. The fogged spot over the knee in Figure 21 was caused when a used cassette was left in a Bucky tray, and the tray was not moved to the foot of the table when a fluoroscope was activated. The

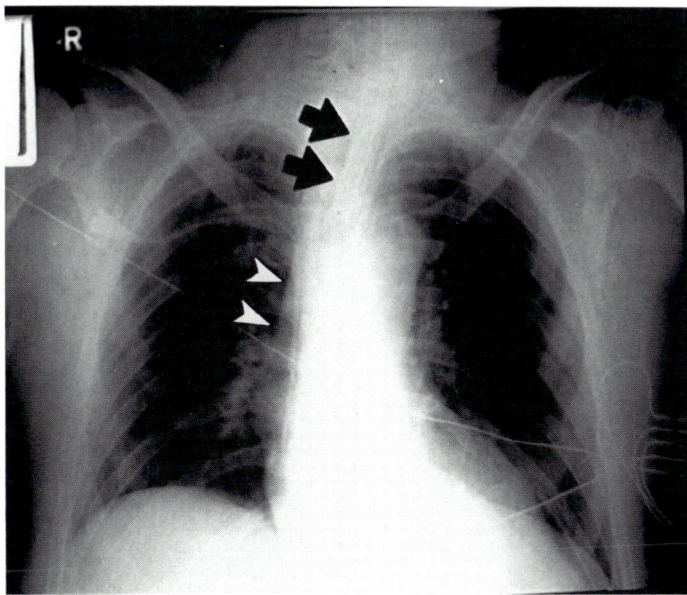

Figure 19. A plastic oxygen hose (dark arrows) and connector (light arrows) hang just over this patient's chest. Their low contrast and slight blur make them difficult to see. These could have been gently pulled to one side without detaching the oxygen.

fogging from scattered radiation has a much more subtle appearance, but can be appreciated by carefully observing almost any lateral lumbar spine view. Figure 104 in Chapter 7 shows the fog line along the back of a lateral lumbar spine radiograph. The tips of the lumbar spinous processes are obliterated by this fog. The scatter radiation producing this fog is created by the raw x-ray beam striking the table behind the patient. By placing a sheet of leaded rubber along the patient's back, the scatter fog can be substantially reduced. With practice, the student can learn to recognize more subtle fog lines on other radiographs.

Double exposures can result in bizarre radiographs such as the strange looking skull and cervical spine in Figure 22. This image resulted when two oblique cervical spine views were taken on the same film, super-imposing the back of the two cranium images and spinous processes. The facial area of the skull and remaining cervical spine were obliterated by the double exposure.

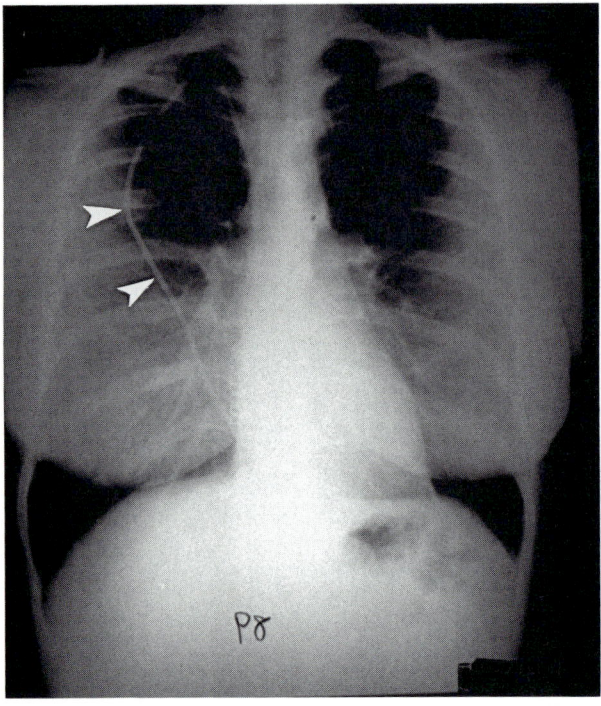

Figure 20. This IV line (arrows) was caught between the patient and the film, presenting a sharp but low contrast image.

MOTION

Movement of any part of the patient, the cassette or the x-ray tube while the exposure is taking place will result in a blurring of the details on the radiographic image. Blur destroys the recognizability of image details. If it is extreme, it can also destroy image contrast, reducing the visibility of details. These effects are fully analyzed in Chapters 13 and 16.

Patient motion is often categorized physiologically into two types: voluntary and involuntary. Voluntary motion is defined as conscious motion involving voluntary (striated) muscles. This does not necessarily imply that the patient intended to move. Involuntary motion is defined as motion caused unconsciously by involuntary muscles such as the heart muscle or the lower muscles of the esophagus once a swallowing action is initiated.

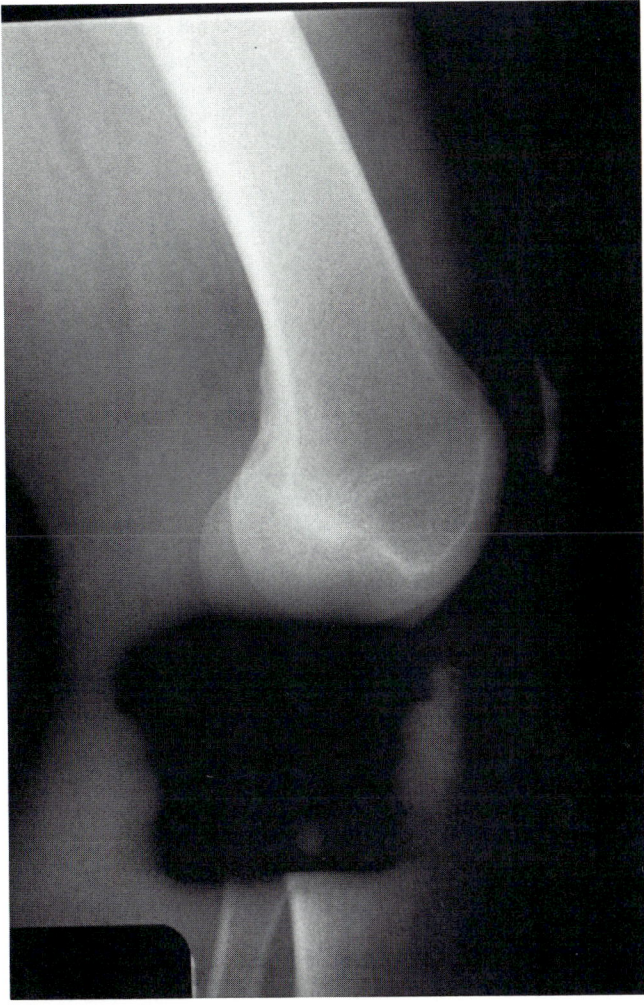

Figure 21. The fogged spot on this lateral knee view was the result of two errors: An exposed film was left in a Bucky tray, then the fluoroscopy unit was activated without moving the tray to the foot of the table.

For the purposes of critiquing radiographs, however, motion is more appropriately divided into four categories as follows:

1. Voluntary motion
2. Breathing motion
3. Peristaltic motion
4. Heart motion

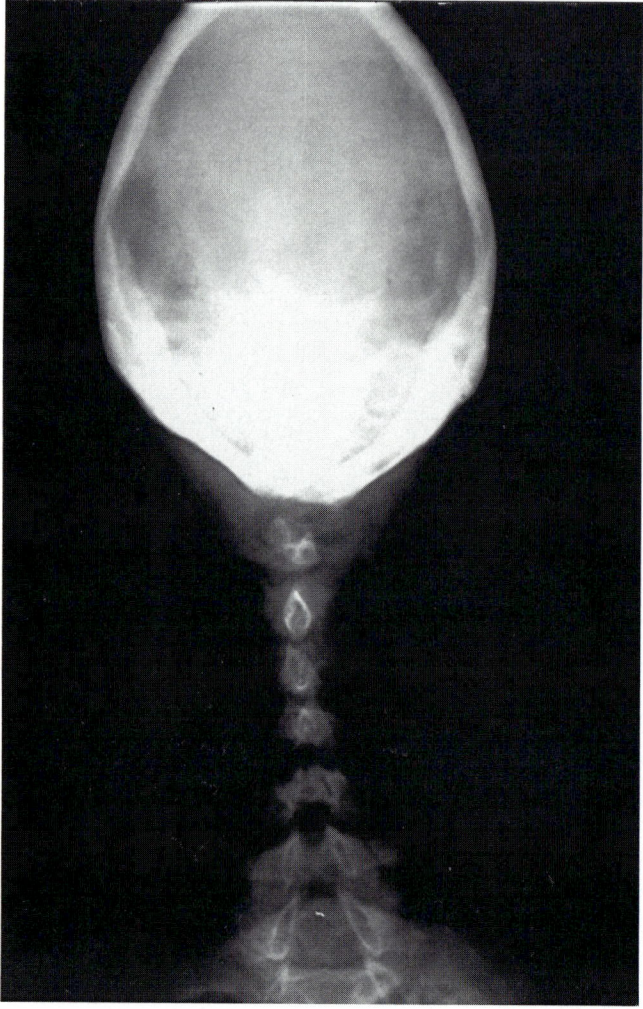

Figure 22. A double exposure resulting from using the same film for two oblique cervical spine views.

Voluntary motion is characterized on an image by a general blurring of an entire limb, the head, or the entire torso. All parts of the anatomical area, the bones, the organs, and the edges of the part itself, appear blurred and indistinct, Figure 23. Frequently patient movement will result in double-images of contrasty anatomy such as the ribs and spine in Figure 24. This type of motion is prevented mainly by clear and thorough patient instructions and by proper immobilization of the part. Breathing motion on a chest or abdominal radiograph can be distin-

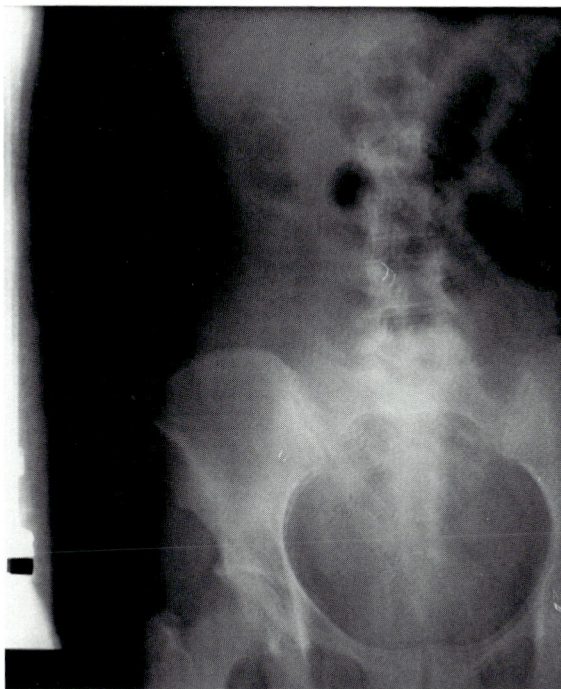

Figure 23. Voluntary patient motion results in blurring of *all* organs and bones in this AP abdomen projection.

guished from general motion. Blurred areas will include the lung markings, the diaphragm, and those organs such as the kidneys and fundus of the stomach which lie immediately beneath the diaphragm as in Figure 25. Ribs may or may not be obviously blurred, depending on the depth of the respiration. The key point is that the bones of the shoulder and the spine will *not* be blurred, nor will the pelvis and organs of the lower abdomen, Figure 25. Breathing motion is primarily prevented by clear and proper instructions to the patient, but with difficult patients the only way of minimizing this motion is by using the shortest possible exposure times.

Peristaltic motion includes any localized movement of the gastrointestinal tract caused by normal digestion or by cramps. Barium or gas in the esophagus, stomach, or a restricted portion of the small intestine or large intestine will appear blurred. It will be noted that other general areas of the GI tract are not blurred, and that bones in the region are not blurred, Figure 26. Peristaltic motion is reduced by proper preparation of the

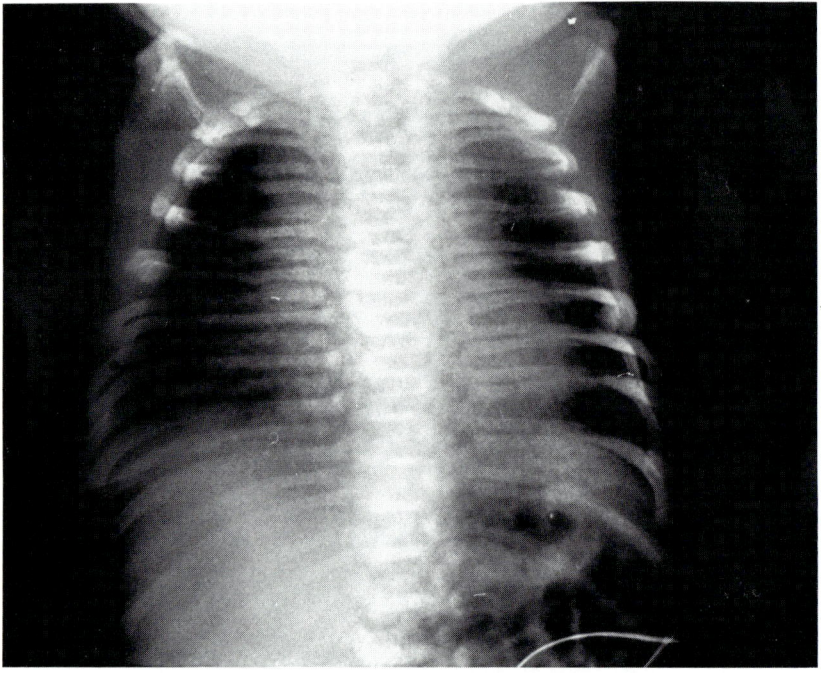

Figure 24. Double images of the ribs and spinal vertebrae due to voluntary motion during a pediatric AP chest projection.

patient for GI procedures, but is reliably controlled only by using the shortest feasible exposure times.

The heart is unique in that it is the only organ in the body which causes continuous involuntary motion. Since the only way to "freeze" this motion and produce a sharp radiograph is by using extremely short exposure times, it can be deduced that any chest radiograph demonstrating obvious heart motion was taken with a long exposure time. The exposure time can be minimized by using the highest available mA station and high kilovoltages (100–120 kVp for grid chests, 80–100 kVp for non-grid chests).

Blurring of the image can also be caused by forgetting to lock the x-ray tube securely in place prior to exposure. Unlocked tubes will occasionally drift across the room due to spring tension, crooked ceiling cranes, and gravity. Such movement will normally be linear, and can result in linear *streaking* artifacts on the image as well as blur. Streaks are caused when high-contrast linear anatomy, such as thin bones or a ureter with an iodinated contrast agent in it, are blurred in the direction of their long axis. Streaking is an expected defect in all linear tomogram images, Figure 27.

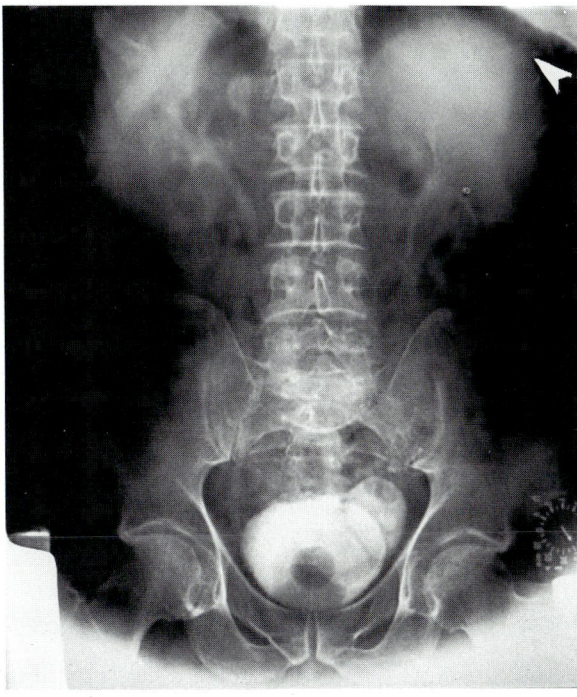

Figure 25. Breathing motion results in blurring of the diaphragm (arrow), kidneys and other organs just below the diaphragm on this AP projection during an IVP series, but all bones and the bladder appear sharp.

It is possible for the film cassette to be moved during an exposure, for example from excessive vibration of the Potter-Bucky mechanism. Such blurring would be difficult to distinguish from patient motion on the radiograph, and must be further analyzed by investigating the equipment.

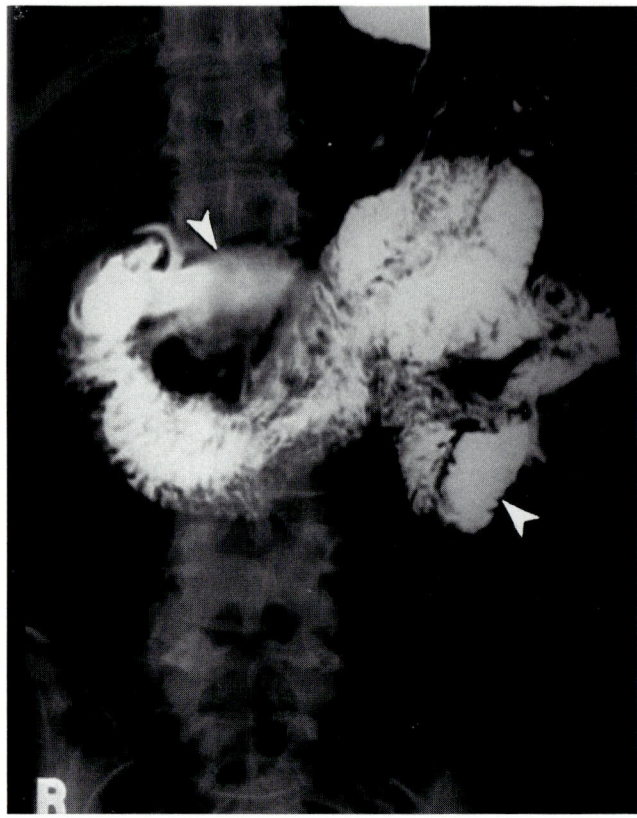

Figure 26. During a small bowel follow through, peristaltic motion blurs the duodenal bulb (upper arrow), while loops of the jejunem (lower arrow) are sharp.

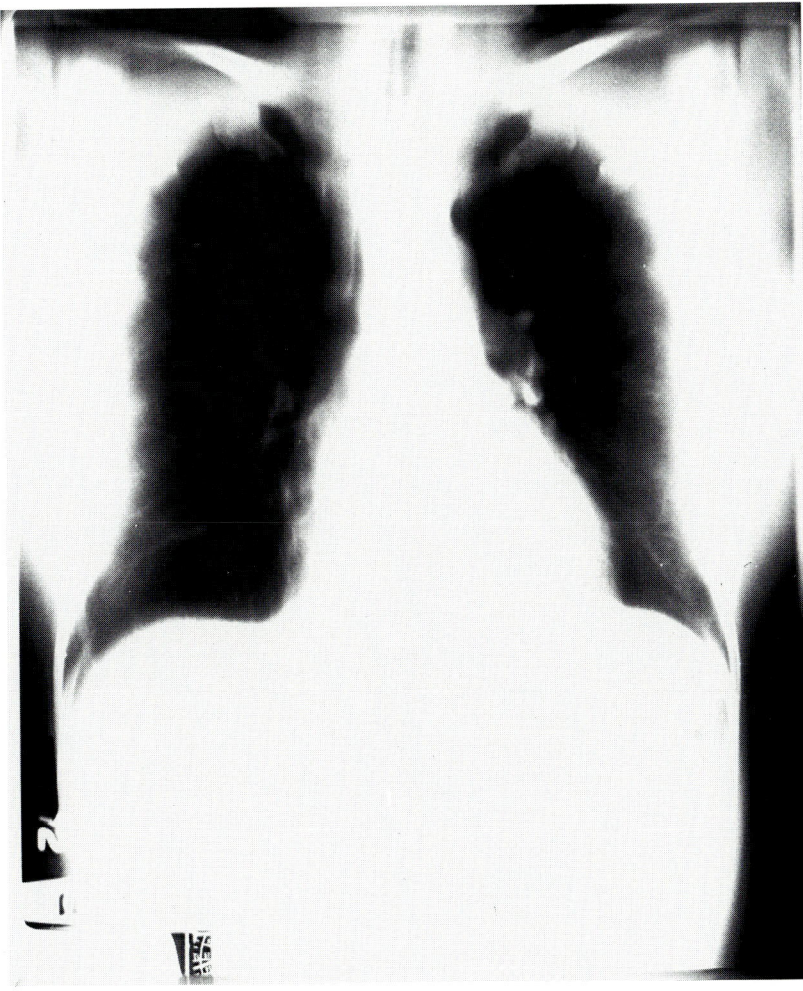

Figure 27. Linear tomogram of the chest showing streaking motion artifacts in the mediastinum, neck and shoulder areas.

Chapter 4

PROCESSING AND FILM HANDLING ARTIFACTS

X-ray film is delicate material and it should not be handled carelessly or roughly. It is sensitive to treatment of any kind, including heat, light, radiation, chemical fumes, pressure, bending, scratching, friction, and static electricity. After a film has been exposed, but prior to processing, it is *eight times more sensitive* to these types of mistreatment than before it is used for an exposure. This means, for example, that an exposed film which is left on the loading counter in the dark room will become fogged eight times faster than an unexposed film left on the counter top. Radiographic film is very expensive, and great care must be taken in its storage, handling, and processing.

STORAGE AND HANDLING

During the storage of unused x-ray film, it must be protected from:

1. Excessive heat
2. Light (of any color)
3. X-rays and other radiation
4. Chemical fumes such as those from processing solutions
5. Pressure

Any one of these phenomena can cause chemical changes in the film emulsion, resulting in image fog such as that in Figure 28. When boxes of film are stacked horizontally, lying flat, the weight of the film produces high pressure on those boxes near the bottom of the stack.

Pressure has a physical effect on molecules similar to heating, as can be seen in the use of pressure cookers. The kinetic energy deposited into the emulsion of the film from pressure can cause chemical changes which effectively expose the film, turning it dark. We also know of a phenomenon called *solarization* in which *excessive* exposure to the film causes a reversal of image formation, making the image turn lighter. Excessive pressure can create a similar effect, causing a light mark against a dark

47

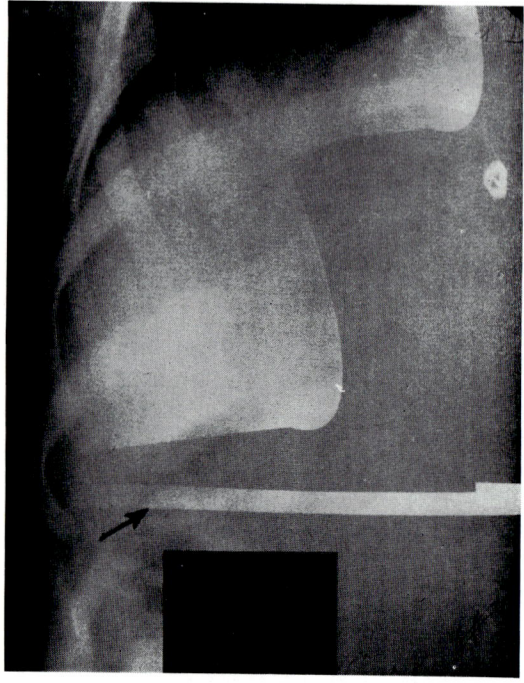

Figure 28. Radiograph made with film previously fogged by radiation. The box of film had been left near a radiation source in storage.

background on the radiograph. Thus, pressure artifacts can be either light or dark, depending on the *amount* of pressure applied. Frequently, pressure marks show up as a light artifact surrounded by a dark "halo" where the peripheral pressure was diminished, as appears in Figure 37. Anything which folds or creases the film can result in different types of pressure marks. A common example is accidentally closing the film bin door on a film.

Another common artifact caused from rough handling is the *crescent mark,* caused when the film is folded or kinked over the end of one's finger. The crescent mark is essentially a pressure artifact. Depending on the amount of pressure applied at the folding point, crescent marks may show as either white marks against a dark background or as dark marks against a lighter background, Figure 29. This is important because dark crescent marks can simulate fractures in bones, and light marks can simulate lesions in the lungs. When the radiologist is unsure about the origin and diagnosis of such an image, a repeat radiograph will be required to "rule out" artifacts as the cause.

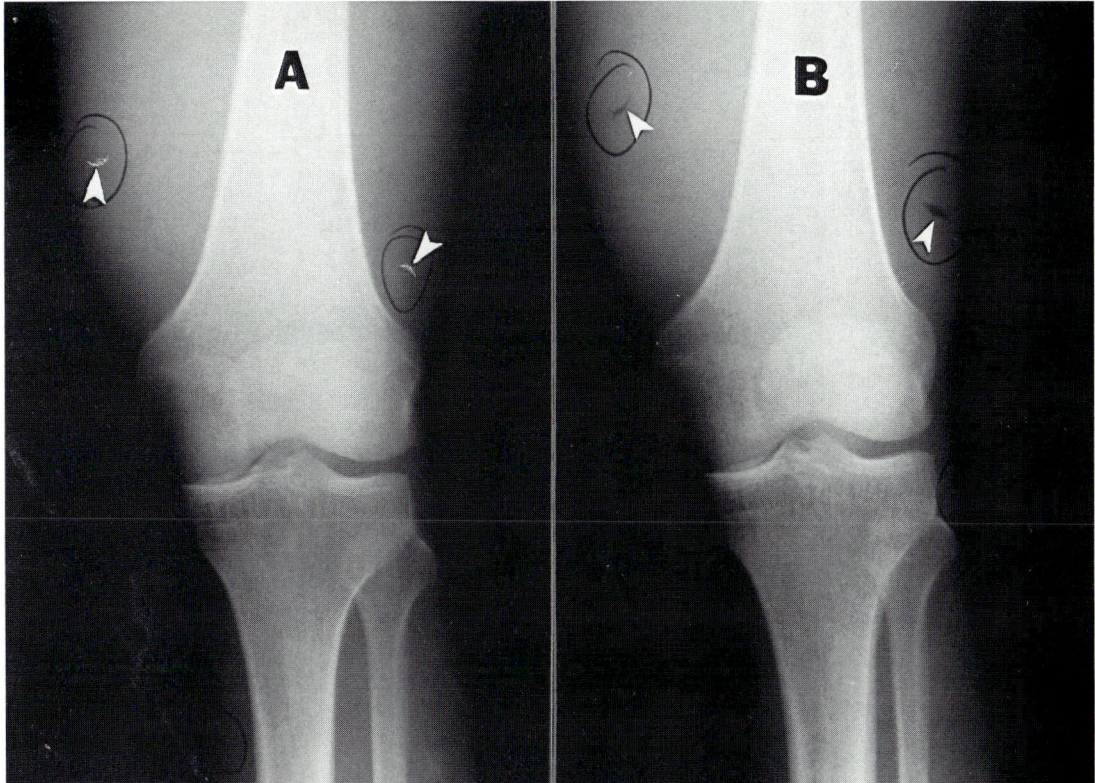

Figure 29. Knee radiographs showing light crescent marks (A) and dark crescent marks (B). The light marks result when higher pressures are applied, but both are from bending the film around fingertips.

Film is sensitive to all colors of light including red light. Darkroom safelights are only "safe" in that this color takes a much longer time to fog the film than blue or white light would. If a film is left on a counter top under safelight illumination for a long period of time, obvious fogging will result, Figure 30. Unfortunately, there are many other causes of film fogging outside of the darkroom. Sometimes the appearance of the artifact allows the cause to be determined, as in Figure 30 where a piece of paper had partially covered the film, but in many cases the fog on the image alone is not sufficient to determine the cause without further information.

Chemical stains are caused on the film whenever *any* liquid, including water, coffee, or processing solutions, is splashed onto the film at any time. A common form of staining occurs with new students who, upon

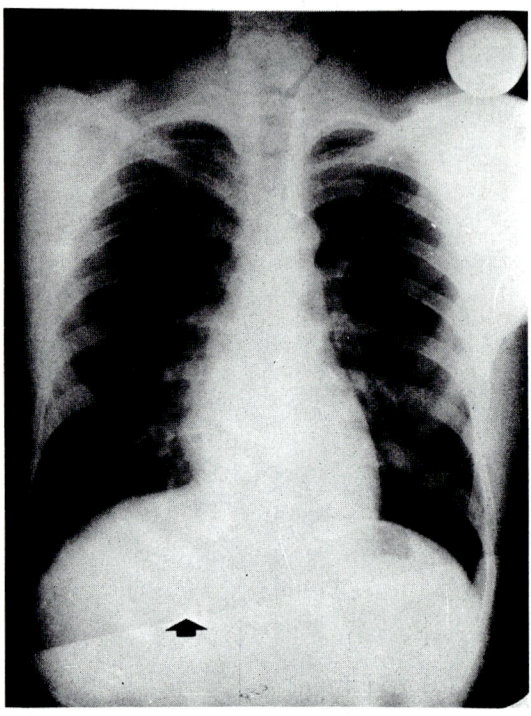

Figure 30. Safelight fog caused when an exposed film was laid on the dark room countertop too long and partially covered by a piece of paper.

realizing that a film is feeding into the processor crooked, pull it back out of the feed rollers to reinsert it, Figure 31. The leading edge of the film may have entered the developer solution by this time, and will drag solution back through the feed rollers and onto the feed tray of the processor, staining the film. The feed tray and feed rollers must be thoroughly cleaned after such an accident. Artifacts involving the feed rollers (or "detection" rollers) always show the broad striped appearance in Figure 31.

Feeding a film into the processor too soon after the last film was inserted may result in the films overlapping each other as they pass through the rollers and solutions. Upon pulling them apart, the two films will usually still be wet with solution in the area of overlap. *If this area is not obscuring the specific anatomy of interest,* the lid and crossover roller rack may be lifted off of the processor and each film reinserted into the *fixer* roller section. This will re-fix, rewash and redry the film, preventing a repeated exposure to the patient.

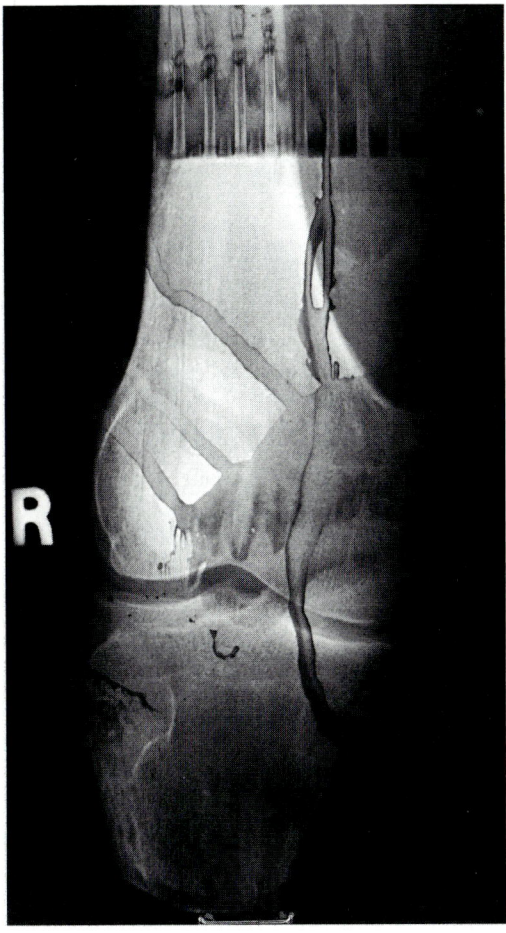

Figure 31. Detection roller marks and chemical splashes caused by pulling a film back out of an automatic processor after its leading edge had submerged into the developer solution tank.

It should be remembered that torn corners from flash cards, cigarette ashes, dirt, or other foreign objects can fall into cassettes while loading or unloading them in the darkroom, Figure 32. Foreign objects lodged between screens will usually show as white artifacts in the image, unless they are thick like a grain of dirt and cause a pressure mark. Frequent cleaning of cassette screens helps prevent this.

Finally, note that some artifacts occur from long-term storage of the film *after* exposure. Eventual shrinkage of the emulsion can cause it to wrinkle, causing the artifact in Figure 33. Cracking of the emulsion occurs when the aging emulsion becomes brittle and then is bent upon

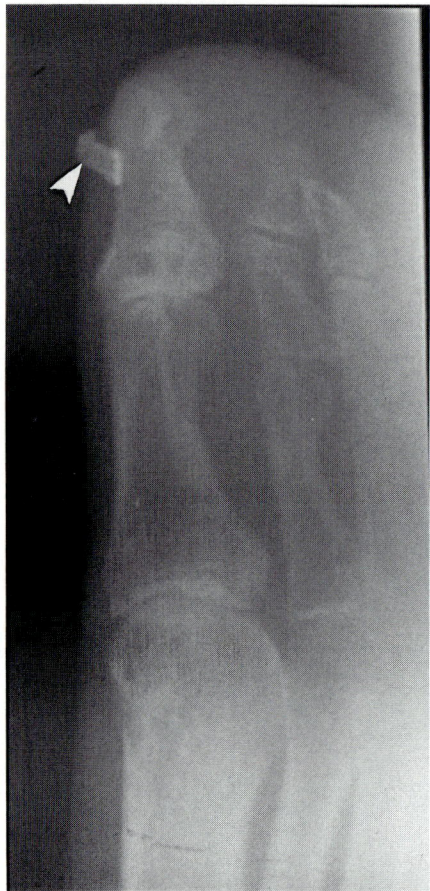

Figure 32. Artifact caused by a small fragment of paper that fell into an open cassette in the dark room and absorbed light from the intensifying screen on subsequent use.

handling. Old films can turn brown due to small amounts of residual developer solution left in the emulsion after processing.

Static Electricity

Everyone has experienced the small shock from a discharge of static electricity upon reaching for a doorknob or other metallic object after walking on a carpeted floor. In daily life, most static electricity charges are built up from friction between two dissimilar substances. The sudden separation or rubbing together of two statically charged objects can also

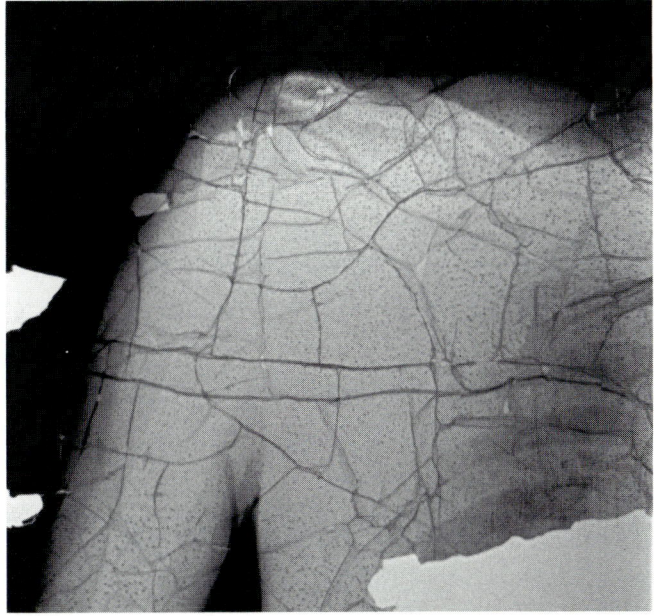

Figure 33. Emulsion wrinkling and deterioration due to long term shrinkage.

result in a discharge of electrons as they "jump" from one object to the other. This discharge may or may not be visible as a spark.

Whenever radiographic film is rapidly pulled from the film bin, roughly pulled from a cassette, or quickly slid across a counter top or processor feed tray, static discharges can result. Also, many types of radiographic equipment (such as "daylight" systems that automatically move film from a chest unit into a processor or angiographic film changers) frequently cause static discharges as the film rubs against conveyor belts, intensifying screens, or other components.

During an electrical discharge, either the movement of the electrons through the film emulsion or light produced from a visible spark will expose the film and turn it black. The blackened artifact will most commonly appear as *tree and crown* marks, or as *smudge and spot* marks. *Tree and crown* static artifacts, Figure 34-A, are believed to be created by invisible discharges of electrons through the emulsion. *Smudge and spot* static marks, Figure 34-B, appear to be caused by the visible light emitted from sparks of static electricity.

Any type of static electricity artifact—pressure, crown, or tree—is more likely to occur when the room air is very dry. To help prevent static

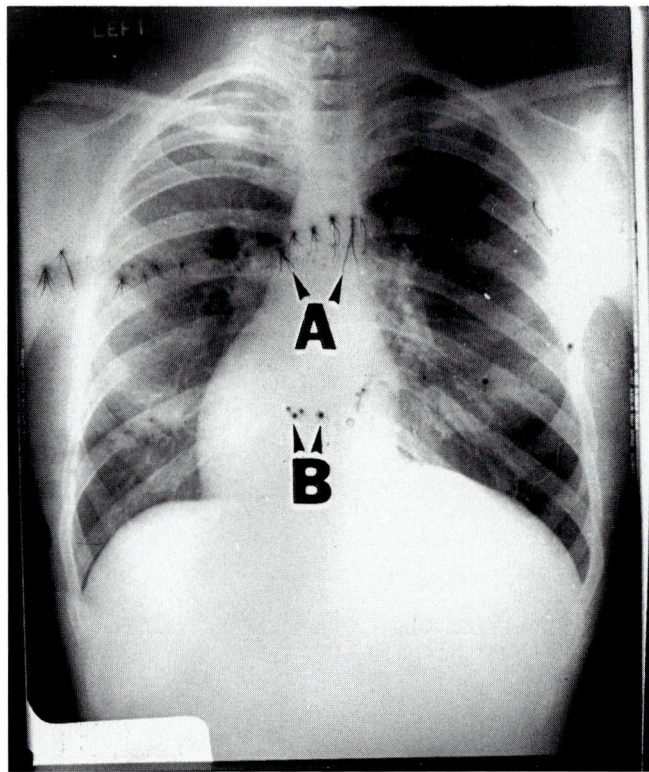

Figure 34. Tree static (A. arrow) and smudge static (B) artifacts.

discharges, film should be stored and handled in an atmosphere with 40 to 60 per cent humidity and a temperature of 50 to 70 degrees Fahrenheit. Film must be handled gently to prevent friction. Also, since lint, dust and dirt can act as electrical conductors and increase the probability of static discharges, screen cassettes should be regularly cleaned using a solution recommended by the manufacturer.

PROCESSING ARTIFACTS

Several artifacts are peculiar to the automatic processors used in modern imaging departments. Scratches appear as clear or *white* lines because emulsion is removed from the film base. When such scratches are straight and run *parallel* to the direction of film travel through the processor, they indicate that some sharp corner of metal or plastic is being brought into contact with the film as it passes through the processor. Common causes include dirt lodged in a dryer tube, improperly seated dryer tubes or roller racks, or misaligned guide shoes in the automatic processor. Guide shoes are curved metal plates in the processor which serve to curl and turn the film as it passes from one set of rollers into the next. Guide shoes are always shaped with *ribs,* Figure 35, so that the wet film does not stick to them. These metal ribs extend slightly beyond the trailing edge of the guide shoe, and can scratch the film. If several scratches are seen toward one side of the film, a guide shoe is crooked. If several scratches are seen across the film at regular intervals about one inch apart, as in Figure 36, then an entire guide shoe has been set at too steep an angle, so that the trailing edge of all of the ribs are scratching the film.

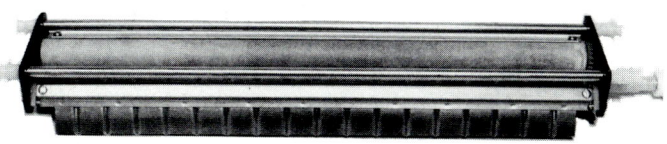

Figure 35. Crossover roller rack from an automatic processor showing ribbed guide shoes (bottom) used to turn film as it travels.

The processor may be accidentally stopped, faulty electrical relays or stripped gears may cause the rollers to hesitate in their turning motion. If a film is in the developer tank when this occurs, white lines are created where each roller touching the film emulsion protects that side of the film from the developer solution. Dark "halo" lines are often seen to either side of each white line; these are caused by the decreased, but still present, pressure against the film at the curvature of the roller. Since some rollers are placed at different intervals than others, these roller lines are not always evenly spaced. The lines will run *perpendicular* to the direction of film travel. This common artifact is demonstrated in Figure 37.

Pi lines are dark linear densities running across the film *perpendicular* to the direction of film travel through the processor. They are the result of crystalized chemical deposits or dirt deposits on processor rollers.

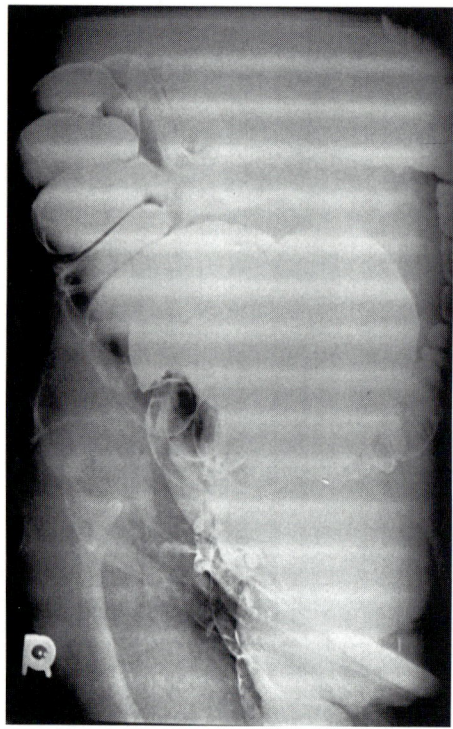

Figure 36. Guide shoe marks. These scratches are from the ribs of a guide shoe seated at too steep an angle in an automatic processor. Guide shoe marks run *parallel* to the direction of film travel, and are evenly spaced at about one-inch intervals.

Each time the dirty roller turns, the pressure of the deposit against the film sensitizes the emulsion and turns it dark. If only one roller is involved, the pi lines will occur at regular intervals, Figure 38. The interval distance between the pi lines is equal to the circumference of the roller that caused them. The circumference of the roller is equal to the mathematical value of pi (3.14) times the diameter of the roller. In other words, to determine the width (diameter) of the roller causing the pi lines, divide the distance between them by three. Often more than one roller is caked with deposits so that an irregular pattern of intervals between the lines is created. It should also be noted that a single grain of dirt embedded in a roller will also create dark spots, rather than lines, at intervals related to pi. These might be more appropriately called *pi marks*.

Uneven or streaky sheen (alternate dull and shiny areas) on the surface of the film may be caused by uneven drying from dirty or improperly seated dryer tubes. Uneven sheen can also be caused by poor

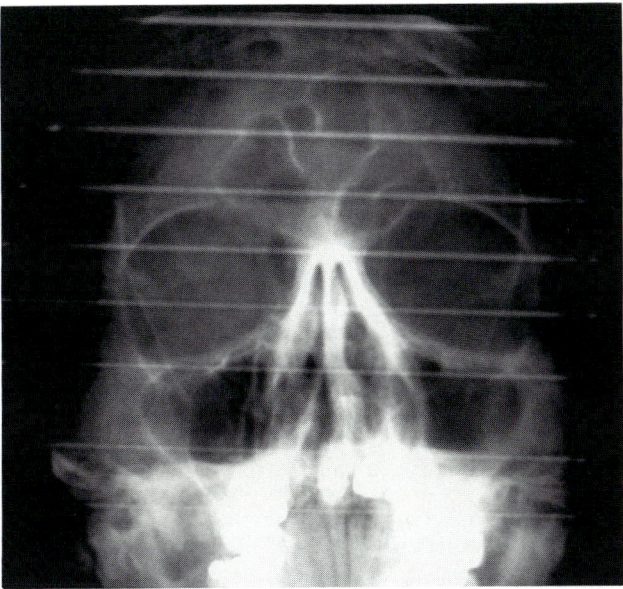

Figure 37. Roller marks due to hesitation or halting of film travel through an automatic processor. Roller marks run *perpendicular* to the direction of film travel. Note the darker halo lines to either side of the white lines, due to lessened but still present pressure at the curvature of each roller.

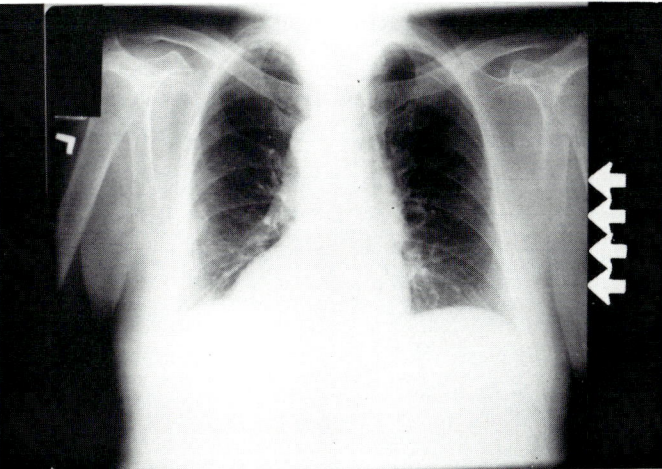

Figure 38. Pi lines caused by crystalized chemical deposits on the rollers of an automatic processor. Pi lines run *perpendicular* to the direction of film travel.

alignment of squeegee rollers in the processor, leaving the film excessively waterlogged in some areas as it enters the dryer section.

Peculiar fogging patterns can be attributed to light leaks in the automatic processor, since the fog will occur in a localized area transversely on the film, but will be found all along the film in the direction of film travel. One of the most common causes of such localized fogging is failure to properly seat the lid of the processor when it is closed. A small light leak on one end of the lid will fog the film in a streaking fashion as the film passes along near the light leak.

Failure of the solution circulation system in an automatic processor will leave the solutions in the tanks unstirred and more concentrated in some areas than in others. This can cause an uneven development of the film, with some areas showing a nebulous lighter density than others.

Frilling appears as a wavy curl along the edges of the film. Some areas of the emulsion can also form *blisters,* or be completely melted away from the film base. Frilling, blisters, and melting are all results of excessive solution temperatures in the processor. Note that when the controlling *thermostats* in a processor malfunction, often the heating elements will stay *on* so that temperatures become excessive.

Reticulation, a network of fine cracks in the emulsion, results from a film passing from a very hot solution into a very cold solution, or vice versa. This effect is uncommon with modern automatic processors, because the solutions share common heating systems.

A speckled or mottled appearance occurs when the processing solutions are dirty, Figure 39. The solution circulation lines have filters in them to remove the dirt and dust that are continually deposited into solutions from entering films. If the filters are absent or allowed to become clogged, the solutions will quickly become contaminated.

REVIEW #1

For each radiograph in Figures 40 through 51, list *all* errors in identification, assessment, labelling, collimation, shielding, motion and artifacts and other general considerations. When you are done, check your answers against the key provided in Appendix 1. The Appendix also provides additional critiques of the positioning and technique employed, if you wish to practice these criteria.

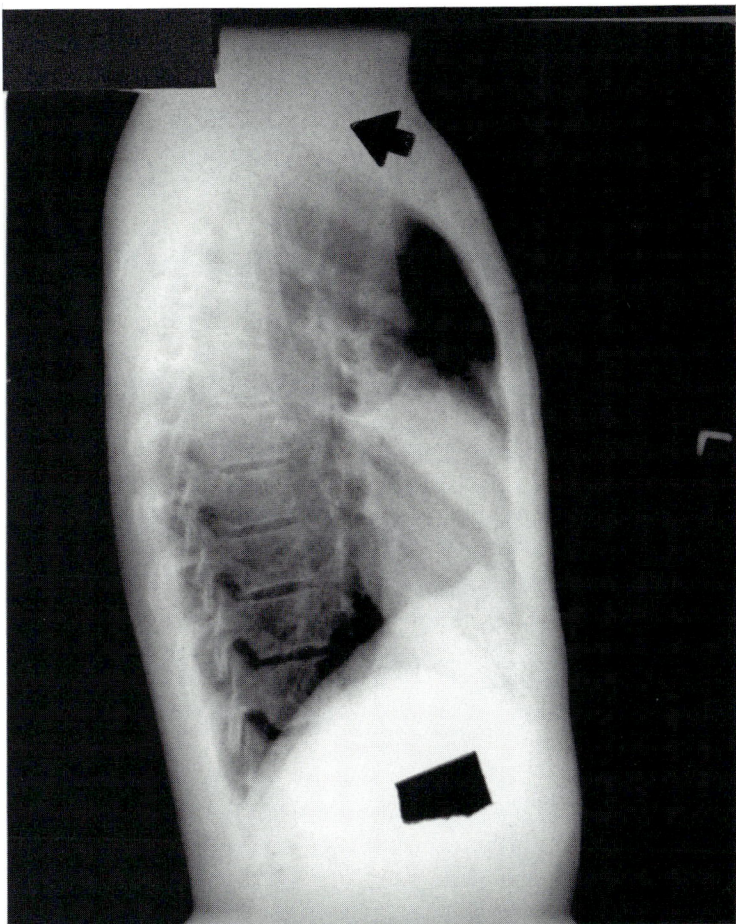

Figure 39. Mottling of the film (arrow) due to dirty solutions.

60

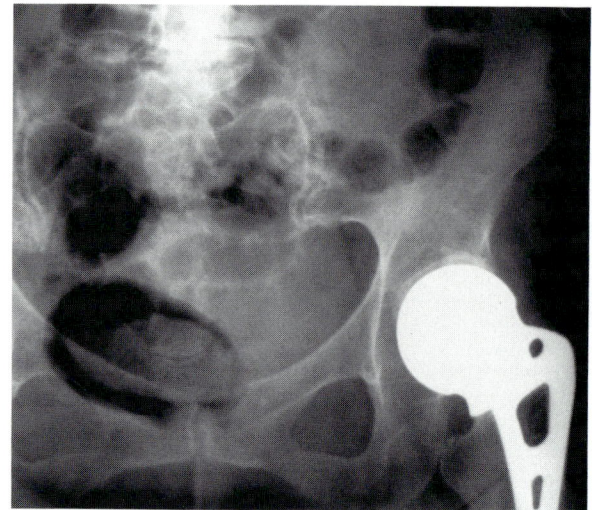

Figure 40.

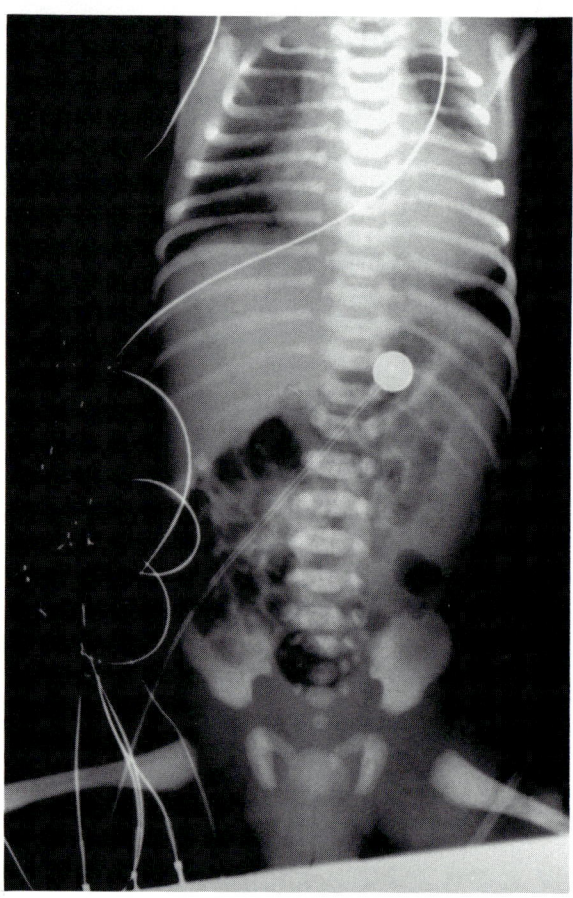

Figure 41.

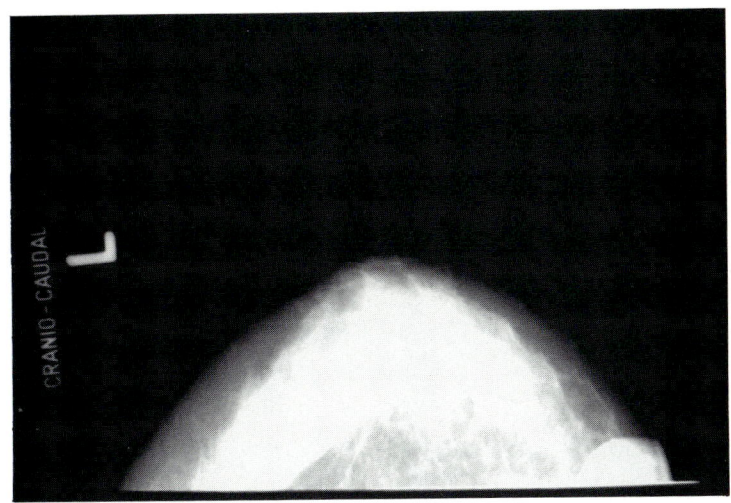

Figure 42.

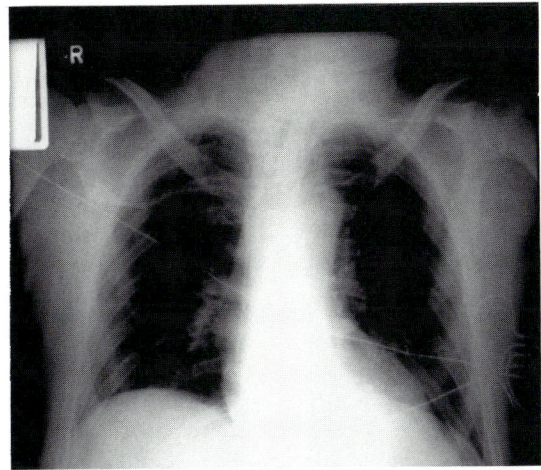

Figure 43.

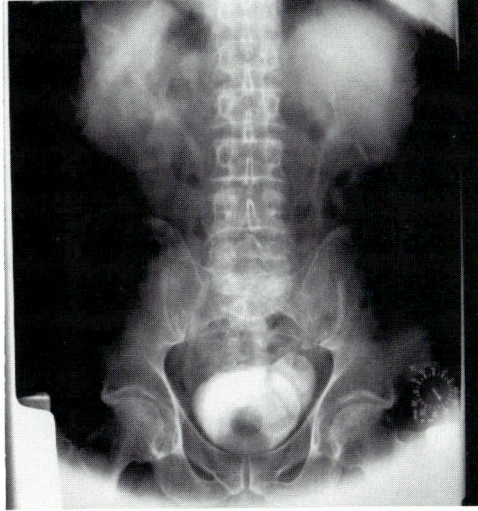

Figure 44.

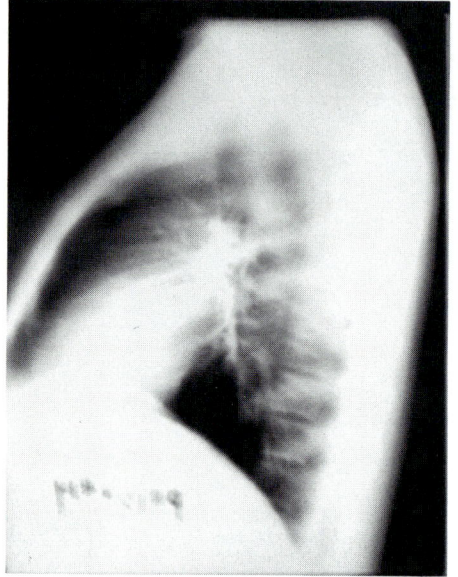

Figure 45.

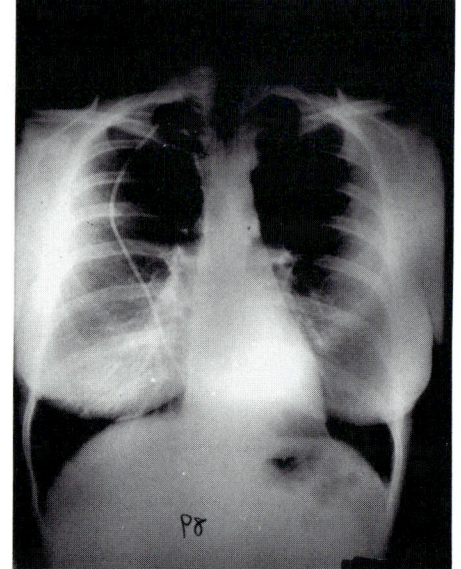

Figure 46.

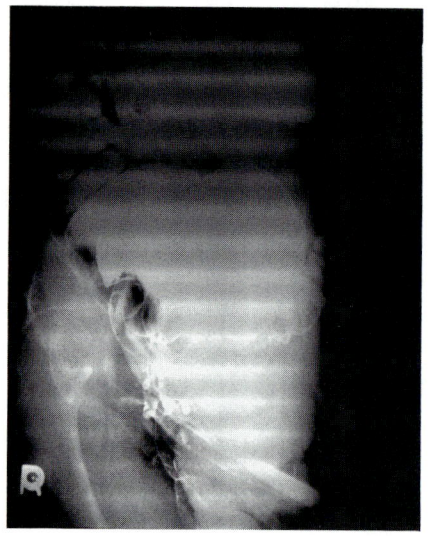

Figure 47.

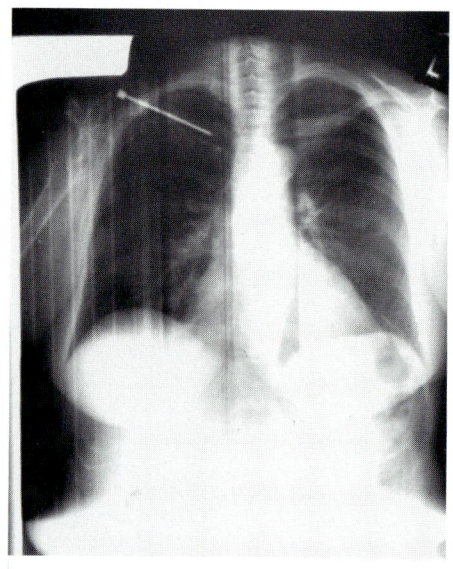

Figure 48.

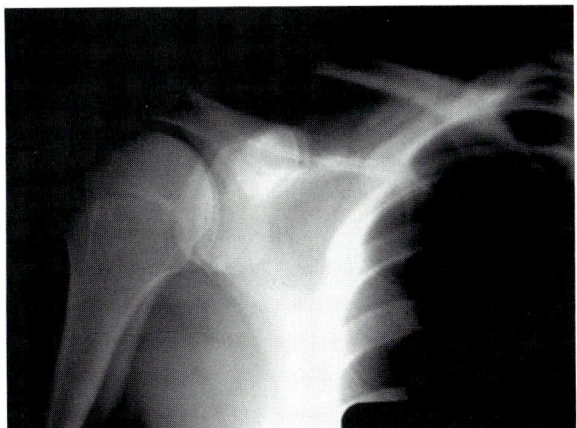

Figure 49.

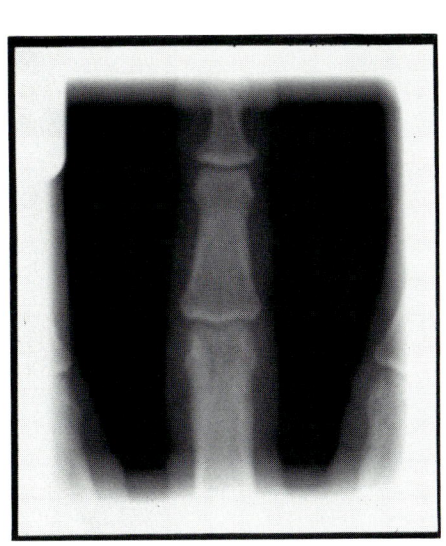

Figure 50.

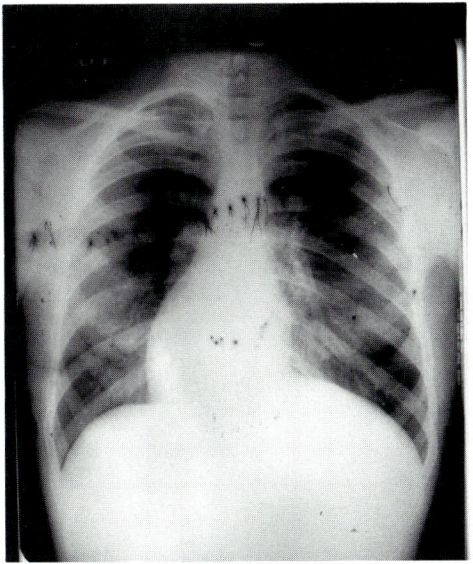

Figure 51.

PART II
POSITIONING QUALITY

Chapter 5

ALIGNMENT AND COLLIMATION

Alignment and collimation includes the placement of the film cassette, the centering of the x-ray beam, and the orientation and size of the x-ray field as indicated by the light field. Any one of these factors may result in the "clipping" or "cut-off" of important anatomy from the final image. Frequently more than one of these factors is involved. For example, the apices of the lungs may be clipped off of a chest radiograph because of a combination of centering slightly too low and collimating the field a bit too small.

Ideally the anatomy of interest is centered within the image field. Yet, a repeated exposure to the patient is *not* warranted on an off-centered radiograph unless the specific anatomy of interest is cut off.

FILM PLACEMENT

Film or cassette placement includes three criteria:

1. *Centering* of the mid-point of the film cassette to the anatomy
2. Proper *orientation* of the long axis of the cassette
3. Placement of the film identification *blocker.*

Most film cassettes are rectangular in shape, and therefore can be oriented either *lengthwise* or *crosswise* in relation to the long axis of the body part being radiographed. *Lengthwise* means that the longer axis of the film is *parallel* to the long axis of the anatomy, whereas *crosswise* indicates that the film is *perpendicular* to the longer axis of the anatomy. Even though a cassette is properly centered to the anatomy, cut-off can occur when it is not oriented properly lengthwise or crosswise.

Figure 52 shows a PA chest radiograph that was taken with the film cassette placed lengthwise in relation to the torso. Note that the costophrenic angles of both lungs are cut off laterally (along the sides). This film was centered to the chest, but should have been placed crosswise for this very broad-shouldered patient. This is the exception, however, rather than the rule—most chest radiographs should be done lengthwise with the blocker at the top. "Long" lungs are much more common than "broad" lungs. Figure 53 shows the result of placing the cassette crosswise on a rather tall patient: the costophrenic angles at the bottom of the lungs are cut off. This mistake is often made on obese patients, whose lungs are actually *smaller* than average due to the encroachment of fat. Crosswise placement of the film is indicated on big-boned, broad-shouldered patients rather than on patients who are simply obese.

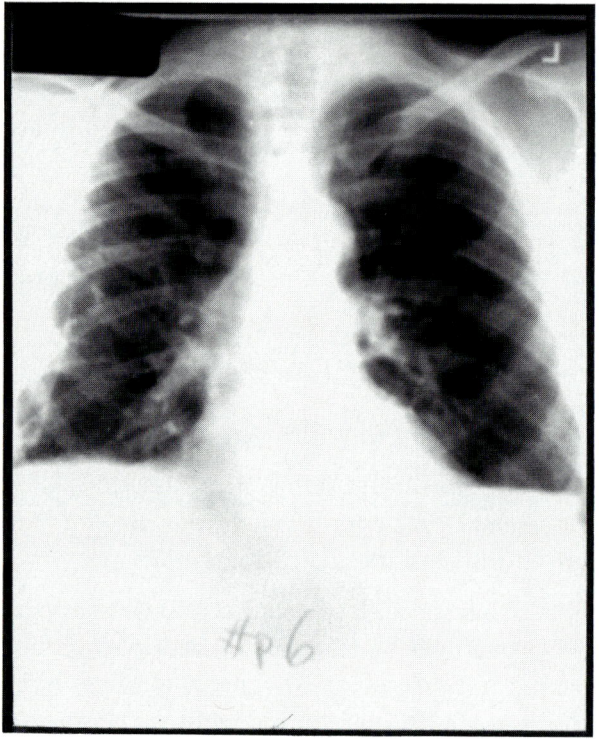

Figure 52. Lengthwise placement of film cassette on broad patient, clipping off both costophrenic angles of the lungs laterally. Cassette should be placed crosswise.

In determining corrective action for a repeated exposure, a simple test can be made to decide if the film should be reoriented crosswise or lengthwise: Find any other film of the same size and hold it up by the original radiograph. Hold it crosswise alongside to see if the lung fields will fit vertically, or hold it lengthwise along the bottom to see if the lungs will fit side-to-side, Figure 54. On rare occasions, you will find that

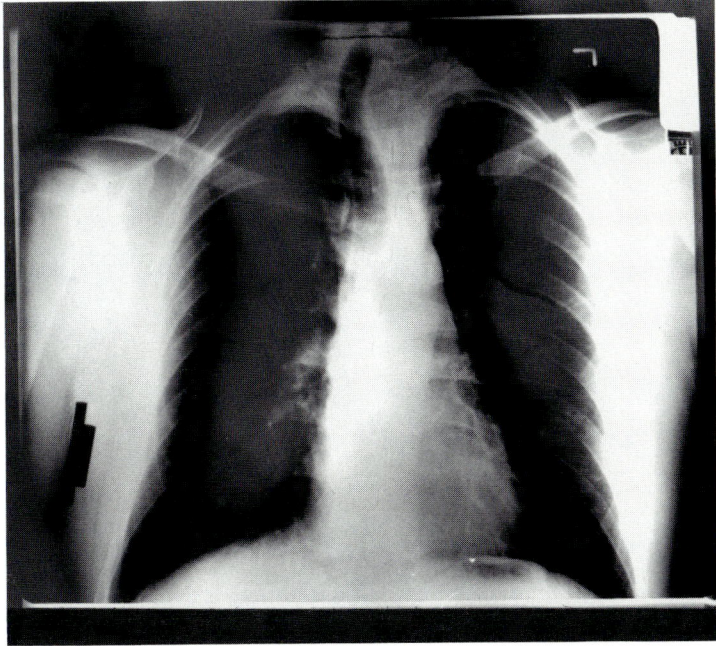

Figure 53. Crosswise placement of film cassette on tall patient, cutting off both costophrenic angles of the lungs inferiorly. Cassette should be placed lengthwise.

the patient is so large that the lungs will not fit either way. If no larger film size is available, two separate exposures will need to be made, one centered high and one low. This approach is preferred over centering one for the right lung and one for the left, because different levels of inspiration would result when comparing the two lungs.

Whether taken with the cassette crosswise or lengthwise, *the cassette blocker should always be placed at the top for chest radiographs,* for the very simple reason that the lung fields are most narrow at the apices. Figure 62, and Figure 4 in Chapter 1 illustrate that no matter what specific corner of the cassette or orientation the blocker is placed in, the upper corners of the field provide large triangular areas without anatomy of interest (lung fields, heart or mediastinal structures) present. The blocker may intrude into the bones and soft tissues of the shoulder area, as long as it does not obscure the upper lung fields. Figures 55 and 56 demonstrate the risk of placing the blocker at the bottom, whether the cassette is crosswise or lengthwise. For chest radiography, never place the blocker at the bottom of the film.

By the same logic, blockers *should* always be placed at the bottom for *abdominal* radiographs, including urography and barium enema proce-

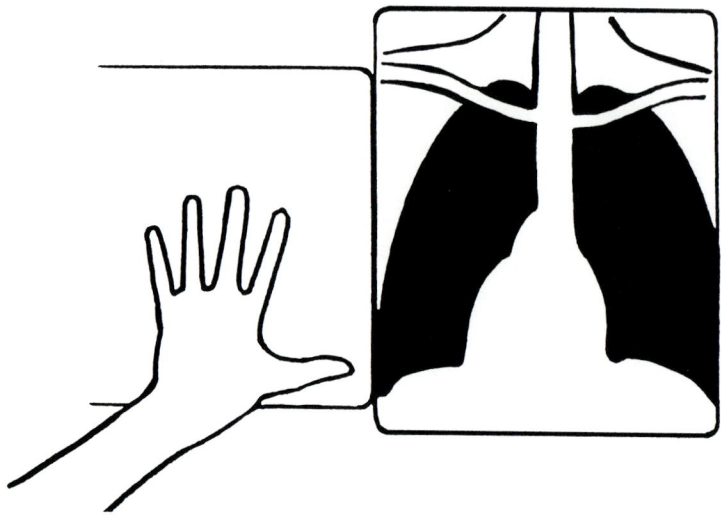

Figure 54. Use of a piece of scrap film to determine whether patient's lungs will fit vertically on a film placed crosswise. In this case, the lungs were clipped with the film lengthwise, but should fit with careful crosswise placement on repeating the exposure. In similar fashion, a scrap film can be held underneath the original radiograph to see if the lungs will fit side-to-side with lengthwise cassette placement.

dures. The pelvic bones are not of interest on these procedures, whereas the abdominal viscera which is of interest is narrowly encapsulated in the pelvic region. Placing the blocker at the top risks getting it over the flexures of the colon, the spleen, the liver or the diaphragm, organs that may show pathology.

Blocker placement is not crucial for many radiographs such as sinuses, skulls and most extremities, as there is about the same risk of super-imposition over anatomy of interest regardless of the particular placement. Nonetheless, at least two guidelines are in order: First, if it does not matter anatomically where the blocker is placed, it is a professional courtesy to the radiologist to place it at the *top* for lengthwise views in order to have the patient information upright and legible without having to flip the film upside-down. Second, blocker placement must always be determined with cassette centering in mind: If you tend to center the cassette relatively low, place the blocker at the bottom. If your tendency is to center the film high, place the blocker at the top. Figure 57 is a crosswise view of the clavicle with the blocker superimposing the sternal extremity of the clavicle. In this case the radiographer should have either centered the film more medially or placed the blocker laterally. Either correction would have avoided a repeated exposure.

All of these guidelines regarding blocker placement are also appli-

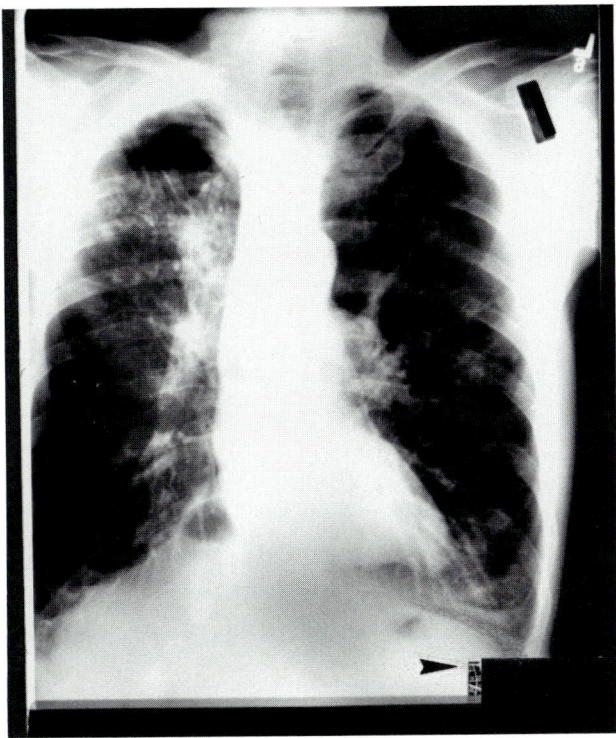

Figure 55. Blocker placed down with cassette lengthwise, superimposing costophrenic angle of left lung inferiorly. (Also the film was not centered to the patient side-to-side, clipping the right lung laterally.)

cable to the placement of right and left markers and other markers on the radiograph. Figure 58 illustrates some views in which there are areas on the film that are clearly safer for marker placement. For example, realizing that the C-spine often runs diagonally across the film in an oblique position, the marker should be placed either in the *upper posterior* corner of the cassette or in the *lower anterior* corner. This rule also applies to the lateral "spot" radiograph of the lumbosacral junction (L5–S1), in which the spinal anatomy runs diagonally across the film—marker placement should be in the upper-posterior or lower-anterior corner.

Figures 59 and 60 demonstrate simple off-centering of the film cassette in relation to the anatomy. One can always eliminate cassette orientation (lengthwise or crosswise) as the cause of such cut-off by examining the amount of space left on the film at the other extreme of the anatomy. For example, compare Figure 59 with Figure 53. In Figure 59, the costophrenic angle of the left lung is slightly clipped, yet more than five inches of film remain above the lung apices at the top. This is a simple case of center-

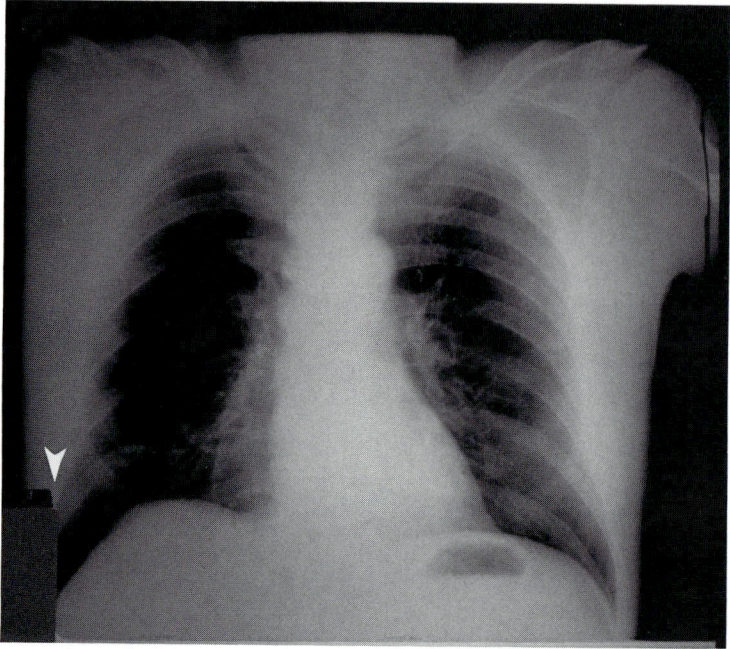

Figure 56. Blocker placed down with cassette crosswise, superimposing blocker over costophrenic angle of right lung laterally.

ing the film too high, whereas in Figure 53 the clipping of the lungs was due to placing the film crosswise rather than because of poor centering.

In Figure 55 the film was off-centered side-to-side, clipping the side of the right lung. Observing the available space to the patient's left, there appears to be room to simply recenter the film side-to-side, still placed lengthwise. This film does not, however, need to be recentered *vertically*. Rather, the blocker should be placed up.

Figure 60 is an AP projection of the lumbar spine taken on a 10 by 12 inch film. Although the centering was done "by the book" (an inch above the iliac crest), this patient's atypical bony structure resulted in the blocker being placed over the first lumbar vertebra. Even if the blocker were placed down, a repeated projection should be centered still higher, since L-1 is nearly clipped at the top of the film.

CENTRAL RAY LOCATION AND COLLIMATION

When x-ray fields smaller than the film are used, as in taking two or more exposures on one film, cut-off of the anatomy can occur due to

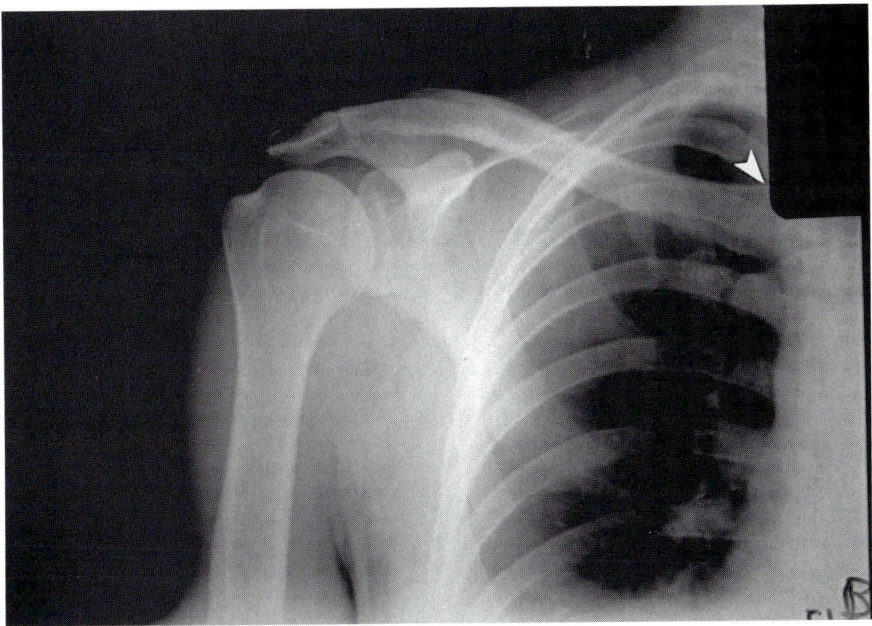

Figure 57. PA Clavicle projection with blocker placed medially and film centered laterally. The blocker superimposes the sternal extremity of the clavicle.

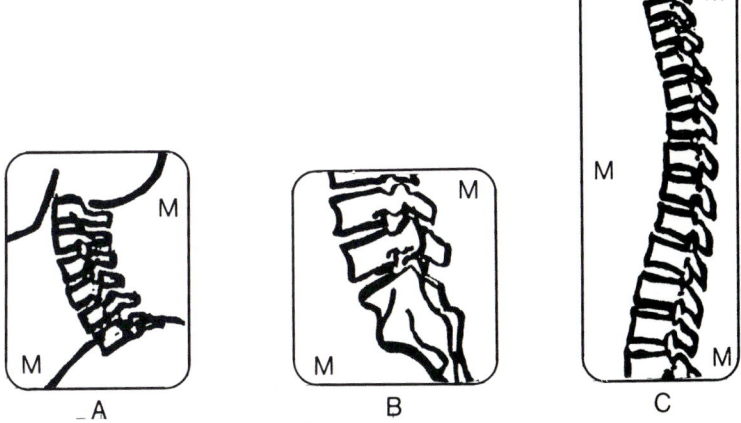

Figure 58. Diagrams of typical spine views in which safe areas for marker placement (M) can be clearly designated. For oblique and lateral C-spines and lateral lumboscacral joint views, upper-posterior or lower-anterior placement. For lateral T-spine, upper or lower posterior corner, or mid-film anteriorly.

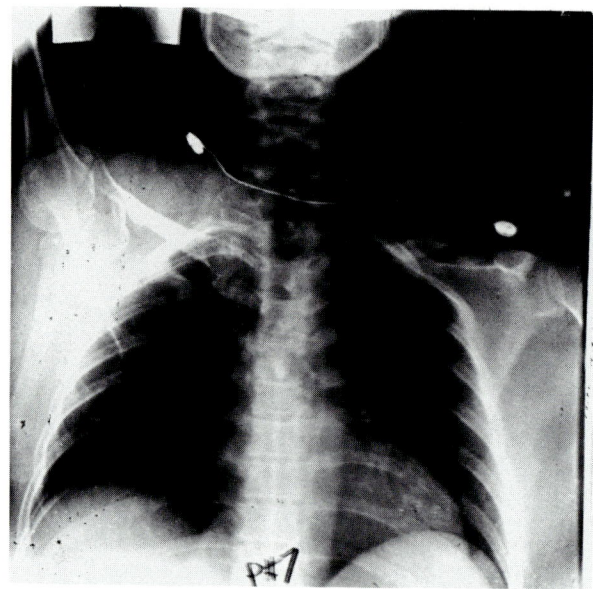

Figure 59. AP projection of chest on a 14 by 14 inch film, with cassette centered much too high, clipping left costophrenic angle.

off-centering of the x-ray beam, as in Figure 61. When a the radiograph is completely covered by the radiation beam, so that no collimation edges are seen, one cannot evaluate with certainty the location of the central ray that was used.

Many newer collimators have lead markers at the exact midpoints of each shutter edge, which cause a short white line to be recorded at the edge of the field. These white lines can be seen at the edges of Figure 1 in Chapter 1. Such markers allow the location of the central ray to be determined on the radiograph, by drawing lines intersecting the marks.

In Figure 61 no centering marks are visible. However, one edge of the x-ray beam is recognizable at the bottom of the image by its blurry appearance, with unexposed film below it, while more than an inch of film is exposed beyond the tip of the thumb. The proximal portion of the metacarpal bone of the thumb was clipped, not by the edge of the film, but by the edge of the x-ray field. Both the film and the field are centered too distally, but in this case it is the centering of the field (the central ray) which is the worse of the errors.

In Figure 62 there is not an excess of film space above the patient's shoulders, yet the costophrenic angles of the lungs are clipped off by the edge of the x-ray beam, with three inches of unexposed film below.

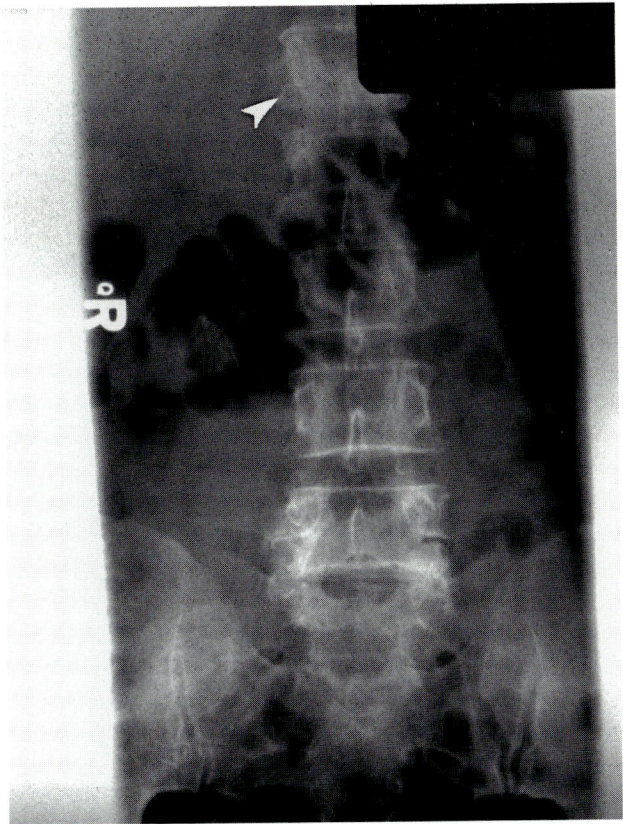

Figure 60. AP projection of lumbar spine nearly clipping top of first lumbar vertebra at top of film and with blocker over L-1. For this patient, film centering is too low.

There are two possible causes: The light field may have been properly collimated crosswise to 14 by 17 inches, in which case it must have been centered three inches higher than the film. Or, the light field was centered slightly higher than the midpoint of the film and collimated so as not to show any light on the wall above the film. This second scenario would be a case of overcollimation resulting in cut-off of anatomy.

Overcollimation can only be determined when the field size is smaller than the film size. If all four borders of the collimated field area are seen on the radiograph, the location of the central ray can be reasonably determined by (physically or mentally) drawing two diagonal lines connecting the opposing corners of the field to make an "X", Figure 63. Generally, if the central ray (the crossing point of the "X") was centered properly to the anatomy of interest, then any cut-off of the anatomy would have to be due to overcollimation or inaccurate collimation.

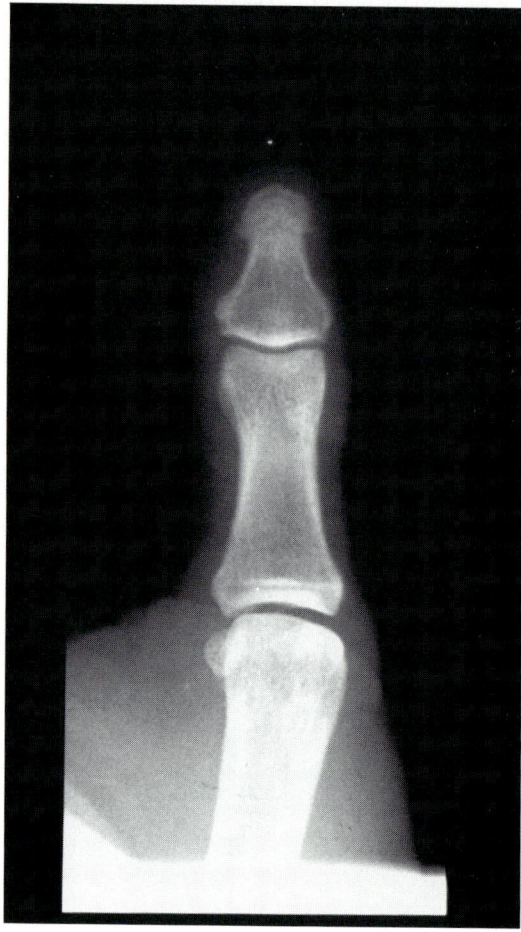

Figure 61. PA thumb projection centered too distally with x-ray field clipping proximal first metacarpal.

Inaccurate collimation refers to the possible slippage of one of the shutters in the x-ray collimator, resulting in a lop-sided x-ray field as in Figure 64.

In the context of film evaluation, the use of sheets of leaded rubber to mask off portions of the film may be considered as a form of "collimation." Sheets of lead are very handy for this purpose, because the edge of the lead is totally reliable as the edge of the field. The edges of the projected light field themselves are not reliable as accurate indicators of the edge of the actual x-ray beam, as they are typically one-half inch (and can be much more) out of alignment with the true beam. This is due to the fact

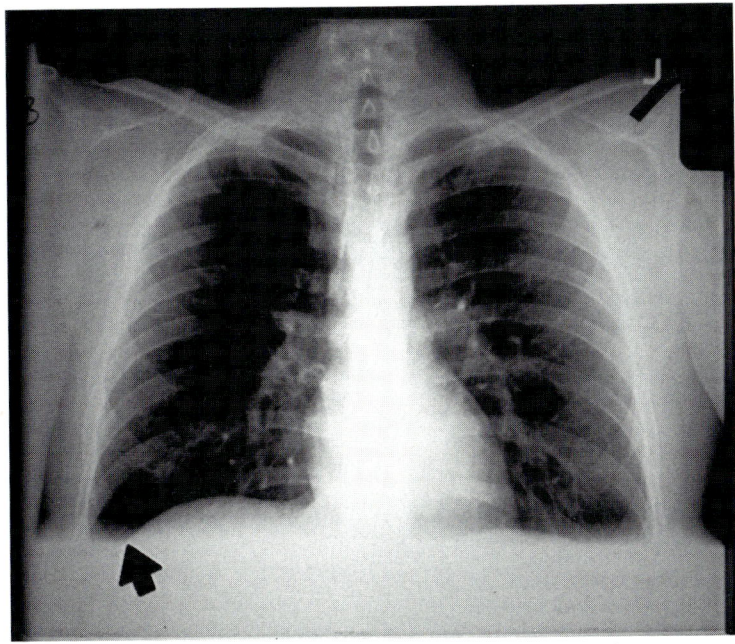

Figure 62. Overcollimation and high centering of light field combine on this PA chest projection to clip off the costophrenic angles. The film cassette was properly centered to the patient.

that the light field is projected from a reflecting mirror within the collimator and a light bulb mounted to the side, whereas the x-ray beam itself is projected straight through the collimator from the x-ray tube housing.

The overlapping fields in Figure 65 caused an area of double-exposure that obscures anatomy of interest. This occurred because the radiographer assumed that the edges of the light field were accurate. The solution to this type of overlap is to *always use lead sheets when the collimated fields result in a "tight fit"* for the anatomy.

On a radiograph, a sheet of leaded rubber can be distinguished because of its sharp, clear edge and near-total absorption of the x-ray beam. The edge of the x-ray beam itself, on the other hand, always includes a certain amount of *beam penumbra* or blurriness. These differences are illustrated in Figure 66. When using lead sheets, one can "trust the shadows" implicitly. The lead can be moved up very close to the shadow of the anatomy in the light field, and as long as the edge of the lead does not get over the shadow of the body part, it will not obscure the resulting image. Generally, when using lead sheets, open the collimated light field so that

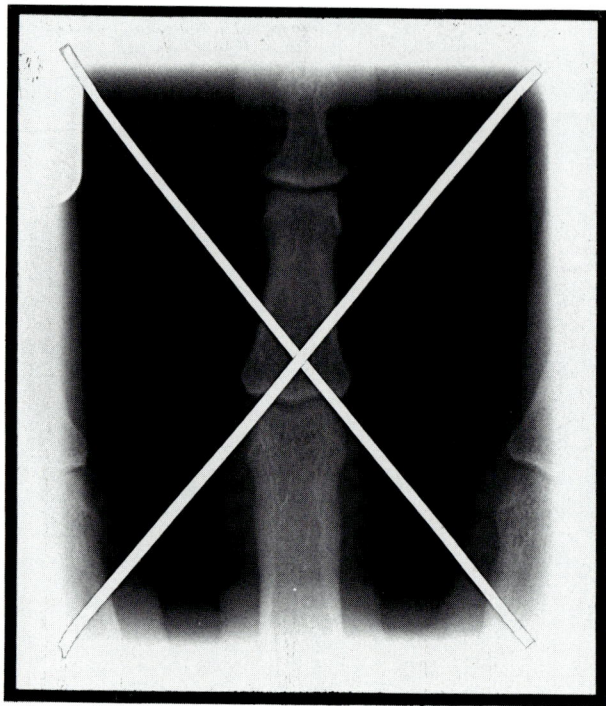

Figure 63. Method for locating the central ray when all four edges of the field are included on the film. Since this view was centered close to the PIP joint, the cut-off is primarily due to overcollimation rather than to centering.

the light overlaps the lead sheets by about one-half inch. The light field will always be larger than the area unmasked by lead.

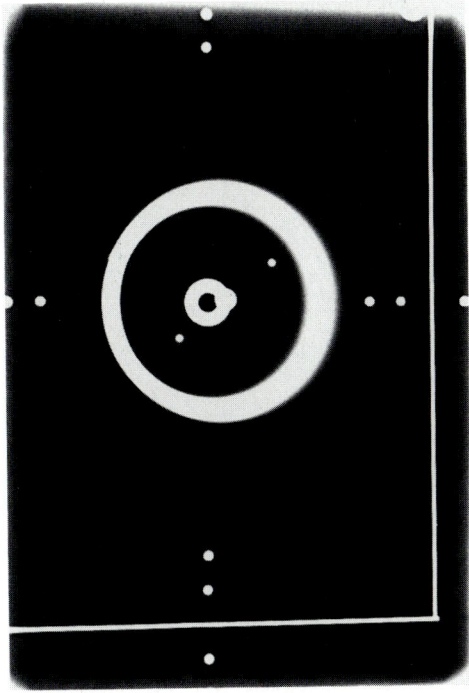

Figure 64. Example of collimator test showing slippage of shutters and a resulting lop-sided field. The exposed area should be aligned with the lead marking lines to which the light field was opened. Note that the lengthwise dimension is off more than the crosswise.

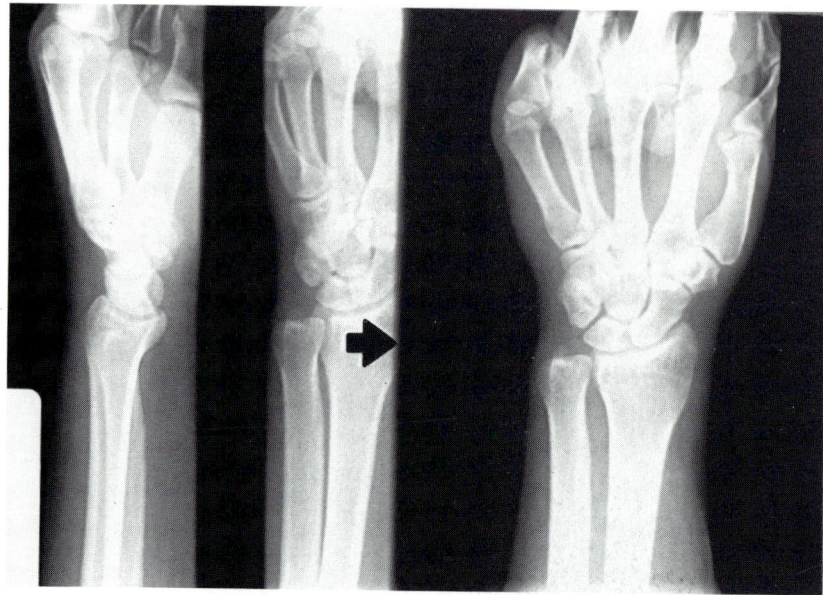

Figure 65. Failure to use lead sheets and inaccurate light field edges resulted in the actual x-ray field used for the PA wrist view overlapping anatomy in the adjacent oblique view.

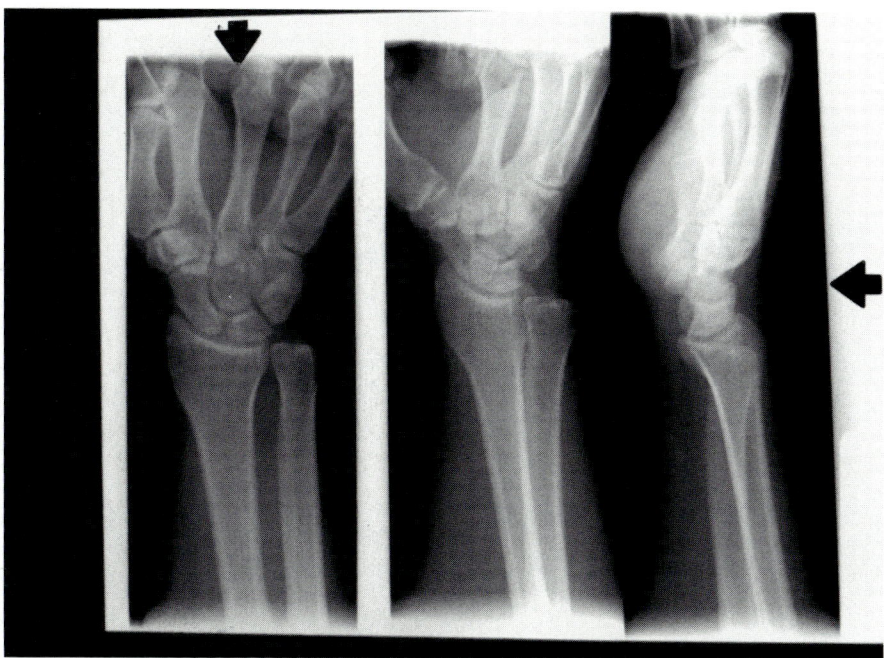

Figure 66. Use of lead sheets allowed plenty of room to fit three wrist views on this 10 by 12 film. Edges of x-ray beam (arrow at top left) are recognized by their blurry appearance as compared to the sharp edges of the lead sheets (right arrow).

Chapter 6

CRITERIA FOR EVALUATING POSITIONS

Radiographic positioning uses body part movements, x-ray beam alignment and beam angles in order to achieve the following four goals:

1. Produce a sharp, clear image by placing the specific anatomy of interest closer to the film
2. Reduce magnification of the image by placing the body part closer to the film
3. Reduce distortion of the shape of the image by centering and placing the anatomy of interest as nearly parallel to the film as possible
4. Maximize the visibility of the anatomy of interest by desuperimposing (removing) other contrasty overlying structures from overlapping it.

There are three general types of body part movements that are utilized in accomplishing the above objectives. These body movements can be listed as:

1. rotation
2. flexion/extension
3. tilt/abduction/adduction

When the rotation, tilt, or flexion/extension of the body part is not close to that prescribed by a positioning textbook, other anatomical parts can overlap and obscure the anatomy of interest, or the projected image might be blurred, magnified, or distorted because the anatomy of interest was placed at a distance or at an angle from the film.

ROTATION

Rotation is defined as a turning motion centered around an axis or pivot. Most body parts have a clear long axis, one dimension (height, width, or depth) that is longer than the other two. The long axis of the body itself is considered to be a midline running from head to toe, thus a turning of the body or head to the left or right is properly referred to as rotation. Nearly all radiographs are hung for viewing so that the long axis of the anatomy runs vertically up and down. Therefore, rotation movements will cause a side-to-side shifting of specific anatomical parts against background anatomy. Comparing Figures 67-A and 67-B, this side-to-side shift from rotation is demonstrated. Specified amounts of rotation produce oblique views which may best desuperimpose obstructing anatomy from the anatomy of interest. But, for routine frontal and lateral projections, any rotation is undesirable.

FLEXION/EXTENSION

Flexion refers to a bending motion of a joint whereby the angle formed between the two limbs is reduced or closed, such as the closing movement of the elbow when one "flexes his arm muscles." For the spinal column and head, flexion is *forward* bending. Extension is the opposite of flexion. Extension refers to the straightening movement of a joint whereby the angle formed between the two limbs is increased or opened. For the spinal column and head, extension is a *backward* bending movement. On *frontal* views, flexion or extension will result in a vertical upward or downward shift of specific anatomical parts against the background anatomy. Comparing Figures 67-A and 67-C, this vertical shift due to flexion/extension is demonstrated. The proper amount of flexion or extension of the body part is essential on all *frontal* views.

TILT, ABDUCTION, AND ADDUCTION

The word *tilt* will be used in this book to refer to a sideways leaning of the head to the right or left. The equivalent movements in the extremities are *abduction* and *adduction*. *Abduction* refers to the movement of a limb sideways *away* from the central axis of the body. *Adduction* refers to the movement of a limb *toward* the central axis of the body. Similar lateral stress movements of the foot are referred to as *inversion* (medial stress) and *eversion* (lateral stress). On *lateral* radiographs, tilt, abduction or adduction movements cause specific anatomical parts to shift vertically up or down against the background anatomy. Proper tilt, abduction or adduction is essential on all *lateral* views.

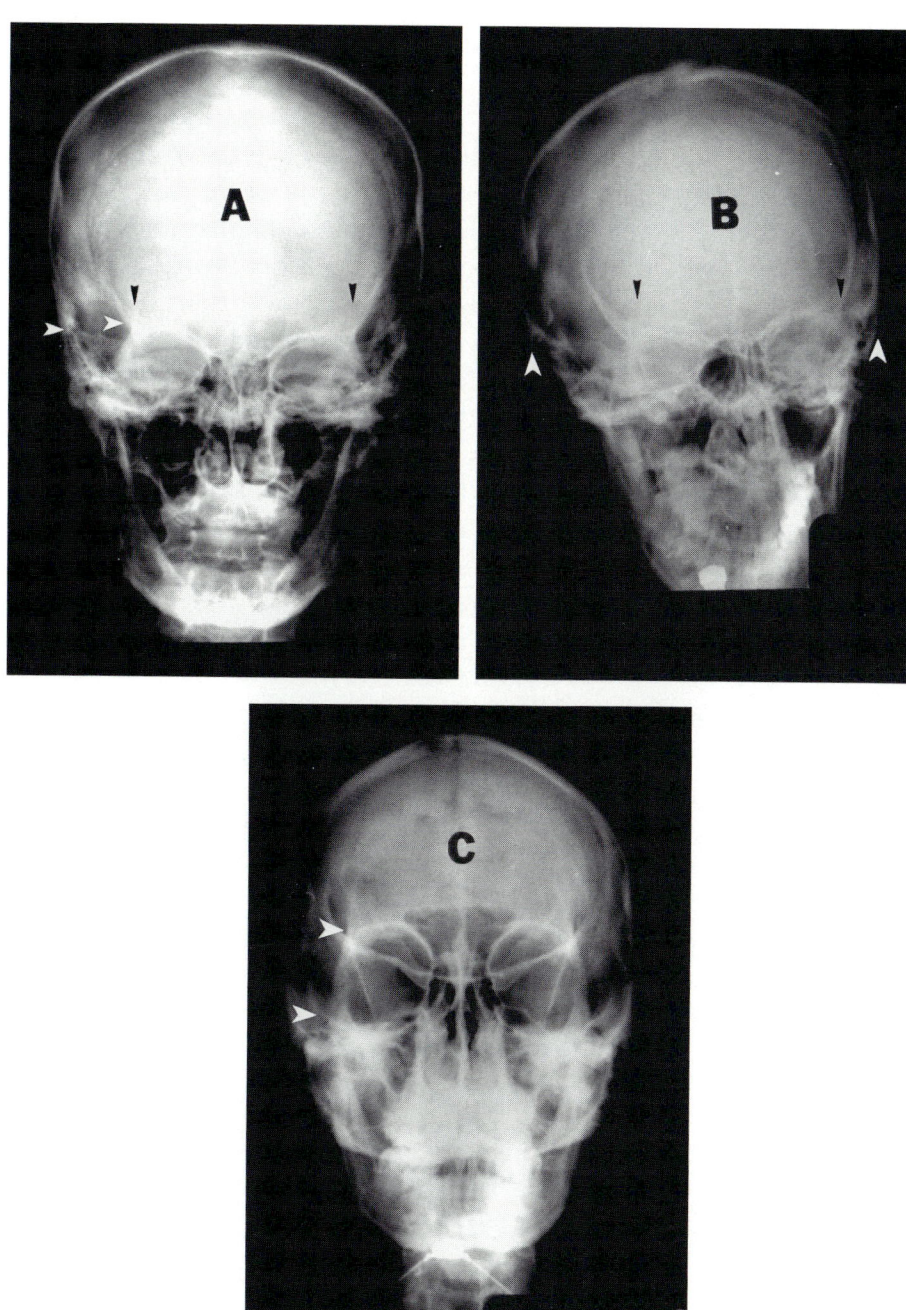

Figure 67. Directions of anatomical shift for rotation and flexion/extension movements from a frontal viewpoint. Comparing *A* and *B*: When rotation occurs (B), the lateral rims of the orbits (black arrows) shift side-to-side in relation to the sides of the skull. Comparing *A* and *C*: With extension movement of the head (C), the petrous ridges shift downward in relation to the orbits (horizontal white arrows). Flexion would shift the petrous ridges upward in relation to the orbits.

An important point of clarification for all body part movements is that they consistently relate to the dimensions of the *body* itself rather than the dimensions of the radiograph or the viewpoint of the observer. For example, observe the radiograph in Figure 68, a submentovertex projection of the skull which is poorly positioned. Is this position rotated? Many radiographers at a glance will call this position rotated, when in fact there is no rotation at all, but a *tilting* of the head. For the sake of clarity, we must be consistent in our terminology. The trick is that most of us are not very used to the axial (through the long axis) viewpoint of the projection in Figure 68. Just because the viewpoint or projection has changed, this does not and should not change the definitions of rotation, tilt or flexion/extension as they relate to the body itself. Figure 69, also using a submentovertex projection, shows true rotation of the head—a turning movement upon its axis.

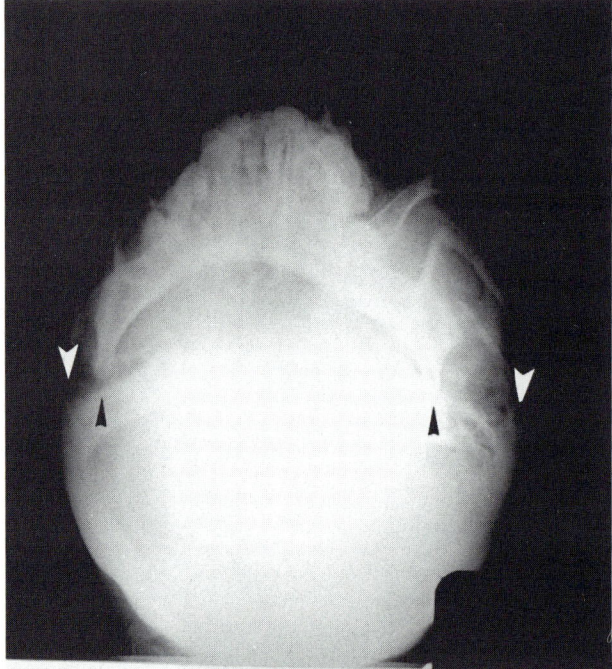

Figure 68. Submentovertex projection of the skull showing head tilt. Tilt shifts the rami of the mandible (arrows) side-to-side in relation to the sides of the skull. On axial views, head tilt is often mistaken for rotation. This view shows some flexion and tilt, but no true rotation.

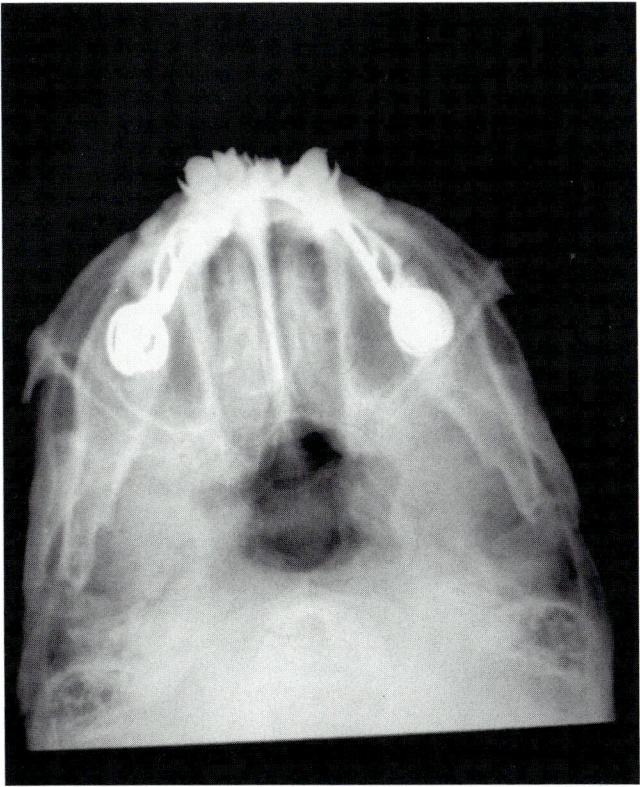

Figure 69. Submentovertex projection of the skull showing true rotation. No head tilt is present, so that the mandible (arrows) is aligned with the sides of the skull.

ANGULATION OF THE X-RAY BEAM

Cephalic or caudal angulation of the x-ray beam serves the same positioning function as certain body movements and is radiographically equivalent to them. When the patient is in a supine or prone position for a frontal type of projection, a cephalic angle of the central ray would be equivalent to flexion or extension of the body part. For example, on an AP view of the cervical spine, angling the x-ray beam cephalic allows one to see up under the chin. Extending the head also allows one to see up under the chin. Similarly, the Waters projection for the sinuses with the patient prone can be accomplished either with a 37-degree caudal angle or with a 37-degree extension of the head.

In lateral positions, angling the tube caudal or cephalic would be equivalent to lateral bending, tilt, abduction, or adduction. For example, angling caudally over the top of the upside shoulder for a cervicothoracic view would be equivalent to depressing the upside shoulder (a tilting movement). During positioning for a lateral skull view, when the head is tilted, the x-ray beam can be angled until it is parallel to the interpupillary line, cancelling out the tilt to produce a true lateral view, Figure 70.

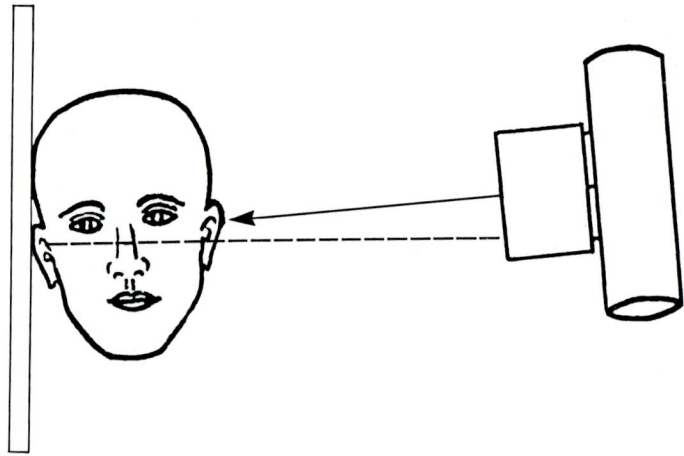

Figure 70. Example of the equivalency of x-ray beam angulation to body movements. In lateral projections, a caudal angle is equivalent to tilt/abduction/adduction motions. Here the caudal angle cancels out the tilting of the head toward the film, resulting in a straight lateral projection.

POSITIONING AIDS AND TIPS

Various shapes of positioning sponges are available which can assist in establishing the proper rotation of the body part. Sand bags, clamps, tape, Velcro™, and numerous other supplies and devices can be used, so long as they do not themselves obscure diagnostically important information. A special precaution is in order regarding the use of sponges: Never assume that the mere use of an angled sponge assures that the body part will lie at the correct angle. Heavy body parts will compress a sponge. Furthermore, often the body part is not slid up snug against the surface of the sponge. Either of these problems will result in the body part lying at a more shallow angle than the sponge itself. Long 45-degree sponges are frequently placed under the patient's torso, but not slid under far enough under the body to place the body flush along the sponge surface, as in Figure 71. The important point is to always consider and measure the body part rotation *as it lies,* and not make any assumptions because of the positioning aids used.

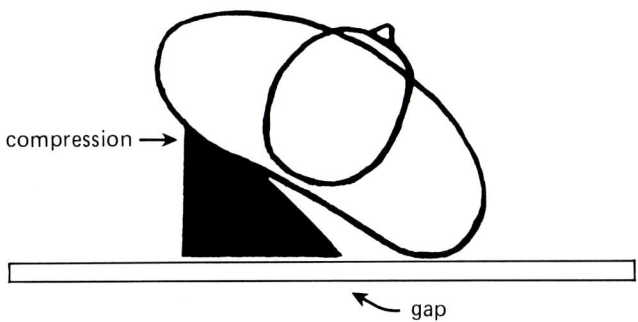

Figure 71. Two reasons why the body cannot be assumed to lie at the angle of a positioning sponge: The sponge compresses, and there is often a gap created when the body is not placed flush against the sponge surface. Both of these result in the body position lying somewhat more shallow than the sponge surface.

For most procedures, *it is essential that the entire length of the body part be rotated by the same amount.* On all oblique views of torso anatomy, both the shoulders and the hips should be rotated at the same angle. Often the upside leg is bent and the hips rolled up to the indicated angle, yet the shoulders are left at a very shallow angle or not rolled up at all. The torso can easily assume a twisted position, but this will result in a view which is rotated at one end or the other.

VIEWS

As distinguished from body movements, the three general classifications of x-ray beam *projections* or *views* can be listed as:

1. Frontal Views
2. Lateral Views
3. Axial Views

All projections including angled views fit into one of these three broad classifications (unless they employ an angle of exactly 45 degrees). The Waters projection of the sinuses uses a 37-degree extension movement and the Caldwell projection uses a 15-degree caudal angle, but both are essentially frontal (front-to-back or back-to-front) projections.

Changing the basic type of view can change the criteria for evaluating body part movements. For example, side-to-side shifting of anatomy on frontal or lateral views indicates rotation of the part, as in Figure 67-B, whereas side-to-side shifting on *axial* views indicates *tilt,* as in Figure 68. (Since only a few projections are made axially, though, it may be said that side-to-side shifting of anatomy indicates part rotation in *most* cases.)

SELECTING ANATOMICAL CRITERIA

What types of anatomy are most reliable and accurate as references on a radiograph to determine if the position is improperly rotated, tilted, flexed, or extended? For any particular view, there are always several anatomical references that may be well used. The very best ones can be selected by using the following four rules:

1. *The selected anatomy should be two identical structures that are normally fixed in place,* and therefore reliable. Parts of the mandible, for example, are less reliable than parts of the cranium, because the mandible is movable and may be cocked to one side. Extremities may be moved. Soft tissue anatomy is not as reliable to be fixed in position as bony anatomy is.

2. *The selected anatomy should have a long axis or edge that lies perpendicular to the direction of expected shift,* Figure 72. For rotation, the expected shift of the two parts would be side-to-side. Therefore, the best anatomy would be something linear running up-and-down. For tilt or flexion/extension, the shift would normally be up-and-down, and the best anatomy would be linear running side-to-side.

3. *The two selected structures should be anatomically as far from each other and from the midline of the body as possible,* Figure 73. When the two structures are close together, it takes a great amount of rotation to obviously desuperimpose them or shift them off of each other. As an example, rotation on a lateral skull is better determined by the greater wings of the sphenoid bone rather than by the posterior clinoid processes. The two clinoids are only one-half inch away from each other, and only severe rotation will cause them to shift in a readily apparent way.

4. *The selected anatomy should be as close to the central ray location of the x-ray beam as possible.* Recall that the central ray is the only "straight"

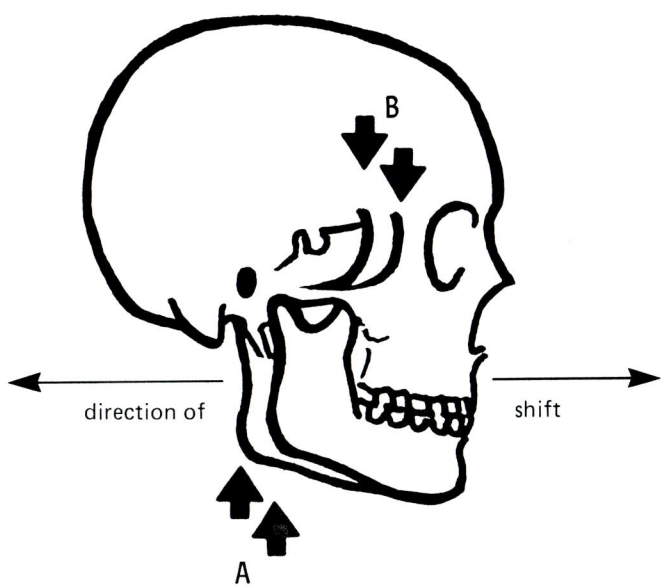

Figure 72. Anatomical criteria used to evaluate a position should lie perpendicular to the expected direction of shift. Here, head rotation produces a side-to-side horizontal shift. Therefore, vertical anatomy such as the rami of the mandible (A) or the greater wings of the sphenoid bone (B) should be used to evaluate head rotation. If two horizontal lines were used, rotation would slide them along on top of each other, still superimposed.

ray. Though a position may be perfect, anatomy placed in the diverging beams away from the CR will be *expected to be desuperimposed and shifted* because of the angle of these beams, Figure 74. The farther the anatomy is from the CR, the greater will be this shift caused by angled beams. Thus, the position may be critiqued as being rotated when in fact it was straight.

Of course, most anatomical parts will not fit *all four* of these rules, but the idea is to select those criteria which fit as many of them as possible. To summarize, the best anatomy to use for evaluating positions on radiographs will be two identical parts that are relatively fixed in location, perpendicular to the expected direction of shift, as far away from each other as possible, and as close to the central ray as possible.

Upon rotating a body part, the distance that the criterion anatomy shifts on the radiograph depends on how far the parts are from each other anatomically. For example, five degrees of body rotation on a PA projection of the chest will shift the ribs, sternoclavicular joints and costophrenic angles about one-quarter inch side-to-side; Yet, five degrees of

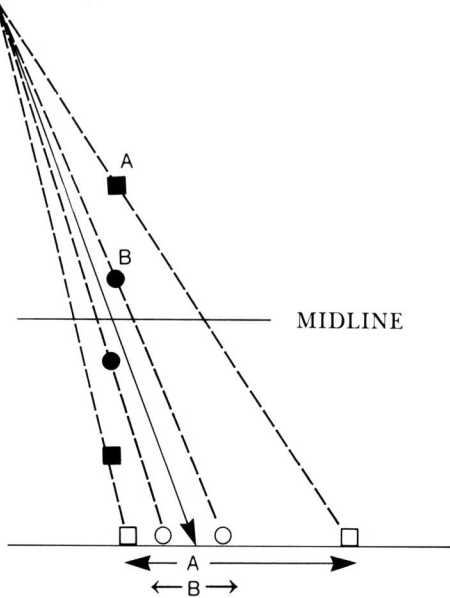

Figure 73. Anatomical criteria which are far from each other and from the body midline will best show body movements. Note that at a given amount of angle or rotation, the images of the squares (A) are shifted much farther apart than those of the circles (B).

body rotation on the *lateral* projection of the chest will shift the ribs and costophrenic angles one full inch. This is because the chest is wider side-to-side than it is thick front-to-back. The lateral ribs are about eight centimeters farther apart from each other than the anterior and posterior ribs are, Figure 75.

A general rule for chest positioning is that more than five degrees of rotation is repeatable for either the PA or the lateral view. But this five degrees is measured differently on the two views: For the PA projection, the sternoclavicular joints should not be shifted more than *one-quarter inch.* For the lateral view, the posterior ribs should not be shifted more than *one inch.*

Other geometrical factors such as the FFD used will also affect the amount of apparent shift caused from body rotation. At an increased FFD, such as 72 inches versus 40 inches, the amount of anatomical shifting seen on the radiograph is diminished.

Finally, one should never conclude that a radiograph has been incorrectly positioned on the basis of any *single* criterion. *Always observe two or more anatomical criteria to see if they agree.* This is important because

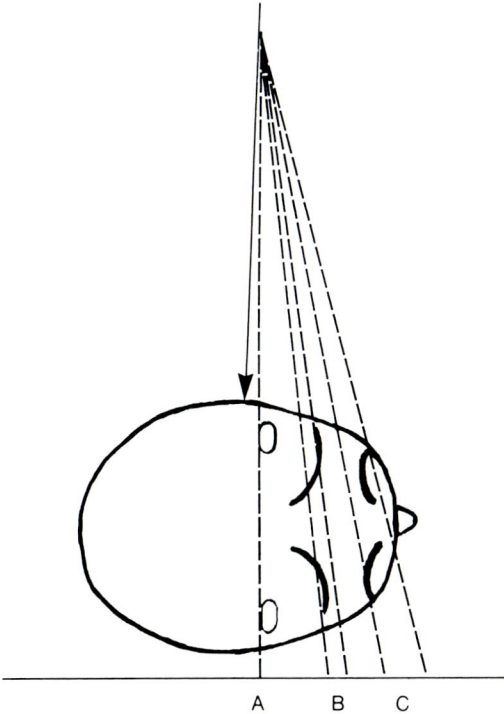

Figure 74. Anatomical criteria selected to evaluate a position should lie as close to the central ray location as possible. To evaluate rotation on a lateral skull, shown here, the rami of the mandible (A) lie very close to the CR (in a side-to-side direction) and make good criteria. The greater wings of the sphenoid bone (B) should also be close together. Note that the rims of the orbits (C) are far enough from the CR that diverging rays in the x-ray beam should be expected to project them off of each other. While the orbital rims make good criteria for rotation on a lateral facial bone projection with the CR centered to the malar bone, they do *not* make good criteria for the lateral skull where the CR is much farther posterior.

some pathological conditions, such as scoliosis, might result in what appears at a glance to be a rotated view, while observing other parts of the image would confirm that the position was as correct as possible under the circumstances. Always use more than one anatomical criterion for confirmation.

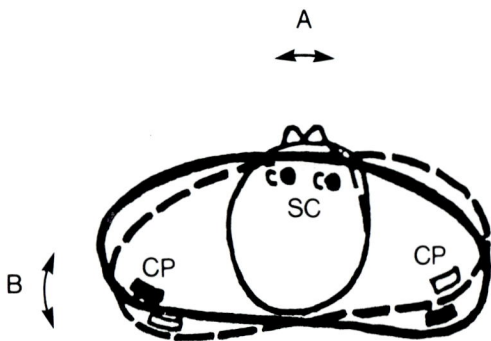

Figure 75. Different views may have different amounts of shift to be expected by a rotational movement. For example, the chest is thicker laterally than it is front-to-back. Five degrees of rotation will shift the posterior ribs and costophrenic angles (CP) one inch on the lateral view, *B*. Yet, on the PA view the same 5 degrees of rotation will shift the sternoclavicular joints (SC) only about one-quarter inch, *A*.

Chapter 7

TORSO POSITIONS

Bony anatomy is always more reliable as a positioning criterion than soft tissue organs. The skeletal criteria for a particular region of the body is shared by any procedures done in that area. For example, the bones of the lumbar spine and pelvis can be used to evaluate *any* abdominal position, including views from IVP, cystogram, barium enema, upper GI or gall bladder series. While attention to the projection of particular organs is sometimes important, by focusing primarily on the skeletal criteria we are able to simplify the rules of film critique. All thoracic procedures can be combined, all abdominal and pelvic views can be combined, and most of the spinal vertebrae can be discussed collectively in selecting criteria to evaluate positioning.

CHEST AND BONY THORAX

Frontal Views

Rotation: For the PA or AP view of the chest or bilateral ribs, the symmetry of the *sternoclavicular joints* is typically recommended as the criterion for rotation. These two joints should be equidistant from the midline of the spine, located by the teardrop-shaped spinous process, as shown in Figure 76-A. Note, however, that in Figure 76-B, although the sternoclavicular joints are only slightly rotated, the bases of the lungs in this view are grossly asymmetrical in length along the diaphragm. (The heart shadow must be ignored and the lung bases measured from the midline of the spine.) SC joints only indicate rotation of the *shoulders.* It is possible to have the shoulders straight and the hips crooked, resulting in rotation only at the bases of the lungs. For a perfectly straight view, the costophrenic angles of the lungs should also appear equidistant *from the midline of the spine.* On normal patients, this is achieved by ensuring that one foot is not placed in front of the other.

On the PA view of the chest, how much rotation is enough to warrant a

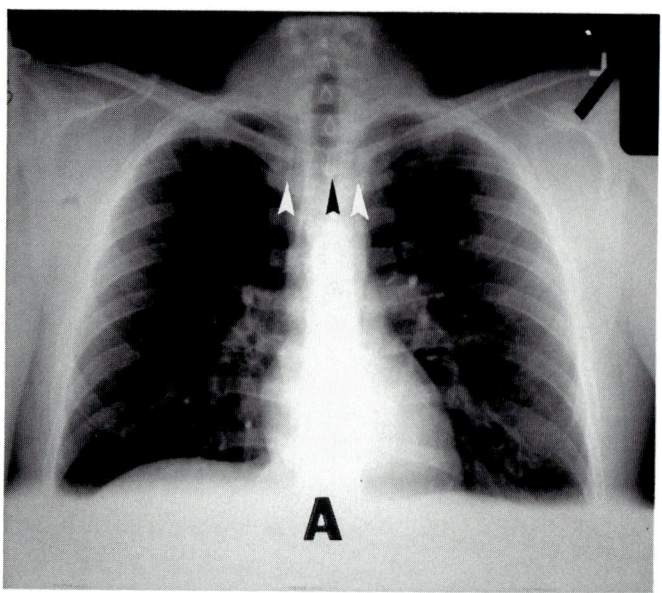

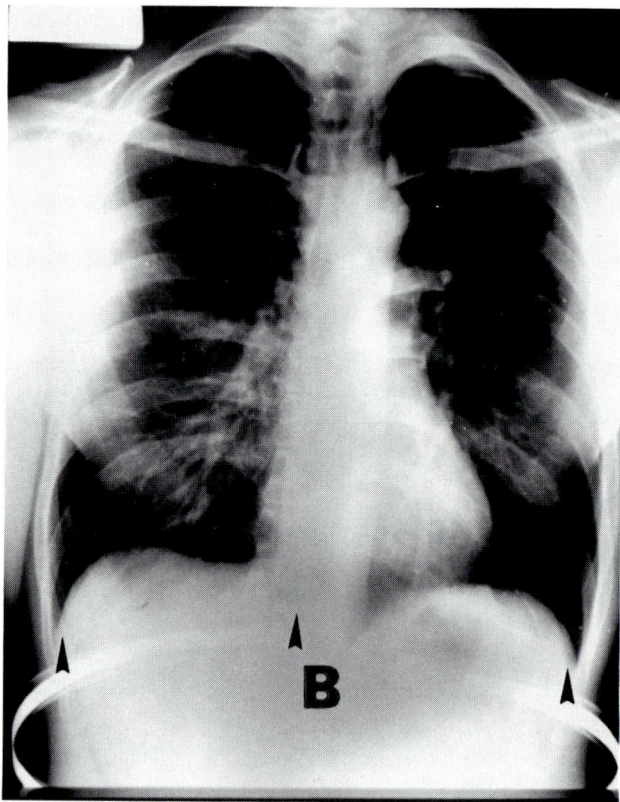

Figure 76. Rotation on PA chest views. *A* shows *shoulder* rotation, in which the sternoclavicular joints (white arrows) are not equidistant from the spinous process of T-3 (black arrow). *B* shows *hip* rotation in which the two costophrenic angles are not equidistant from the mid-spine (arrows). (*A* also shows cut-off of the lower lungs due to a combination of centering high and over-collimating.)

repeated exposure? There is great variation in the distance from the mid-spine to the sternoclavicular joints, depending on the thickness and size of the patient. On average, the SC joints are approximately ¾ inch to either side of the mid-spine. *One-quarter inch* of sideways shift for these joints equates to about five degrees of rotation in the shoulders. With five degrees of rotation, one SC joint would be about ½ inch from the spinous process, while the opposite joint would be an inch from the mid-spine. For normal anatomy, any more rotation than this (¼ inch of shift) would be repeatable.

Note that the spine itself can be used to indicate rotation on frontal views of any torso anatomy, by checking if the spinous processes lie in the middle of the vertebral bodies. This is fully discussed in the "spine" section that follows.

Shoulder Rotation. Ideally, the scapulae should be completely desuperimposed from the lung fields for a PA chest projection. This is accomplished by rotating the patient's shoulders forward until both are in contact with the table, chest board or cassette. In practice, the medial borders of the scapulae may superimpose the upper lateral lung fields along the inner borders of the ribs by a small amount. But, more than one-half inch of such superimposition, as shown in Figure 77, implies an inadequate effort in rotating the shoulders forward, and is repeatable. Compare Figure 77 with Figure 76-A, in which the scapulae are completely rotated out of the lung fields.

(This rule is not practical for chest views taken in *AP* projection, such as portable chests, because it is difficult to rotate the shoulders forward while lying on one's back. Portable chest views are therefore expected to show overlapping of the scapulae and the lung fields.)

When *both* shoulders are rotated forward equally, this helps to eliminate any rotation of the chest itself and the sternoclavicular joints will be symmetrical. If one scapula overlaps the lung field more than the opposite one, then both shoulders were not rotated forward *evenly*.

Angulation and Flexion/Extension. Routine chest and rib views require no angulation of the x-ray beam. On frontal views, the medial aspects of the *first three posterior ribs* will be demonstrated *above the clavicles* as shown in Figure 76-B. On some patients the third rib will be partially covered by the clavicle as in Figure 76-A. For intentional *lordotic* views of the chest, a proper angle of the x-ray beam or extension of the spine will produce a view with the clavicles projected over the medial aspects of the *first posterior ribs* and completely above the *apices of the lungs.*

It is common when performing *AP* chest projections, such as "stretcher

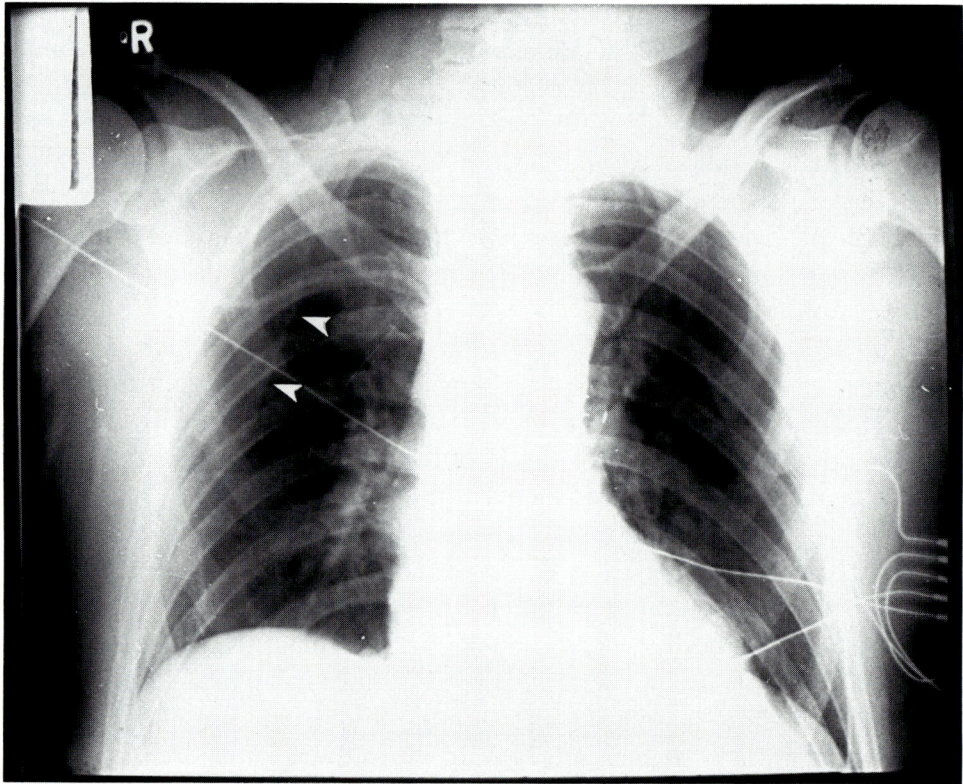

Figure 77. Scapulae superimposing lung fields due to failure to rotate shoulders forward. Arrows show medial border of right scaula.

chests" or portable chests, to obtain *improper lordotic* views from insufficient *caudal* angulation of the x-ray beam. Such views will demonstrate the clavicles above the posterior third ribs and tend to cause a "straightened out," linear appearance to the posterior ribs from the distortion of their normal curvature, as in Figure 78. This problem is avoided by ensuring that the central ray is angled sufficiently caudal to be perpendicular to the mid-axillary line of *the patient* rather than perpendicular to the film, bed or stretcher.

Small children's skulls are much larger in proportion to their bodies than those of adults. It does not take very much flexion or extension of the neck to get the chin or the occipital bone of an infant over the apices of the lungs, Figure 79.

When lying an infant on it's back, the large cranium resting against the table often forces the chin into a flexed position, superimposing it

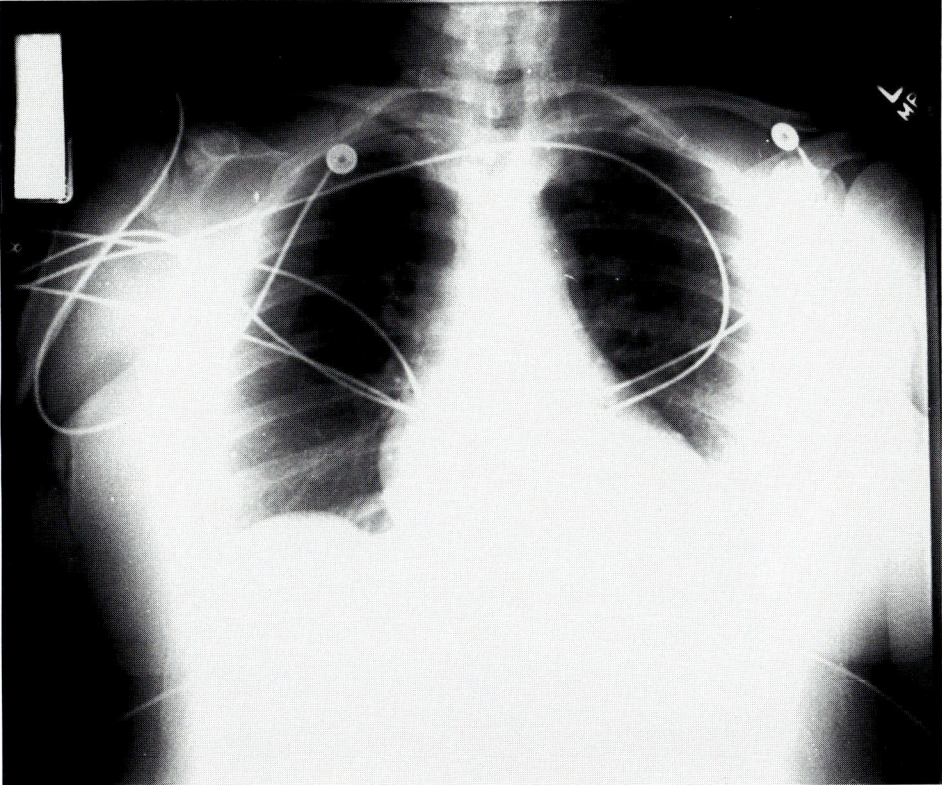

Figure 78. Lordotic chest view caused by failure to angle beam caudally on a portable AP projection with patient sitting. Note clavicles projected over first pair of ribs and "straightened out" appearance of posterior ribs. (Also shows unnecessary amount of lead wires over lung field.)

over the lung fields. To avoid this (as well as to avoid a lordotic projection), place a 10–15 degree angle sponge on top of the cassette with the thickest end under the baby's shoulders, allowing the head to fall gently back *onto the film.* (Dropping the head off of the sponge *and* film, or using a thicker sponge, may hyperextend the head and injure the child. Be cautious.)

Respiration. Normal frontal views of the chest on adult patients should be on full inspiration, with *10 posterior ribs* showing in the lung fields. To consider a rib as being in the lung field, at least the medial one-half of the posterior rib should appear above the diaphragm. This same rule applies for above-the-diaphragm projections of the ribs. Figure 80 is an example of inadequate inspiration, and shows how to count the ribs.

100

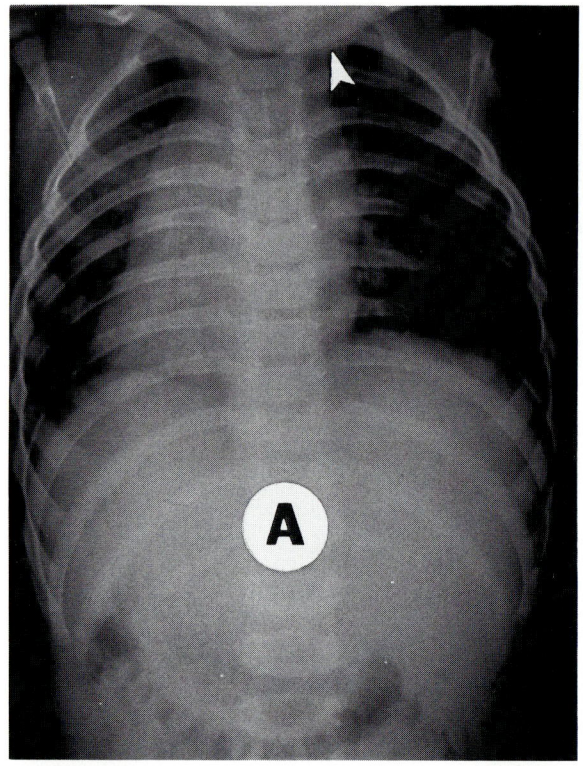

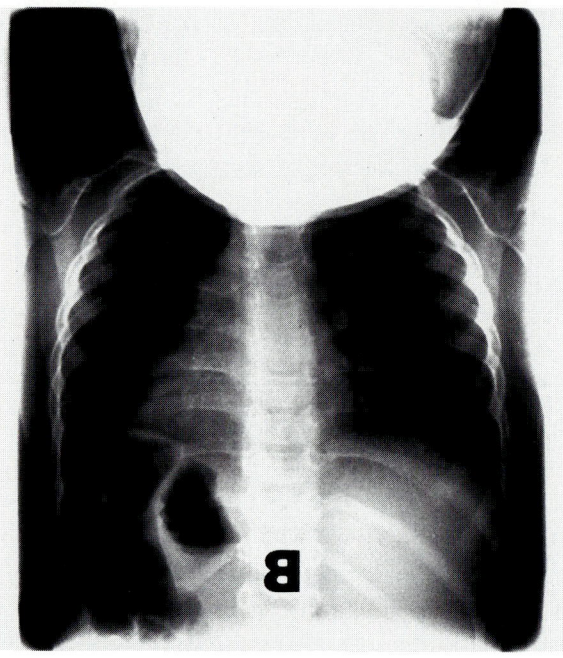

Figure 79. Typical problems with chest radiography on infants. *A* shows infant's chin over lung apices caused by resting proportionately large head on cassette. *B* shows occipital bone over apices when head was hyperextended.

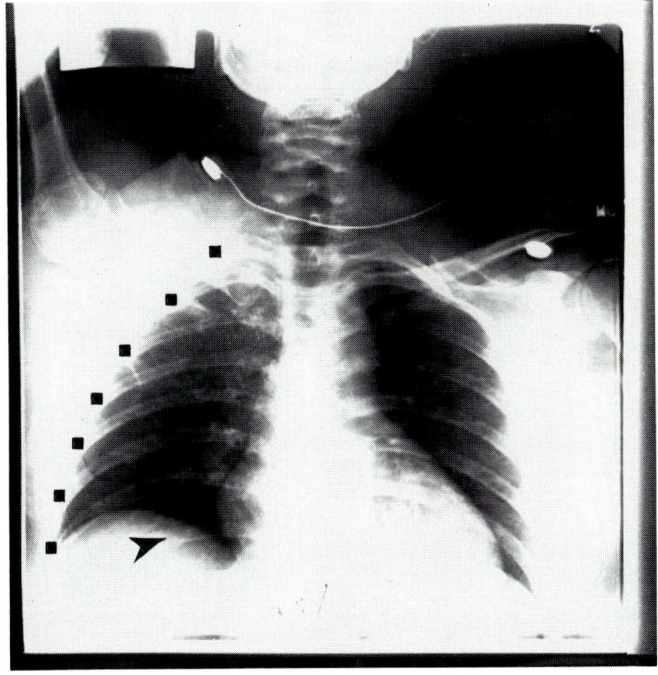

Figure 80. Inadequate inspiration on frontal chest view. Marks show how to count the posterior ribs with the medial portion of the eighth rib (arrow) showing above the diaphragm for a total of eight. Ten ribs indicate a good inspiration on adult chests. (Also, top of cassette was placed so high that the left costophrenic angle is slightly clipped.)

For *infants* in general, nine ribs above the diaphragm is adequate. For *premature* and *newborn* infants, eight ribs is adequate.

Technique

When adequate penetration (kVp) is used for chest radiography, details of the thoracic spine and medial ribs will be *just visible* through the heart shadow, as in Figure 76. Proper density will then also demonstrate the soft tissue markings in the lung fields. A chest radiograph is repeatable any time that the *mediastinal* structures are obliterated by inadequate penetration or density, leaving the heart and spine area with a "white" or clear appearance. Figure 81 illustrates improper chest techniques.

Lateral Views

Rotation. The lateral view of the chest has no pairs of reliable anatomy close to the central ray. In assessing rotation, we are limited to using anatomy along the back of the chest, which is less variable than the anterior chest wall. Two criteria which serve well in this area are the

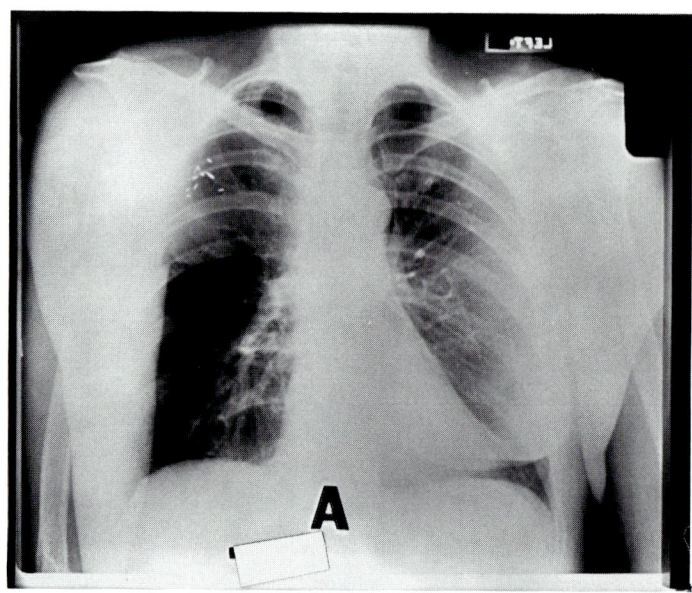

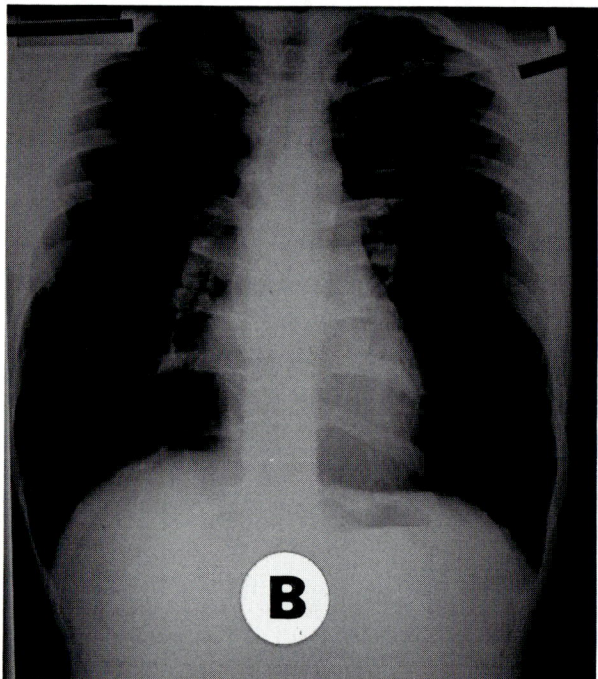

Figure 81. Extremes in chest technique. *A* is underpenetrated since the spine cannot be seen through the heart shadow. *B* is too dark in the lung fields. (Note that *B* is also centered low, placing the cassette blocker over the right lung apex.)

posterior ribs and the *posterior costophrenic angles of the lungs.* The right and left posterior ribs should be superimposed directly on top of each other, and the right and left costophrenic angles should also directly superimpose each other. Figure 82 shows that when the lateral chest view is rotated, a "space" of lung field will appear between the sets of ribs, usually with one set of ribs showing the circular on-end appearance from looking "down the barrel" at them. As a rule of thumb, *if this space is more than two finger-breadths (about one inch) wide, the view should be repeated.* On lateral views, one inch of shift between the ribs indicates about 5 degrees of rotation, since one side shifts forward by ½ inch and the opposite side shifts backward ½ inch. The posterior costophrenic angles in Figure 82 are shifted by the same amount as the ribs, and are reliable indicators of rotation.

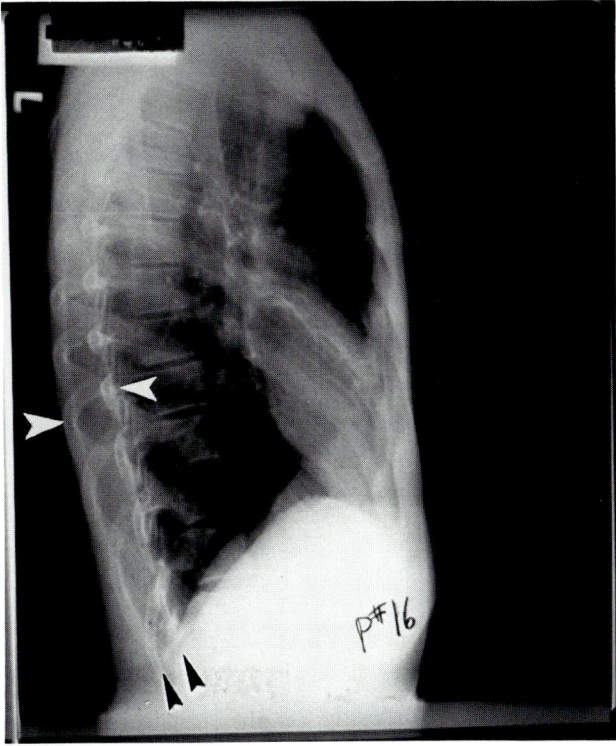

Figure 82. Rotation on lateral chest, detected by shifting of two sets of posterior ribs (white arrows) and two posterior costophrenic angles (black arrows). This amount of rotation is passable but borderline: Any more would require a repeat.

Note that there is a normal "lung space" that lies behind the spine, between it and the posterior ribs. Some patients have very curved ribs so that this space is large, an appearance that can be mistaken for rotation even though the posterior ribs are exactly superimposed, Figure 83. Be careful not to mistake this normal space behind the spine as a space between the two sets of ribs.

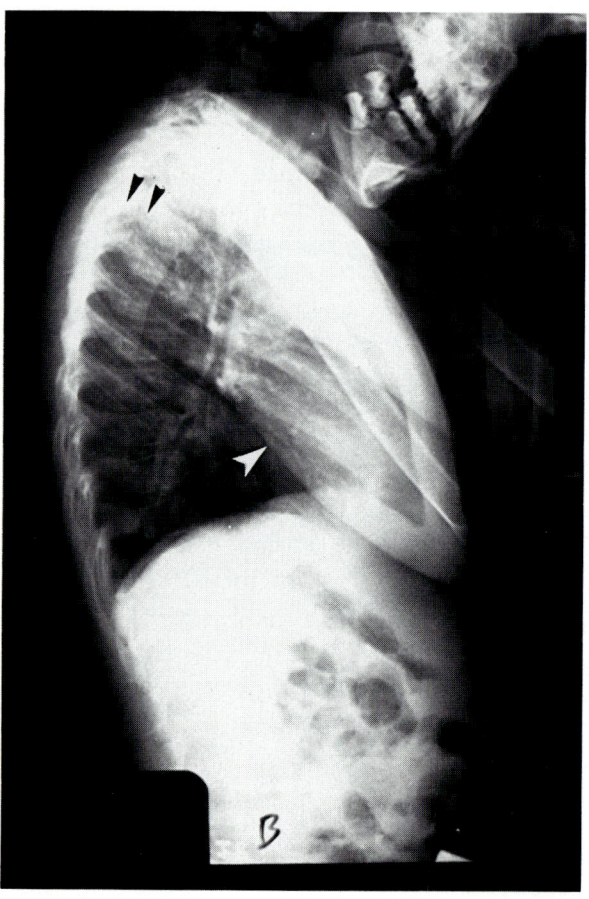

Figure 83. Normal lung space behind vertebral bodies (black arrows) on a perfectly straight lateral chest view. Insufficient abduction of the arms resulted in the arm shadow (white arrow) obscuring the lung field.

Again, the spine itself can be helpful as discussed later in this chapter.

Flexion/Extension. During lateral chest projections, a common error is to fold the patient's *hands* on top of his head, rather than his *arms*.

Views like that in Figure 83 can result, with arm tissue superimposing the lateral lung field. Whenever possible, the patient's *forearms* should be crossed over his head.

Asking the patient to keep his chin up also helps him to stand straight, and on large patients this can make a difference in fitting the lung fields on the film. In Figure 84 a large patient's *anterior* costophrenic angles were clipped off when he leaned back upon taking a deep breath, extending the spine. Patients must be observed carefully *as* they follow breathing instructions.

Respiration. The same rule used for the PA chest, of demonstrating ten ribs above the diaphragm, also applies to the evaluation of adequate inspiration on the lateral chest view, but one must observe the position of the uppermost *peak* of the dome of the diaphragm and count the number of posterior ribs which lie above that point, as shown in Figure 84.

Oblique Views

Rotation. When a proper 45-degree oblique view is taken of the chest or ribs, the posterior ribs on one side will appear to be *one-half* as long as those on the opposite side, as in Figure 85. Also, the sternum will be shifted so that there is a 2–3 inch space between it and the spine. When the rotation is *too shallow,* the space between the sternum and spine will be less than two inches and the foreshortened lung will not yet be reduced to one-half. When the rotation is *too steep,* the foreshortened lung will be reduced to less than one-half the width of the opposite lung, and the view will begin to take on a distinct rotated *lateral* appearance.

For coned-down oblique views of the right or left ribs, the posterior ribs on the side of interest are laid out roughly parallel to the film, so that they appear long and somewhat straightened, while those on the opposite side are foreshortened and very curved. For *posterior oblique* positions, the side of interest is the *downside.* For *anterior oblique* positions, the side of interest is the *upside.* Ideally, on the side of interest the heads of most of the ribs will not superimpose the bodies of the vertebrae. If they do, the position is too *steep.*

Decubitus Views

Decubitus views of the chest should meet all of the criteria for routine frontal views. In addition, it is essential that the arms be placed above the patient's head so there is no chance of superimposing them over the lung fields. If the interest is in ruling out *fluid levels* of any kind, the

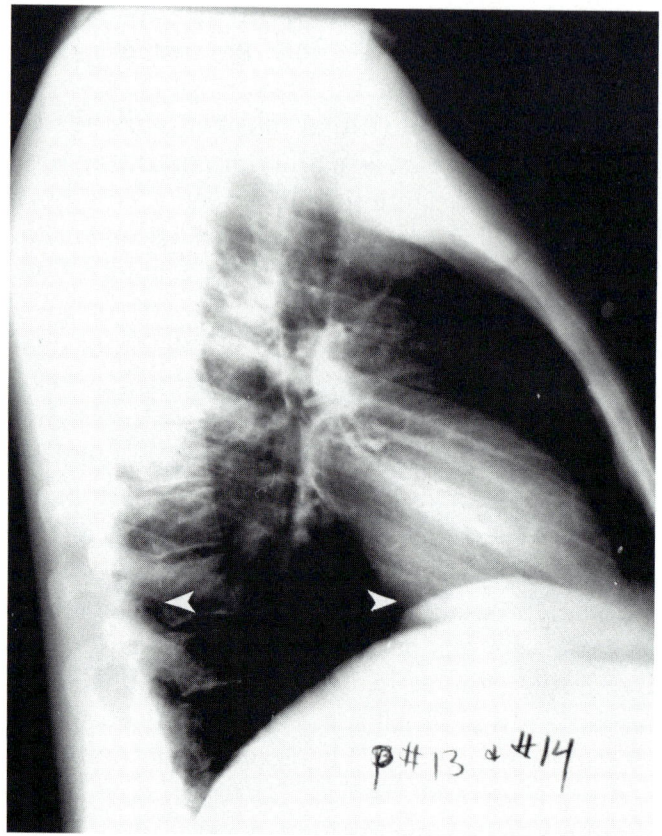

Figure 84. Large patient who leaned back on inspiration, causing the *anterior* costophrenic angles to be clipped. (Arrows mark the level of the diaphragm, which should fall below the posterior tenth rib to indicate adequate inspiration.)

downside should be the side of interest and must be completely demonstrated within the view. If *free air,* such as a pneumothorax, is to be ruled out, the *upside* should be the side of interest and must be included. Generally, both lungs should be included if possible.

Sternum and SC Joints

Oblique View

Rotation. The right anterior oblique position of the *sternum* or of the *sternoclavicular joints* should be a shallow 15–20 degree angle of rotation. This ideally projects the sternum *just off of the spine,* and over the heart shadow, Figure 86. If there is more than *one inch* of space between the

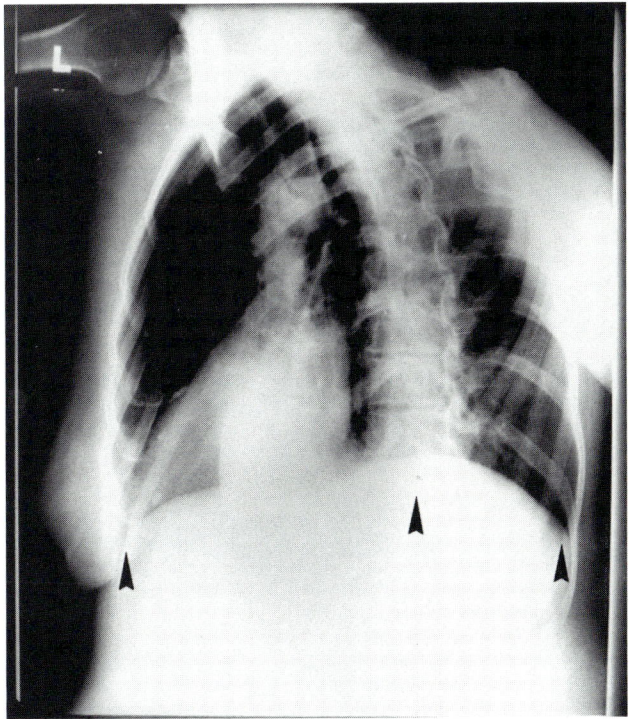

Figure 85. At 45 degrees of rotation, one hemidiaphragm is twice as long as the opposite (arrows). The ribs also appear twice as long as the opposite side and take on a straightened appearance.

sternum and the spine, as in Figure 87, the position is *too steep*. If *any portion* of the sternum (including the broad manubrium) overlaps the spine, the position is *too shallow*.

Respiration. For oblique views of the sternum, shallow steady breathing is recommended, which will demonstrate blurred trabecular soft tissue markings of the lung fields.

Lateral View

Rotation. The lateral view of the sternum should show the sternum squarely sideways, with no rib shadows extending in front of it.

Technique

For the thin ribs or sternum, a lower penetration technique is required when compared to chest radiography. Using 70–76 kVp will produce high contrast visualization of these delicate bones, as in Figure 86.

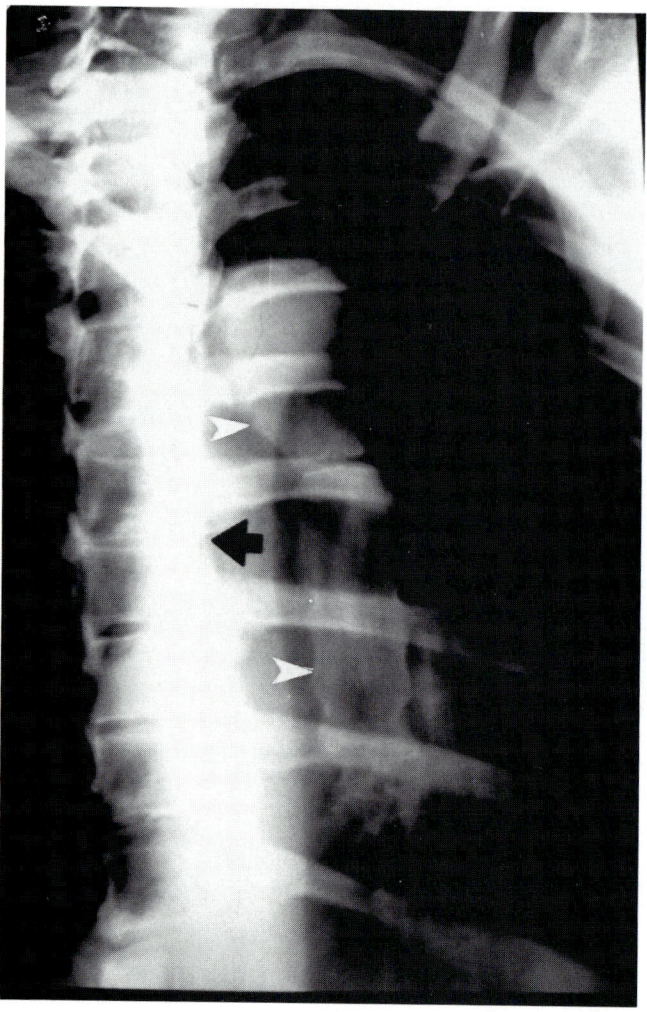

Figure 86. Proper amount of rotation for PA sternum projection. Manubrium and gladiolus of sternum (white arrows) are just clear of the spine (black arrow).

ABDOMINAL AND PELVIC VIEWS

Frontal Views

Rotation. The easiest and most reliable criteria for determining rotation on *any* abdominal views, including urography (IVP) and barium enema radiographs, are the bones of the pelvis. The flat *alae, or crests, of the iliac bones* lie at an oblique angle, extending laterally as they project

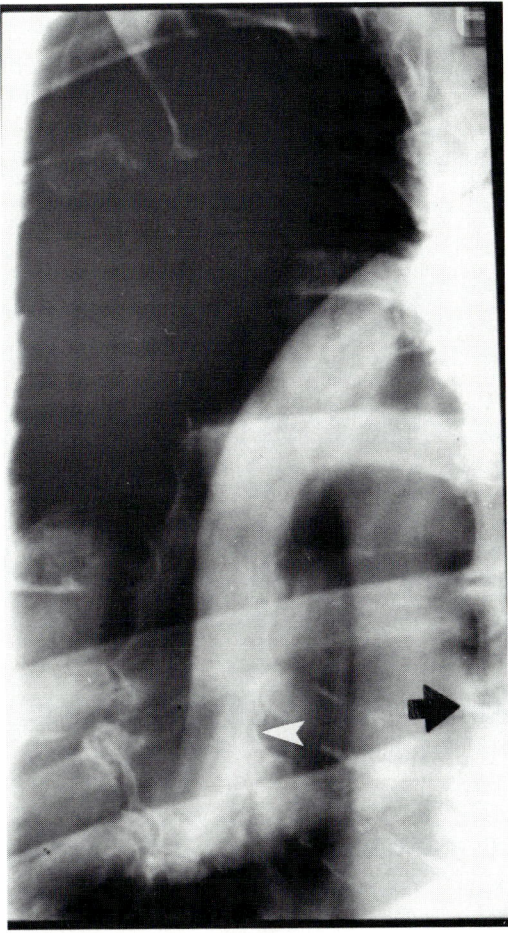

Figure 87. Too much rotation for PA sternum projection, with four inches from spine (black arrow) to sternum (white arrow).

forward. Figure 88-C shows how, if an abdominal view is rotated, one crest will always appear *narrower* than the opposite crest due to fore-shortening distortion. With rotation, the foreshortened crest has been placed more *perpendicular* to the film, and the opposite crest lies more *parallel,* which lays it out flat and makes it appear broader. Note that the broader crest also will begin to roll around behind the fifth lumbar vertebra, so that on the radiograph it appears to run into the spine, Figure 88-C. When an abdominal or pelvic radiograph is unrotated, the iliac crests will appear symmetrical and there will be a small space between them and the fifth lumbar vertebra symmetrically on both sides as shown in Figure 88-A.

Figure 88-A also shows that, whenever the ischium bones are included on an abdominal radiograph, rotation can be further confirmed by observing the symmetry of the *obturator foramina.* These are the oval spaces formed between the pubic bones and the ischia to either side. They lie at an oblique angle *opposite* to the iliac crests, extending *medially* as they project forward to meet at the symphysis pubis. This anatomical relationship between the iliac crests and the obturator foramina is diagrammed in Figure 89. When the right iliac crest is foreshortened and narrow, the right obturator foramen will appear more open and broad, while the opposite foramen becomes narrow and appears to close, Figures 88-C and 90-A.

Generally, when the patient is in a rotated *supine* position, *the upside iliac crest will be foreshortened, but the upside obturator foramen will be opened up as shown in Figure 89-A.* (In a rotated *prone* position, the downside crest will be foreshortened, and the downside foramen will be opened.)

The appearance of the spine may also be useful in critiquing frontal views of abdominopelvic anatomy, as described in the next section.

Oblique Views

Rotation. Both the iliac crests and the obturator foramina lie at about 35-degree angles from the coronal plane of the torso on average, so that 35 degrees of rotation opens the foramen and 55 degrees places the crest on end, as diagrammed in Figure 89. There is considerable variation in the angle of the iliac crests, and it should be remembered that generally the crests on the male pelvis lie at a steeper angle than those of the female pelvis. But by combining the appearance of the crests with the appearance of the obturator foramina, these two criteria together are very useful in assessing pelvic rotation.

Figure 90 analyzes the general appearance of the upside iliac crest and obturator foramina at various degrees of rotation for posterior oblique projections. At 25 degrees of rotation from a supine position (*A*), the upside crest is somewhat foreshortened and the upside obturator foramen is open.

Thirty-five degrees of rotation will fully open the upside obturator foramen, with the downside foramen quite foreshortened as shown in *B.* Note that the upside iliac crest is foreshortened and takes on a crossed-over or looped appearance, but it is not yet on end.

At forty-five degrees of rotation (*C*), the upside crest now forms a narrow looped appearance and is almost on end. Fifty-five degrees of

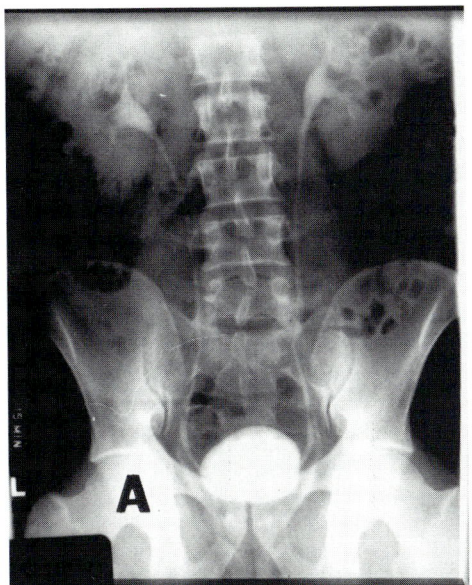
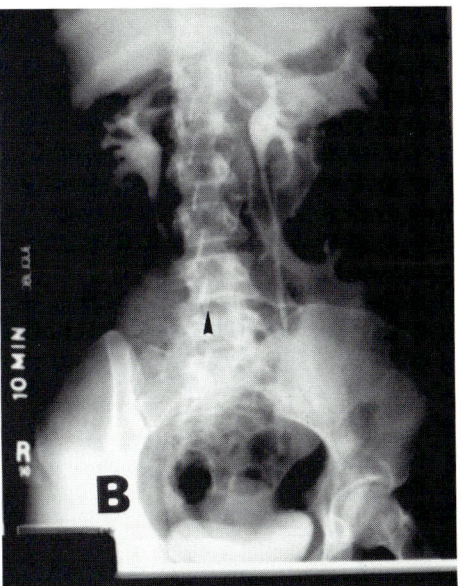
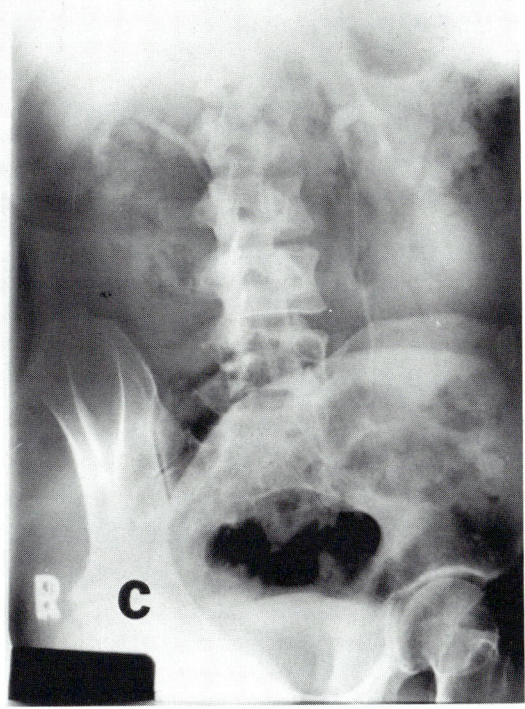

Figure 88. Abdominal projections during IVP. *A* is a non-rotated frontal view showing symmetrical iliac crests and obturator foramina (arrow). *B* shows 20–25 degrees of rotation with narrowing of upside iliac crest and good visibility of urinary system. Downside kidney is in profile (on end) and upside kidney lies parallel to film. Spinous processes (arrow) are shifted off-center. *C* shows 35 degrees of rotation with looping of upside iliac crest. Upside ureter overlaps spine, and ureteral filling is poor. Compare to Figure 90. (Note that *A* is mismarked, since the lower kidney is on the *right* side, and that *B* is centered too high, clipping the floor of the bladder.)

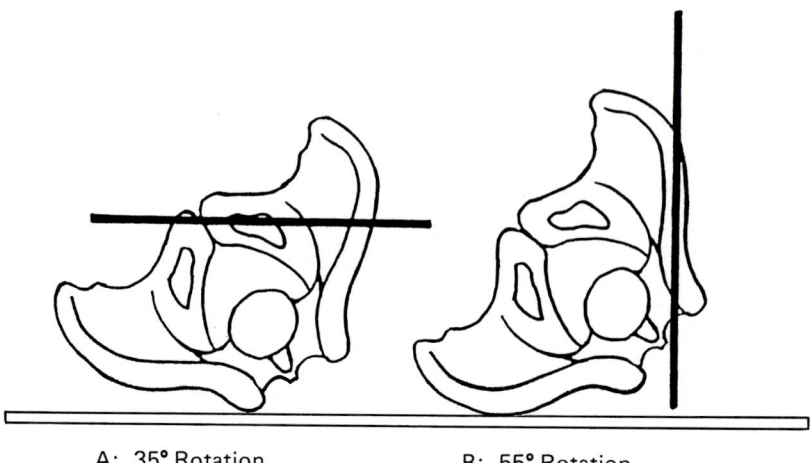

A: 35° Rotation   B: 55° Rotation

Figure 89. For the average pelvis, 35 degrees of rotation (A) places the upside obturator foramen parallel to the film, opening it fully. (Note curvature of the upside crest, which is projected into a looped appearance shown in Figure 90-B.) At 55 degrees of rotation (35 degrees from lateral), the upside crest is placed on end, perpendicular to the film.

rotation places the upside iliac crest fully on-end as in *D*. At this steep obliquity, the upside obturator foramen closes off and neither foramen is visible.

In summary, the upside obturator foramen is most open at about 35 degrees of rotation, while the iliac crest is placed completely on end at 55 degrees of rotation (35 degrees from a lateral position). Oblique views of the kidneys and ureters during an IVP series are usually taken at 25–30 degrees of rotation, and the pelvis would appear similar to *A* in Figure 90. Obliques for a barium enema series might appear more like *B*, with some looping of the crest. Oblique views for a lumbar spine should be done at precisely 45 degrees, and the upside crest should be narrowly looped as in *C*.

Other Considerations for Supine, Upright and Decubitus Views

Centering. For abdominal radiographs generally, one should try to include all anatomy from the diaphragms to the pubic bone. On larger patients this is not always possible. In most cases, such as the *"KUB"* or the *scout* radiograph for an IVP, *it is of greater diagnostic interest to include the entire bladder than to include the upper poles of the kidneys.* Therefore, if the patient has a long torso, *be sure to include the upper rim of the pubic symphysis on the radiograph.* Then take additional radiographs if requested

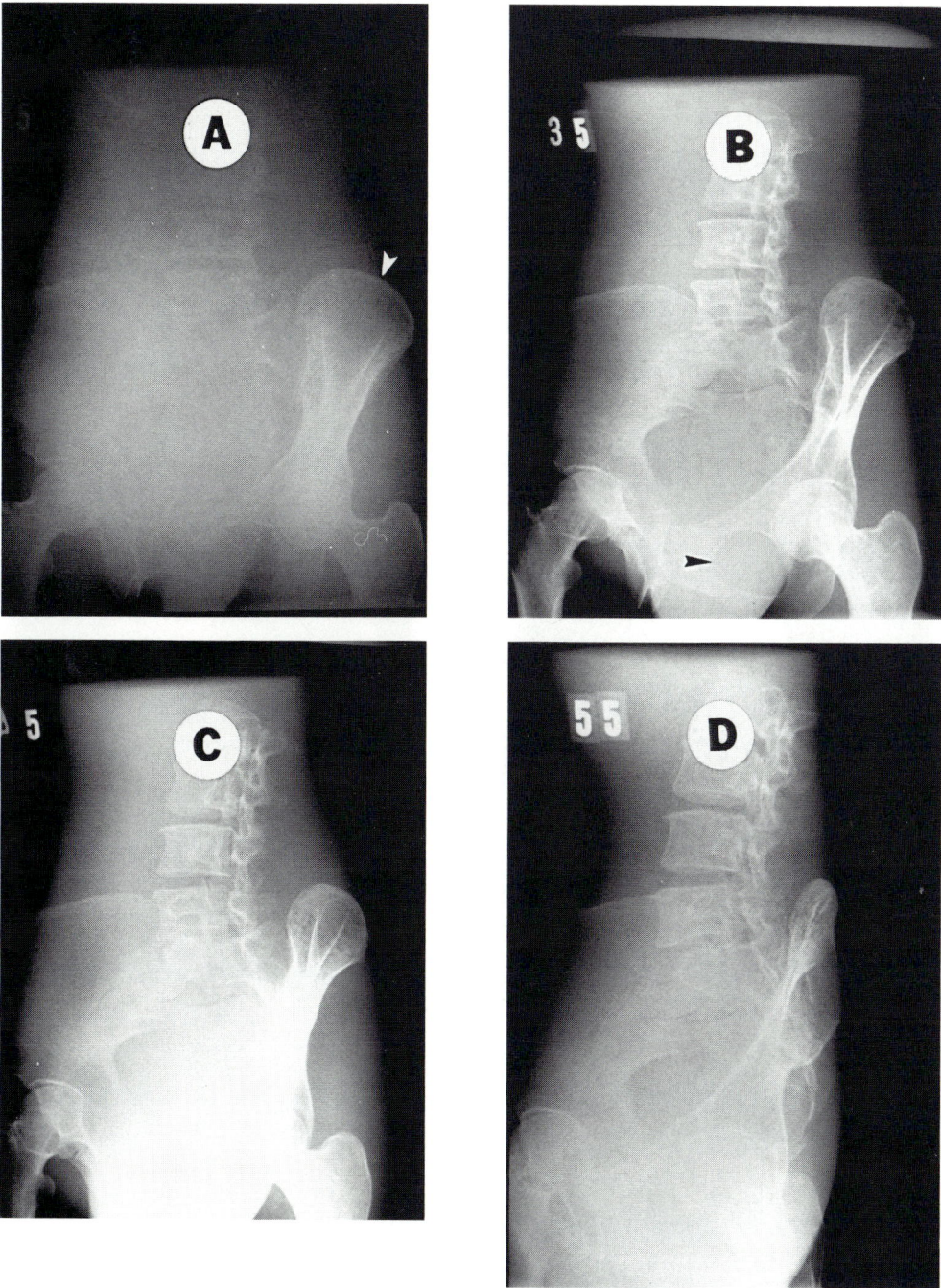

Figure 90. Pelvic phantom showing various degrees of rotation from a supine position. At 25 degrees (A), upside iliac crest (arrow) foreshortens. At 35 degrees (B), upside crest takes on looped appearance, while downside crest crosses over spine. The upside obturator foramen (arrow) is fully opened. At 45 degrees (C), crest is nearly on end and obturator foramen is obscured. At 55 degrees (D), upside crest is fully on end.

to include the upper abdomen. Figure 88-B is an example of clipping the floor of the bladder from centering too high.

One exception to this rule would be those radiographs taken, during the first five minutes of an IVP series, which must be centered to include the entire kidneys. After five minutes, the interest shifts to the distal ureters and bladder as they fill with contrast agent, and once again the top edge of the symphysis should be included. The worst centering error is shown in Figure 91-A, where an attempt to "split the difference" in centering on a large patient resulted in clipping off *both* the top of the pubic symphysis and the diaphragms, ensuring a repeated exposure.

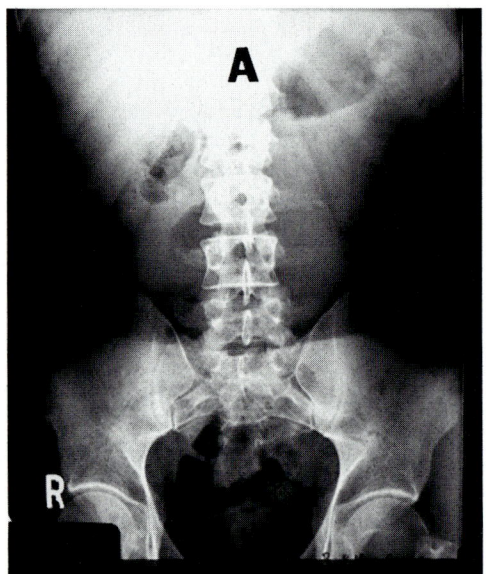
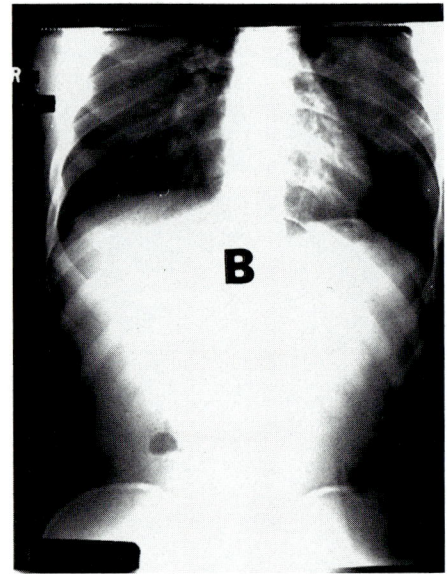

Figure 91. Abdominal centering errors. The supine KUB in *A* has clipped *both* the symphysis pubis and the diaphragms. It should be centered low enough to include the top edge of the pubis. In *B* an upright view during an acute abdomen series is centered much too high. Centering 3–4 inches above the crest is required to include the entire diaphragm.

In order to demonstrate any free peritoneal air rising up under the diaphragm, all upright views of the abdomen must include both entire hemidiaphragms. This requires centering *three to four inches above the level of the iliac crests,* depending on how tall the patient is. Some positioning texts recommend a centering point two inches above the crests, but this is often not high enough to include both entire diaphragms. Figure 91-B demonstrates the opposite case—it is centered nearly seven inches above the iliac crests.

Most *decubitus* views of the abdomen are taken to rule out free abdominal air. Therefore, in addition to the preceding criteria, collimation and centering must be such that the *upside* of the abdomen is the side of interest and is completely included in the view.

Angulation for Upright and Decubitus Views. In nearly all cases, upright or decubitus views of the abdomen are ordered specifically to demonstrate the presence of abnormal air/fluid levels within the abdomen. Even without contrast agents, air/fluid levels are apparent at the bottom of gastrointestinal air bubbles, especially the air bubble characteristically found in the fundus of the stomach. But the presence of any free gas or fluid levels *outside* the gastrointestinal system, within the peritoneum or abdominal cavity, is abnormal and critical to diagnosis. In order to show air/fluid levels, *a horizontal beam must be used.*

Acute abdomen series including an upright view are routinely ordered on emergency patients who are in a very weakened condition. To lessen the chance of having the patient faint or fall during the upright view, radiographers often elect to stand the radiographic table up 10 or 15 degrees short of vertical, so that the patient can lean back a bit for support. In this case, the x-ray beam should *not* be angled caudally in order to place it perpendicular to the film. *The central ray should be kept horizontal, even though this results in an angle to the film.* Figure 92 illustrates the reason why: Air/fluid levels may not be visible if the tube is angled, leading to a misdiagnosis. The horizontal surface of a small amount of fluid will only be demonstrated when the beam is kept horizontal.

Technique

Technique on all abdominal and pelvic views should be set for optimum penetration of the *bones,* showing the spinous processes and pedicles visible *through* the bodies of the vertebrae, yet with relatively high contrast.

Sacroiliac Joints

Oblique Views

Rotation. The proper amount of rotation for views of the sacroiliac joints is 25–30 degrees, so that positioned correctly, the upside iliac crest will take on a crossed over or looped appearance just as discussed under

116

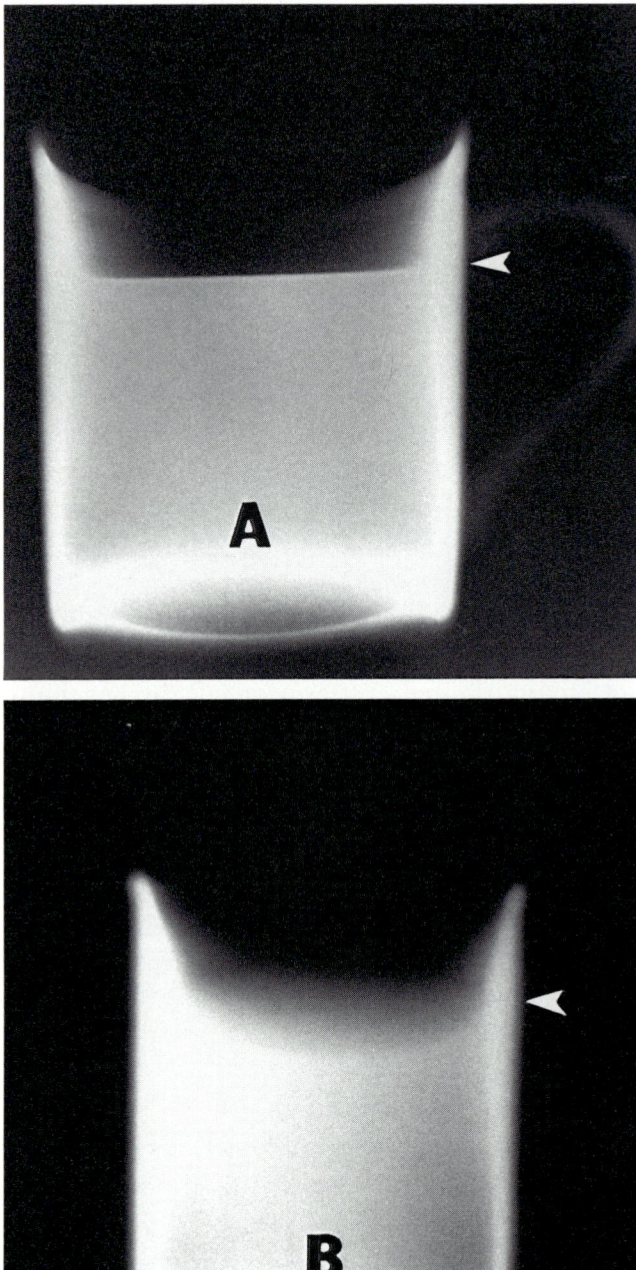

Figure 92. Radiographs of a mug of water demonstrate the absolute necessity of a horizontal beam for upright abdomen views even if the patient and film are not fully upright, in order to demonstrate abnormal fluid levels. The mug and film were tilted 15 degrees on both views. *A* employed a horizontal beam and demonstrates a clear fluid level. In *B*, the beam was angled 15 degrees caudally to place it perpendicular to the film, resulting in poor visibility of the fluid level. In real anatomy, the visibility might be diminished to the point of missing the fluid level in diagnosis.

the section on abdominal and pelvic views, and as shown in Figure 93-A. Note that the anterior and posterior openings to this deep joint appear as *two* dark lines on a radiograph. With correct positioning the lower two-thirds of these lines come together and superimpose.

Figure 93-B shows how too *steep* an oblique (40–50 degrees) places the crest on end and closes of the SI joint.

ABDOMINAL VISCERA

When coned-down views of abdominal organs are made, the only bony anatomy references may be the spine and the ribs, to be discussed shortly. Among the soft tissue organs, the only ones that are easily indicative of position are the kidneys, the stomach and duodenum, and the various parts of the colon which must be filled with contrast agents or air to visualize.

Gastrointestinal Procedures

Rotation. In an upper GI series, a 30–45 degree *LPO* position opens the C-loop of the duodenum somewhat. The duodenal C-loop is opened best with a very *steep* LPO or RAO position (about 60 degrees), Figure 97. For the RAO view during a cardiac series, 45 degrees of rotation demonstrates the esophagus in between the spine and the heart, as in Figure 94. If the esophagus overlaps the spine, the position is too shallow. For a barium enema series, a 30–35 degree LPO position opens up the loop of hepatic flexure of the colon, and the cecum frequently superimposes the rectosigmoid colon.

In a 30–45 degree *RPO* position, the body of the stomach is laid out parallel to the film on an upper GI series, and the loop of the splenic flexure (the higher of the two flexures) opens up for a barium enema series. Since the RPO is the *only* position during a barium enema which opens the splenic flexure, this view should be centered 4 inches above the iliac crest to ensure that this flexure is included as in Figure 95.

Angulation for Sigmoid Colon. The only common angled view of abdominal anatomy is that of the sigmoid colon during for a barium enema, which employs a 35-degree cephalic angle of the CR. This angle serves to desuperimpose the flexures of the sigmoid colon from the proximal rectum and distal descending colon as in Figure 96.

Other Considerations. Generally, centering and collimation on all

118

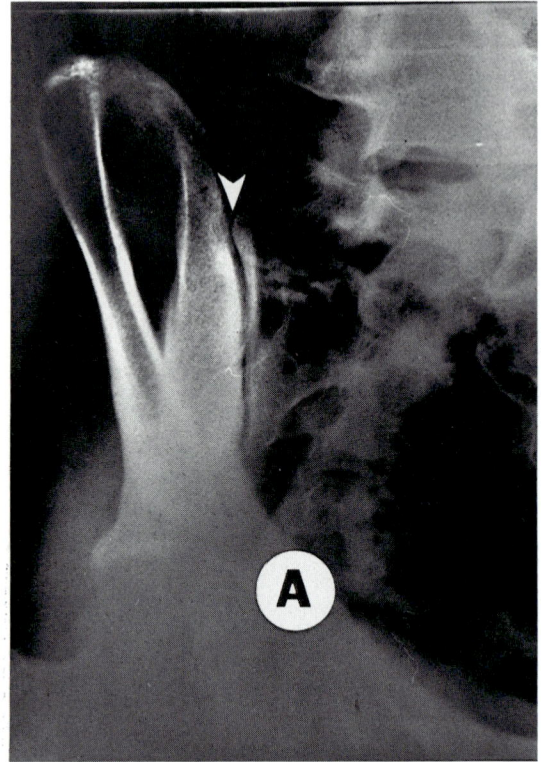

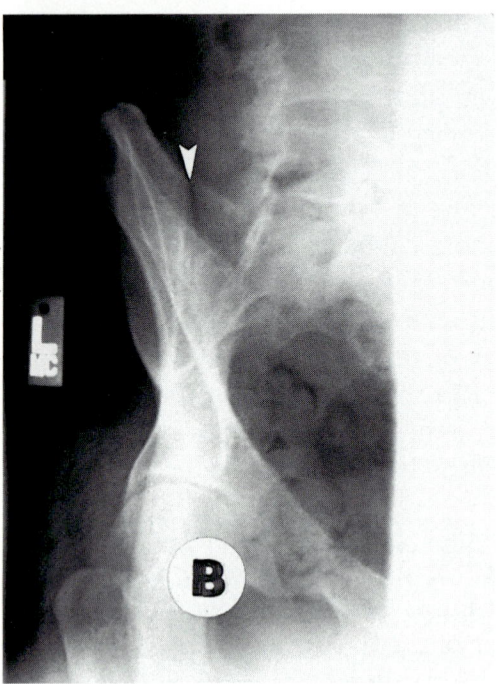

Figure 93. Proper 25–30 degrees of rotation (*A*) opens sacroiliac joint (arrow). Steep rotation past 40 degrees (*B*) closes off joint.

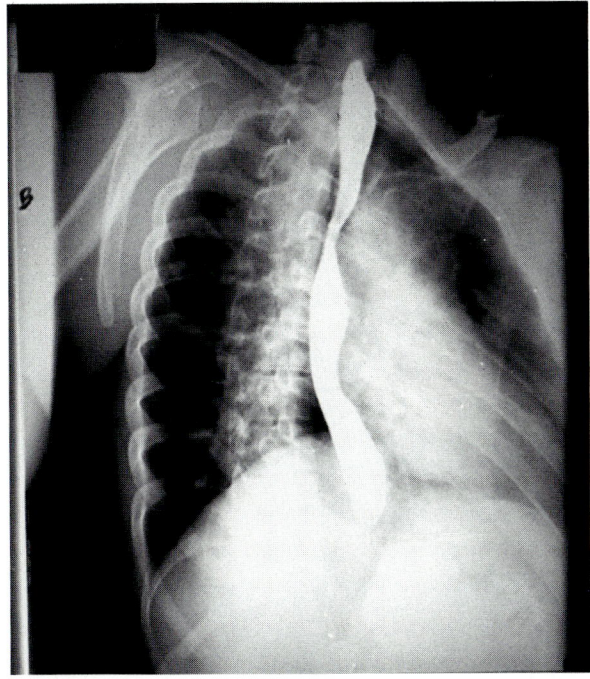

Figure 94. During cardiac series, 45 degrees of rotation places esophagus between spine and heart.

views of the stomach should be such that the C-loop of the duodenum is included as well as all portions of the stomach itself as in Figure 97.

Beside the above overview, good positioning texts describe other important anatomical relationships, such as the placement of barium or air, in recognizing different positions. Our purpose here, however, is to *critique* the positions. Because of the great variation in location and shape of soft tissue organs, they are not very useful for film critique. The appearance of the spine and other bony anatomy is a more reliable indicator of the exact body position.

It should be noted, however, that the presence of any distinct fluid levels indicates that a horizontal x-ray beam was used. The position can then be recognized as either an upright or a decubitus position by remembering that fluids will settle according to gravity. By remembering that the higher of the two colonic flexures is the splenic flexure on the left, and that the sigmoid colon extends to the left from the rectum,

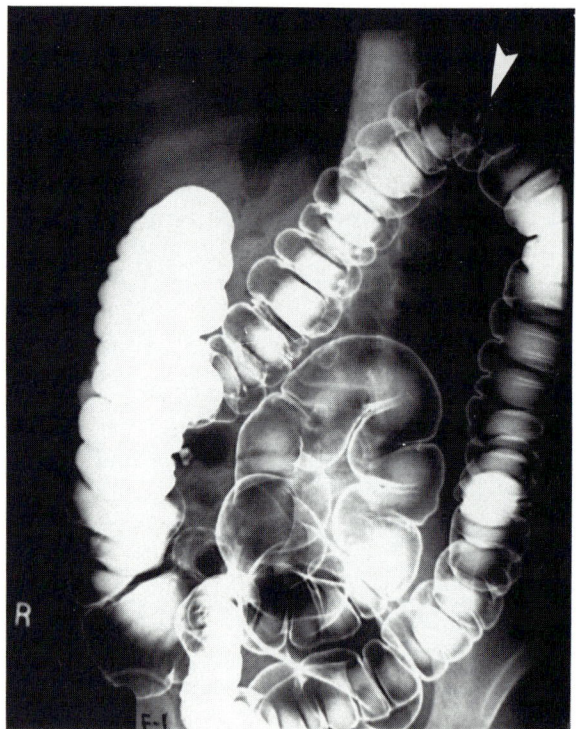

Figure 95. During barium enema, RPO (or LAO) projection should be centered 3–4 inches above iliac crest to include splenic flexure of colon (arrow) which is opened in this position. (Other views in series include distal rectum.) Pooling of barium in ascending colon and rectum (vertical portions of colon) proves that position is *posterior* oblique rather than *anterior* oblique.

one can further determine which specific decubitus position was used as in Figure 98.

Even when a vertical beam is used and no distinct fluid levels are present, one can determine on a double-contrast study with barium and air whether a patient is supine or prone, in RPO or LAO, or in LPO or RAO position by knowing the anatomy and observing the pooling of the barium. In the stomach, the fundus is posterior and pooling of barium there indicates a supine or posterior oblique position. *All of the vertical portions of the colon lie posterior, while the transverse and sigmoid colons lie anterior.* Therefore, pooling of barium in the ascending and descending colon and the rectum indicate a supine or posterior oblique position as shown in Figure 95.

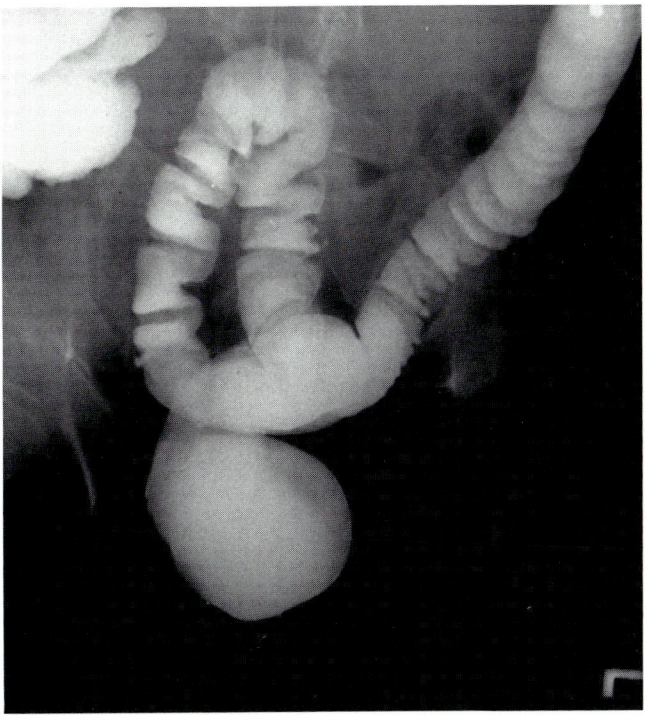

Figure 96. Cephalic angle of 35 degrees used for sigmoid view during barium enema desuperimposes loops of sigmoid colon.

Genitourinary Procedures

Rotation. For renal procedures, in the 30 degree posterior oblique position, the *upside* kidney is placed nearly parallel to the film providing an unobscured view of the ureteral pelvis, and the *downside* kidney is in profile (on end), as in Figure 88-B. In Figure 88-C the renal pelvis and proximal ureter overlaps the spine. If the upside kidney overlaps the spine at all, the position is too *steep*. If the view is under-rotated, the upside renal pelvis will still overlap the hilar tissue of the kidney.

For oblique views during cystourethrography, the rotation of the torso should be somewhat steeper than for renal procedures. Cystograms require from 40 to 60 degrees of rotation for posterior oblique positions, so that the upside iliac crest will be on end and the downside obturator foramen will be closed. For urethrography, male patients often require a similar amount of steep obliquity in order to desuperimpose the prostatic and proximal penile urethra from the bladder floor, but for female urethrog-

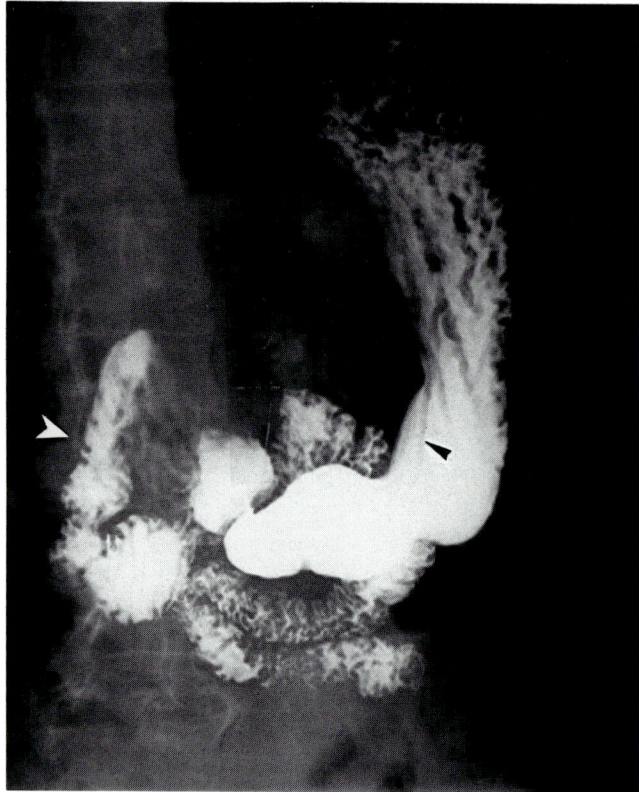

Figure 97. Good centering and collimation for UGI series, including the C-loop of the duodenum (white arrow) and the entire stomach. Kilovoltage should be enough to penetrate *through* the barium bolus and demonstrate pathology or rugal folds as shown here (black arrow). Note that the C-loop is not fully opened at this 35 degrees of rotation. A steeper oblique will open it. Barium pooling in the *antrum* proves that this is an RAO, rather than an LPO, position.

raphy, Figure 99, 35 to 40 degrees of rotation is recommended. This will give the pelvic bones an appearance similar to that of the oblique renal views just described. Centering for the oblique views on a male voiding cystourethrogram must be more anterior in order to be sure to include the entire penile urethra, as in Figure 100.

For more exact estimation of the amount of rotation on these views, use bony anatomy as discussed in the section on abdominal and pelvic views.

Angulation for Cystourethrography. In the supine position, a 5-degree caudal angle of the x-ray beam should be routinely utilized as in Figure 101 to desuperimpose the top edge of the pubic bones from the floor of

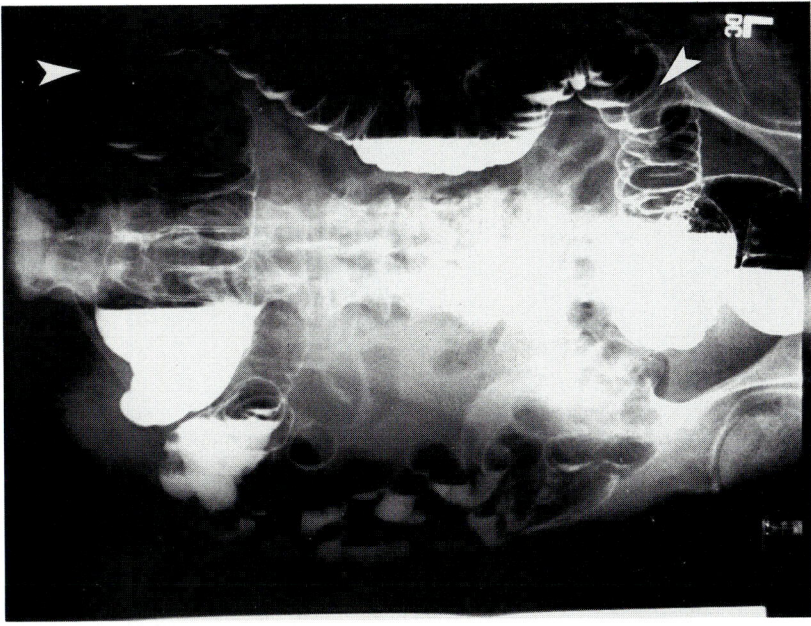

Figure 98. Distinct barium fluid levels attest to horizontal beam projection during a barium enema. Position can be further defined as a right lateral decubitus because splenic flexure and sigmoid colon (arrows), on left side of body, are upside.

the bladder and proximal urethra. When the pubis overlaps the bladder, no angle or insufficient angle was used. Occasionally, more than 5 degrees is required. This caudal angulation may also be used for the AP projection for female cystourethrograms.

Technique and Patient Preparation

Whenever contrast agents are used, the ideal level of penetration (kVp) is such that some details can be seen *through* the bolus of contrast agent. For urography, the distal ureters should be seen coursing *behind* the upper portion of the contrast-filled bladder, and ureteral stones or kinks should be seen *within* the ureters. For barium studies, the folds of the *rugae* should be seen in the stomach wall *through* the barium, as in Figure 97, and pathology such as diverticulae or polyps in the colon should be able to be seen *through* the barium. Any blank "white" appearance of contrast agents indicates that insufficient kVp was used. Generally, 76–80 kVp should be used for iodine agents and 100–120 kVp for barium studies.

For an IVP series, the time elapsed *since the start of the injection* should

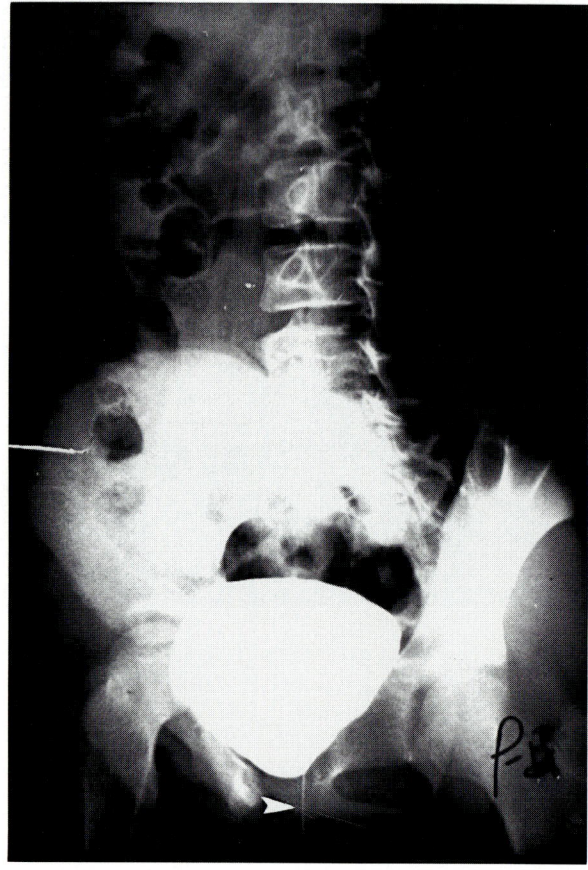

Figure 99. Female cystogram, oblique view with 35–40 degrees rotation (note open obturator foramen), showing iodinated catheter still in place (arrow).

be accurately marked on each radiograph as shown in Figure 88-B. Timing of the exposures is important for any contrast study in order to obtain maximum filling of the organs of interest with contrast agent. Taken too soon or too late, only a small amount of contrast agent will be present as shown in Figure 88-C.

Proper patient preparation cannot be overemphasized. The presence of stool in the colon or food in the stomach can obscure the visibility of biliary or renal anatomy, Figure 102.

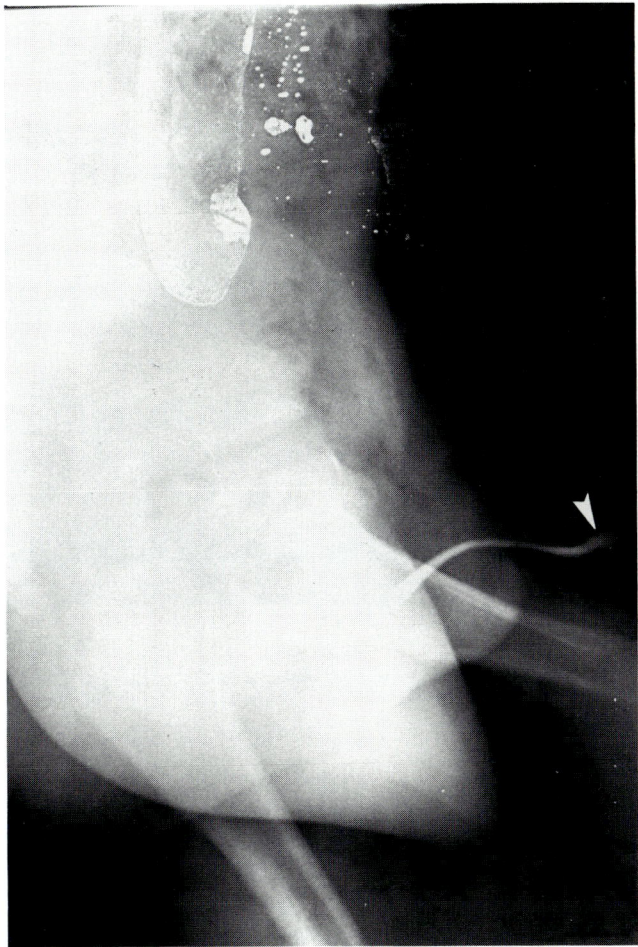

Figure 100. Male cystourethrogram must be centered anteriorly to include entire penile urethra (arrow).

SPINES

The general appearance of the vertebrae can be used not only to critique views of the lumbar, thoracic, and cervical spines, but also to critique any chest or abdominal radiographs that include vertebrae within the field of view.

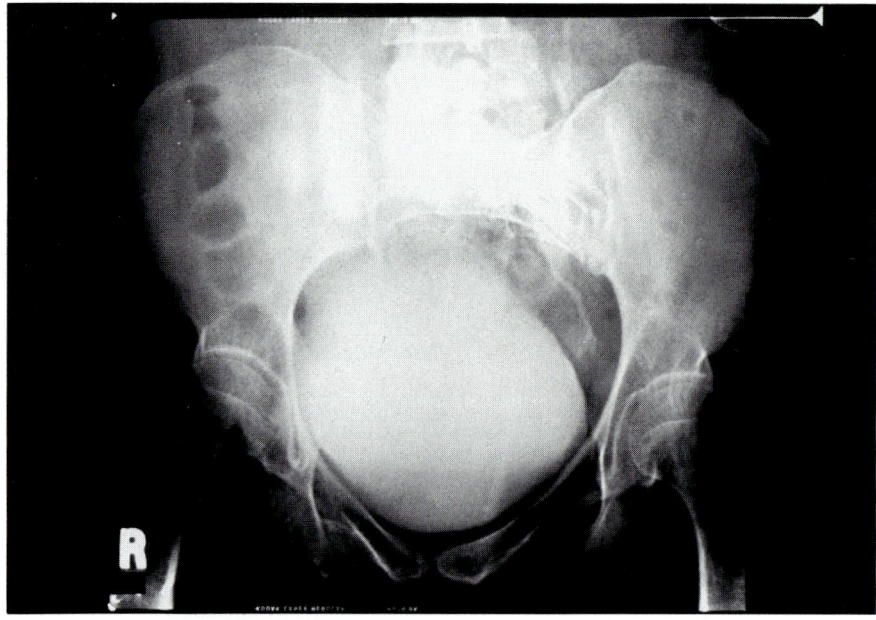

Figure 101. Cystogram with 5 degrees of caudal angle projects upper rim of symphysis pubis below floor of bladder for maximum visualization of bladder.

Thoracic and Lumbar Spines

Frontal Views

Rotation. Although the three portions of the spine each have unique vertebral features, at least two anatomical parts are fairly universal as criteria for critiquing rotation. These are the spinous processes and the pedicles, which are visible on all but the upper cervical vertebrae.

On a straight, unrotated frontal view of most vertebrae, the spinous process can be seen on end as an oval or teardrop-shaped feature exactly in the midline of the vertebral body. Some of the processes are so low that they appear over the intervertebral joint space just below the vertebra from which they arise, while others are right in the middle of the vertebral body, Figure 103. Cervical spinous processes may appear as an inverted "V" rather than as an oval. When the spine is rotated, the spinous processes will appear off-centered within the rectangular vertebral body as in Figure 88-B. In rotated supine positions, the spinous process shifts toward the *upside.* In rotated prone positions, the process shifts toward the *downside.*

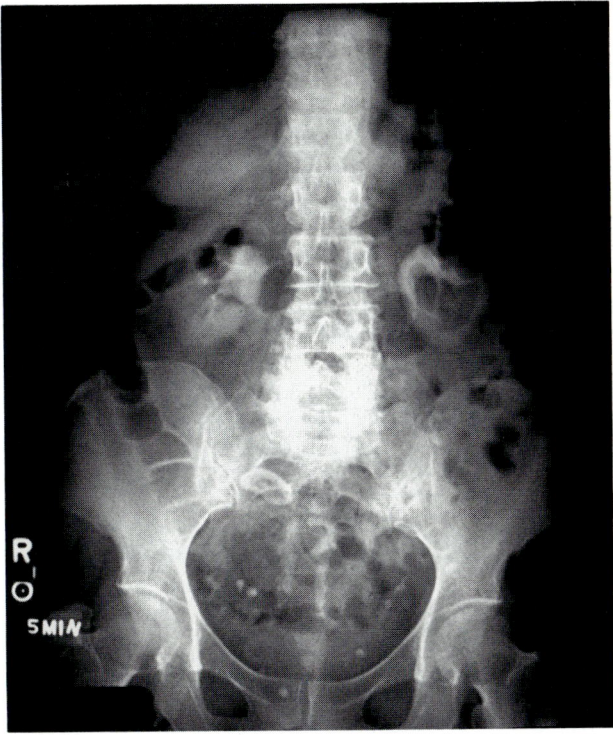

Figure 102. Poor patient preparation results in fecal material and gas obscuring kidneys and ureters during this IVP.

On straight frontal projections, the pedicles of the vertebrae are also seen on end, and appear as oval markings within the vertebral bodies along their side edges. They should be equidistant from the midline spinous process. Often on rotated views, one pedicle is still seen somewhat on end but the opposite pedicle seems to disappear (as an oval feature), Figure 88-C.

In the lumbar spine, the transverse processes are prominent and rotation will cause the appearance of one overlapping the vertebral body more than the other. The sacroiliac joints in the pelvis should also be equidistant from the midline. In the thoracic spine, this same unilateral overlapping effect can be seen with the ribs as one side superimposes the vertebral bodies more than the other.

Scoliosis vs Rotation. Mild scoliosis is a very common condition, and may simulate rotation of the spine when evaluating radiographs. Scoliosis causes a twisting of the spine, shifting the spinous process to one side on an AP radiograph. In most cases, scoliosis can be distinguished

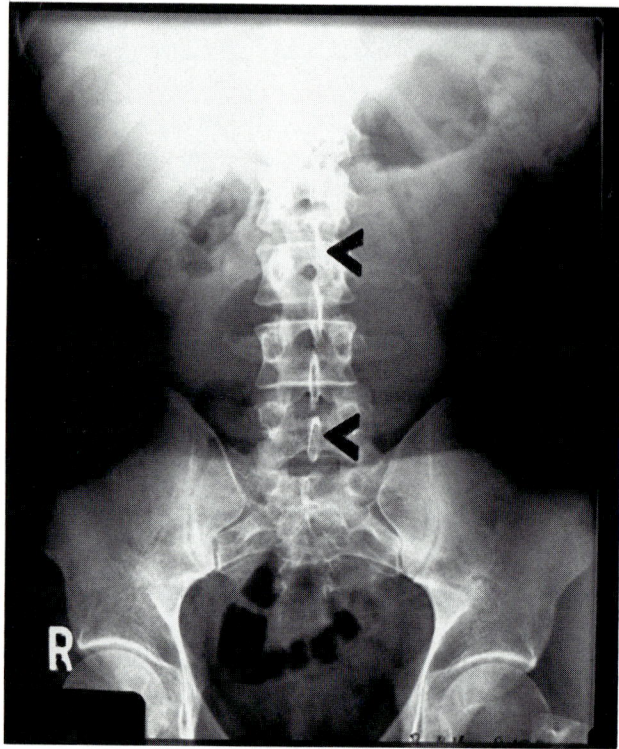

Figure 103. Spinous processes (arrows) of lumbar spine are centered at bottom but increasingly shift toward patient's left in upper vertebrae, indicating rotation of the *shoulders* to the *right*.

because it is *regional.* That is, the spinous processes will appear to begin to rotate and then *return* to straight alignment further down the spinal column, Figures 88-A and 122.

A twisting rotation frequently occurs during positioning, because patients will "favor" an injured hip or shoulder and tend to raise that side off of the x-ray table to relieve pressure. With this type of rotation, however, the spinous processes are seen to become gradually and steadily farther out of alignment toward the hips or shoulders, as shown in Figure 103. This type of rotation is a fundamental positioning error for the radiographer, since in *any* body position the coronal planes of the hips and shoulders must be aligned parallel to each other. A rotated view with hips and shoulders aligned will demonstrate the spinous processes about equally shifted to one side on all vertebrae. It is not possible for positioning rotation to produce the kind of twisting and then returning into alignment that scoliosis can cause.

Angulation, Flexion/Extension and Tilt. For spine radiography, the primary aim of angling the central ray cephalic or caudal, employing spinal flexion, or extending the head is to *desuperimpose* vertebrae off of each other in the *superior/inferior* axis. When this is accomplished, the *intervertebral joint spaces will be opened up* and appear dark. Without exact angulation and flexion/extension, the normal lordotic or kyphotic curvatures of the spinal column cause the bottom edges of vertebrae to superimpose the upper portions of the vertebrae below.

A tube angle is not normally used on the AP thoracic spine, since joints in the middle and lower sections will be opened well. Normal kyphotic curvature closes the upper joints, and a cephalic tube angle may be called for on coned-down views of this area. The AP lumbar spine also uses no tube angle, but in this case the spine can be extended to open the joint spaces better by *flexing the knees and hips.* With the knees bent up off of the table, the lordotic curve of the lumbar spine is lessened and all five vertebrae are better demonstrated.

Lateral Views

Rotation. Lateral views of all spines should show the vertebral bodies clear of any superimposing facets or processes. Fortunately, the posterior surface of the vertebral bodies has a slight indentation in the middle where the spinal cord runs. This results in a slight "heart" shape to the body, with two posterior surfaces. In true lateral position, these two surfaces will be superimposed and appear as one feature. When rotation is present, a double-line will appear along the back of each body as in Figure 104. For the thoracic spine, the superimposition of the right and left posterior ribs can also be referenced as is done for a lateral chest radiograph.

Angulation. On lateral views of the thoracic spine, a cephalic angle of 5–10 degrees is frequently required on broad-shouldered or narrow-waisted patients in order to compensate for the tilt created, place the central ray perpendicular to the spine, and open the intervertebral joint spaces. Patients vary greatly in this respect and on some the T-spine will lie parallel to the table and require no tube angle. When the lateral view shows overlapping of the upper and lower edges of thoracic vertebrae, either the beam was angled and should not have been, or it was not angled and should have been.

For Twining or Pawlow views of the cervicothoracic region, a caudal tube angle of 5 degrees may be needed on patients who cannot adequately depress their upside shoulder.

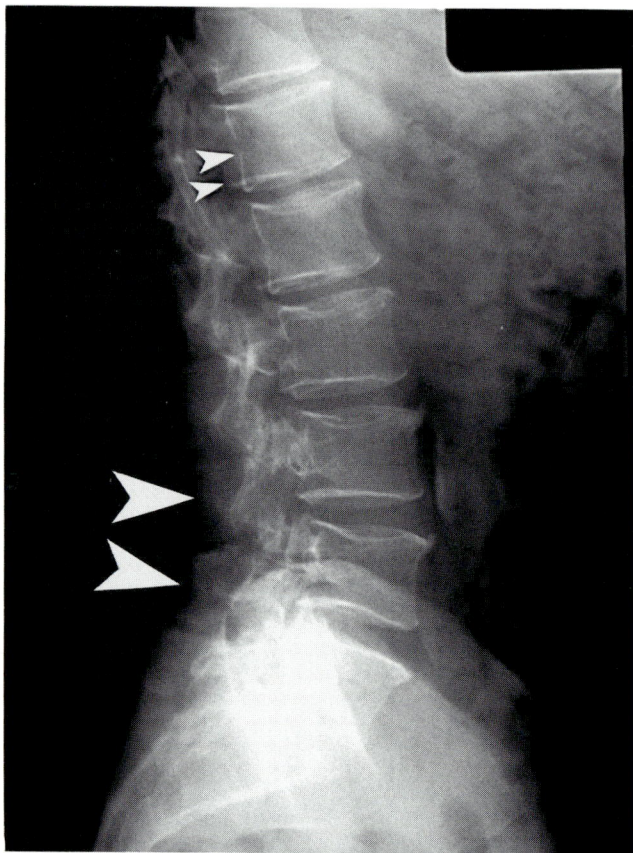

Figure 104. Slight rotation on lateral lumbar spine shows double-edges on posterior vertebral bodies (small arrows, top). Distinct fog line caused from scatter radiation from the tabletop behind the patient obliterates posterior halves of spinous processes (large arrows).

For the lumbosacral joint, the coned-down "spot" lateral view of the joint frequently requires a 5–10 degree caudal tube angle, but *not always*. Nor can it be generalized that female patients require the angle while male patients do not. The only reliable method of determining the amount and direction of beam angle during positioning is to use *palpation of bony landmarks*. The beam can be angled *perpendicular* to a line drawn between the palpated spinous processes of the fifth lumbar vertebra and the lower sacrum, or *parallel* to a line drawn between the two iliac crests or the two posterior superior iliac spines, (these are felt as bony prominences at the posterior end of the iliac crests in the sacroiliac region about two inches to either side of the midline). Direct palpation (feeling for landmarks) will result in much lower repeat rates than any visual estimation or generalized rule.

If the routine lateral view of the lumbar spine is processed and available prior to exposing the L5-S1 "spot", the need for an angle can be determined from it as follows: Remember that when centered at or above the iliac crest, those rays which pass through the L5-S1 joint on the lateral view are diverging, *angled* rays located several inches below the central ray. Therefore, if the L5-S1 joint is opened well on the routine lateral view, a caudal angle is indicated for the "spot" view. When this joint is *not* opened on the routine lateral view, in most cases a *straight* vertical projection is indicated for the "spot".

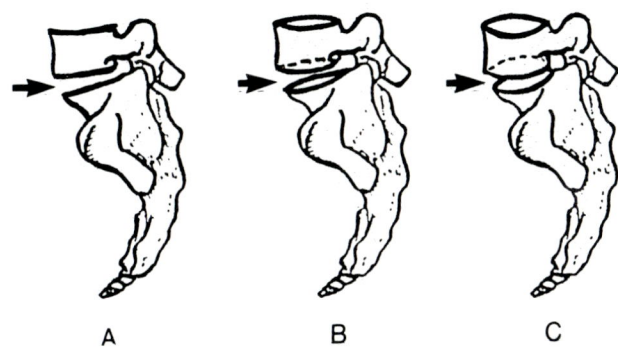

A   B   C

Figure 105. Diagram of appearance of upper and lower surfaces of vertebral bodies as angulation or off-centering close off joint spaces. *A:* joint fully open, *B:* joint partially closed, *C:* joint completely closed. Compare with Figure 106.

Figure 105 is a diagram showing the appearance of the superior and inferior surfaces of vertebral bodies when mild or severe misangulation is used. Figure 106 demonstrates corresponding correct and incorrect lateral "spot" views of the L5-S1 joint. When the joint is completely open, these upper and lower surfaces of the vertebral bodies appear as a straight line or as a very narrow oval.

Note that the views in Figure 106 *B* and *C* are off-centered as well as off-angled, (*B* is centered too high and *C* is centered too low.) Off-centering results in the angled, diverging rays of the x-ray beam passing through the joint of interest (L5-S1), effectively changing the angle of the projection as illustrated in Figure 107. Thus, off-centering can also contribute to "closing off" the joint space.

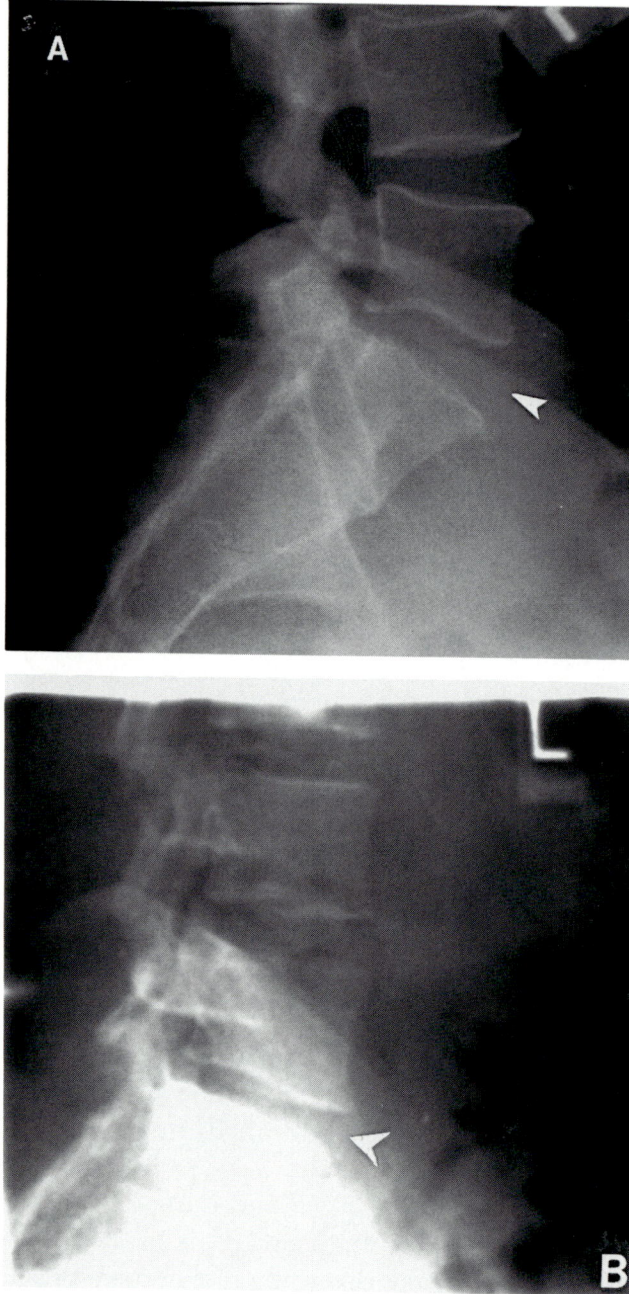

Figure 106. Lateral "spot" views of lumbosacral joint (arrow). View *A* shows correct angle and opened joint. Poor angulation and off centering partially close the joint in *B,* and fully close the joint in *C* which is repeatable.

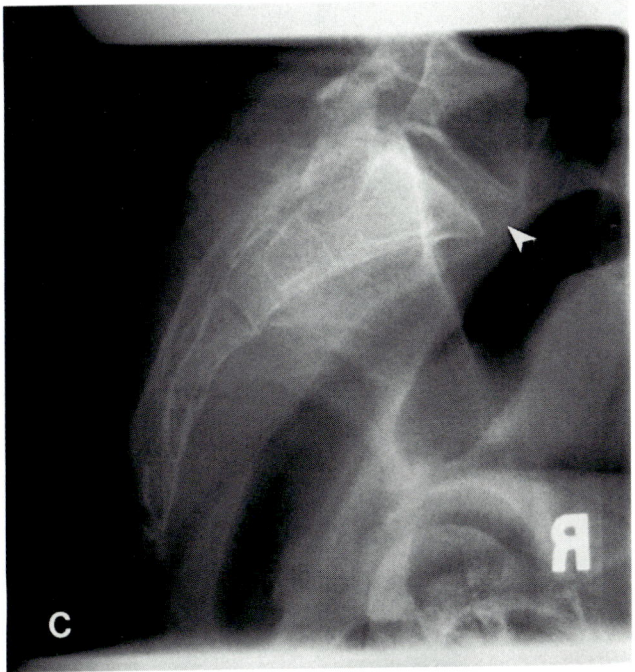

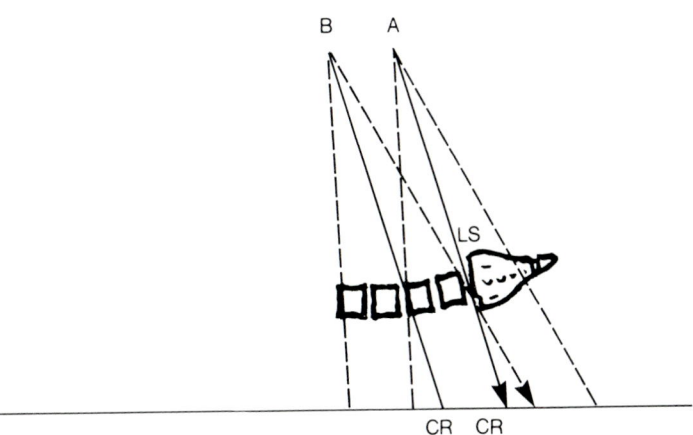

Figure 107. Diagram showing how off-centering contributes to "off-angling", closing off joint spaces. In *A*, the central ray is angled 5 degrees caudal and opens the LS joint space. The same central ray angle is used in *B*, but centering too high for the LS joint results in a diverging beam passing through this joint at an increased angle, closing the joint space.

Oblique Views

Rotation. On good 45-degree obliques of the lumbar spine, the apophyseal joints will open and appear as dark slits running through the vertebral bodies, and the familiar "scotty dogs" will be most recognizable, as in Figure 108. The "eye" of each scotty dog is the *downside* pedicle for posterior oblique positions, (the upside pedicle for anterior obliques). When the apophyseal joint is not dark and this pedicle lies near the anterior edge of the vertebral body, as in Figure 88-B, the body rotation is too *shallow* or *less than 45 degrees.* When the apophyseal joint is not dark and the pedicle lies posteriorly within the vertebral body, as shown in Figure 109, the body rotation is too *steep* or *more than 45 degrees.*

Sacrum and Coccyx

Frontal Views

Rotation. For the AP views of the sacrum and coccyx, the sacroiliac joints should be seen equidistant from the midline spinous processes of

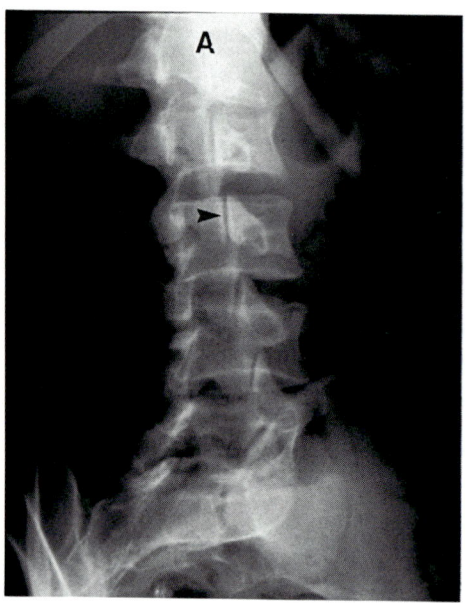
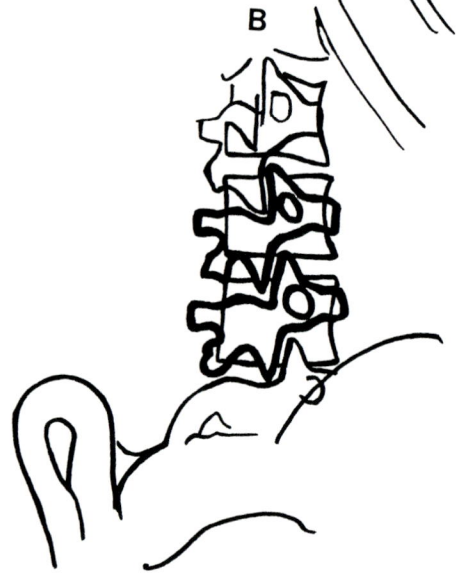

Figure 108. A true 45 degrees of obliquity opens the apophyseal joints of the lumbar spine (*A*, arrow) and demonstrates the popular "scotty dogs", diagrammed in *B*. Note that upside iliac crest is nearly on end. This view is frequently taken with too shallow obliquity, probably because 35-degree obliques are so common in other procedures.

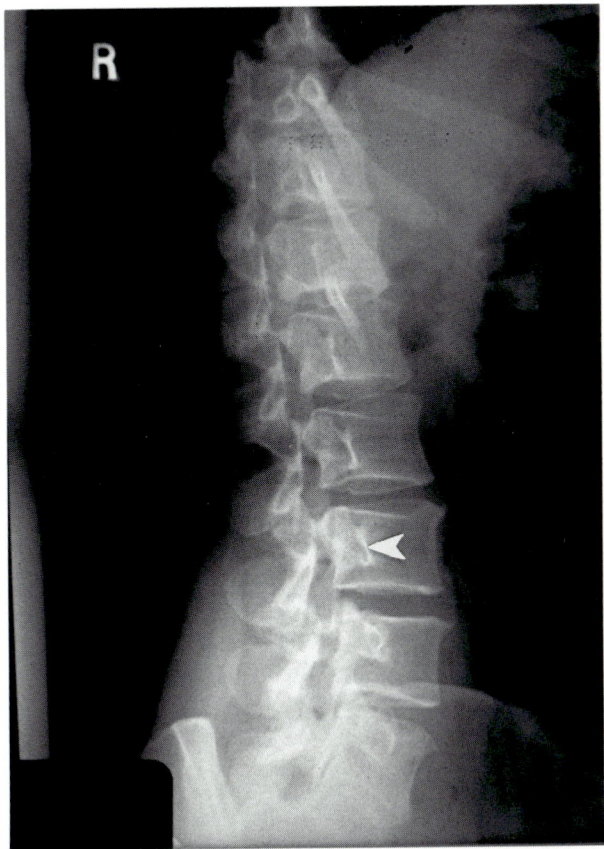

Figure 109. Oblique lumbar spine positioned too *steep,* placing the pedicles (arrow) in the posterior half of each vertebral body.

the sacrum, the obturator foramina should appear symmetrical, and the symphysis pubis will be aligned with the spinous processes of the spine and sacrum in the middle. The easiest way to detect rotation is to observe the symphysis pubis. If the symphysis is shifted to the left of the midline of the sacrum, as shown in Figure 110, the body is rotated to the *left,* and vice versa.

Angulation. The 15-degree cephalic beam angle recommended for the AP view of the sacrum is designed to minimize the foreshortening distortion that occurs when projecting angled anatomy with a vertical beam. With this amount of angle, the fifth segment of the sacrum will just clear the top of the pubic bone as in Figure 110. If too much cephalic angle is used, especially on thicker patients, it can superimpose the

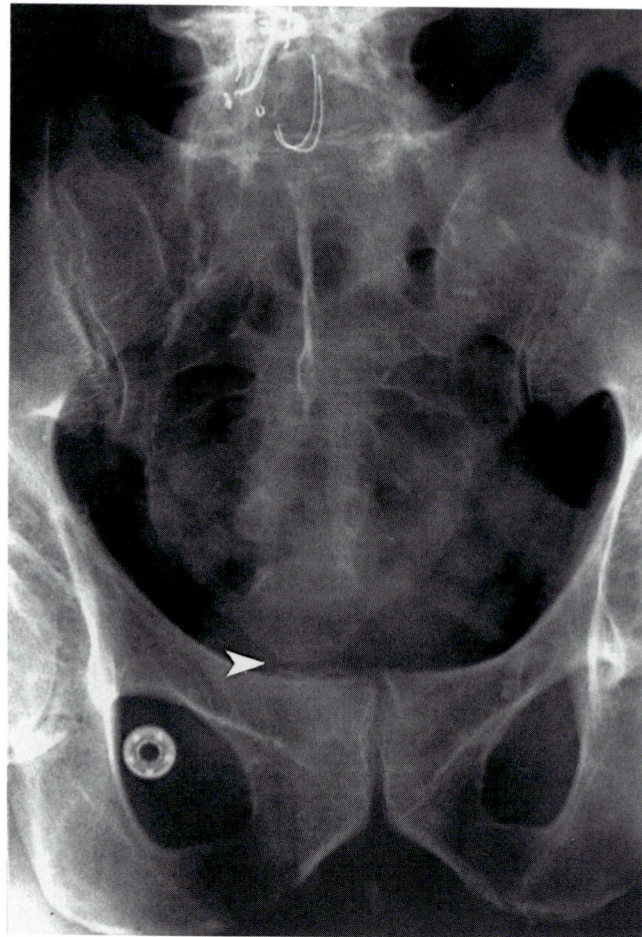

Figure 110. Frontal view of sacrum with correct beam angulation projects upper rim of pubic bones just below sacrococcygeal joint (arrow). Note, however, that symphysis pubis is shifted to the patient's left from the midline of the sacrum and spine, indicating pelvic *rotation* to the left.

pubic bones over the lower sacral segments as in Figure 111. When this occurs, the angle should be reduced. It is common for the sympysis pubis to be projected over the *coccyx,* and this is acceptable, as long as it does not get into the 5th sacral segment.

For the coccyx, with the proper 10-degree caudal angle of the x-ray beam the coccyx will be seen in its entirety above and free of superimposition from the pubic bones, as in Figure 112. If the pubic bones obscure the coccyx, insufficient or no tube angle was used.

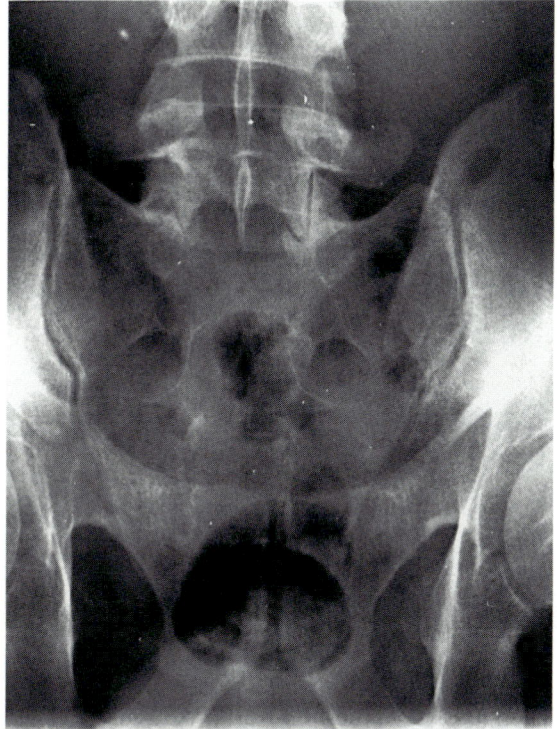

Figure 111. Excess cephalic angulation for frontal view of sacrum projects pubic bones over sacrum.

Lateral Views

Rotation. On the lateral views of the sacrum and coccyx, the posterior margins of the *ischia* should be nearly superimposed.

Cervical Spine

Frontal View

Rotation. For all but the uppermost cervical vertebrae, the spinous processes and the pedicles can be used as rotation criteria just as described for the thoracic and lumbar spines. Instead of the usual teardrop shape, the cervical spinous processes may appear as an inverted "V". When the spine is rotated, the spinous processes will appear off-centered within the rectangular vertebral body, and the pedicles of the lower vertebrae will not be equidistant from the midline, just as shown for the lumbar spine in Figure 88-B. In rotated supine or posterior oblique positions, the

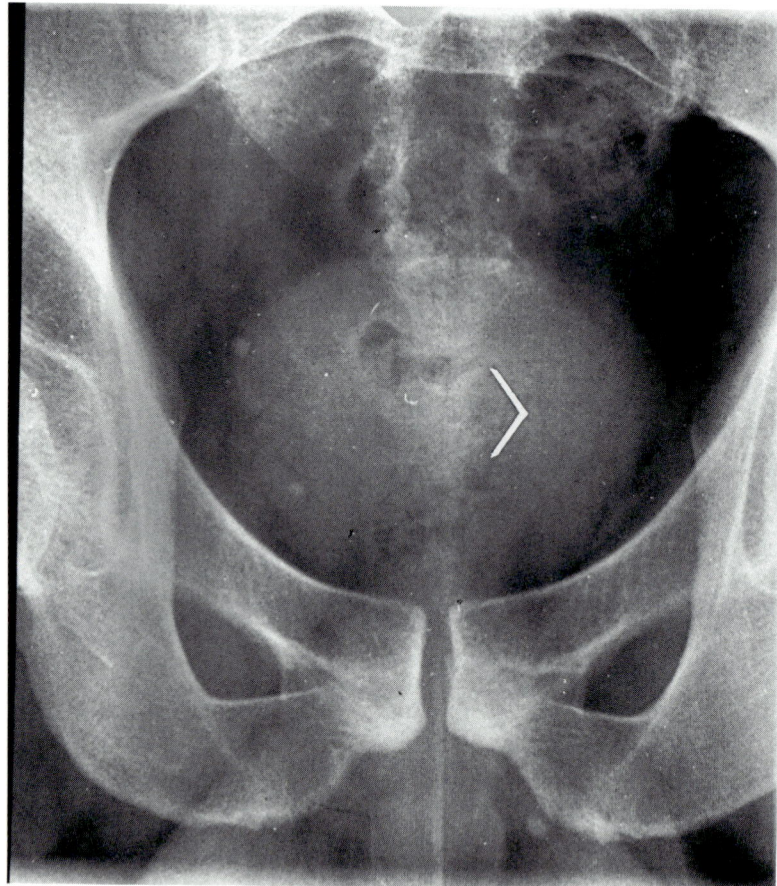

Figure 112. Proper angulation for frontal view of coccyx (bracket) projects pubic bones well below it. Note, however, that in this view the bladder was full of urine creating a fluid density that obscures the coccyx. Patients should void prior to this procedure.

spinous process shifts toward the *upside.* In rotated prone or anterior oblique positions, the process shifts toward the *downside.*

Angulation and Flexion/Extension. The lordotic curvature of the cervical spine causes all but the top two of these vertebra to slant downward, and a cephalic angle of 15 to 20 degrees is required to desuperimpose them. Figures 113 and 114 show the difference in radiographic appearance when no cephalic angle is used: In Figure 113, the joint spaces are not dark and the vertebra superimpose each other, because no angle was used as in Figure 114. Note also that in Figure 113, the chin obscures the 3rd cervical vertebra. This vertebra is *not* demonstrated on the open-mouth odontoid view. Since the AP cervical spine projection is the *only* frontal view of C-3 that the radiologist will be provided with, *this view must be repeated any time that the chin obscures any portion of C-3.* The AP view of the C-spine should clearly demonstrate C-3 through C-7.

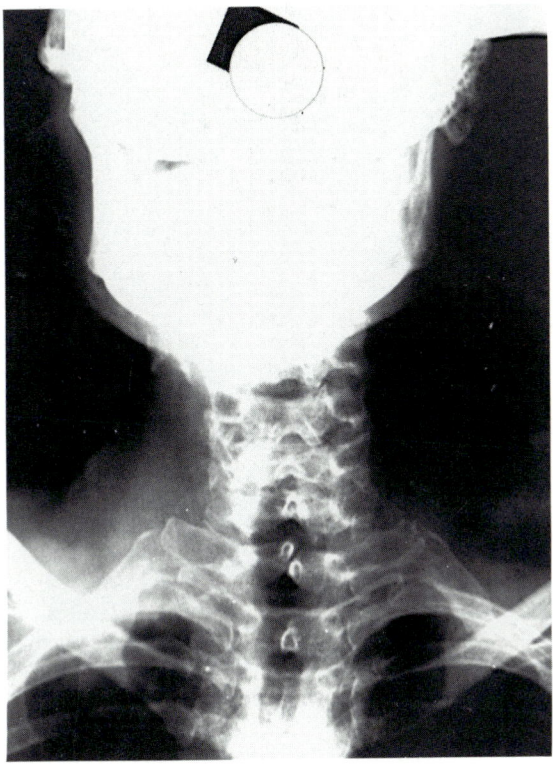

Figure 113. Frontal view of cervical spine. No cephalic tube angle was used. This resulted in closed intervertebral joints (compare with Figure 114). Too much flexion of the head combined with the failure to properly angle the tube resulted in superimposing the chin over the upper *four* cervical vertebrae.

There are two possible causes for the chin being projected into C-3. The first is failure to use a cephalic tube angle as just described. The second is failure to properly *extend* the chin on the AP projection. Adequate extension of the head during positioning is achieved when the under-surface of the body of the mandible is almost perpendicular to the film. In observing the undersurface of this bone, the chin cannot be flexed more than about 10 degrees. If it is, the chin will obscure C-3 as in Figure 113. Of course, these superimposition problems can be caused by a *combination* of inadequate tube angle and inadequate head extension. If

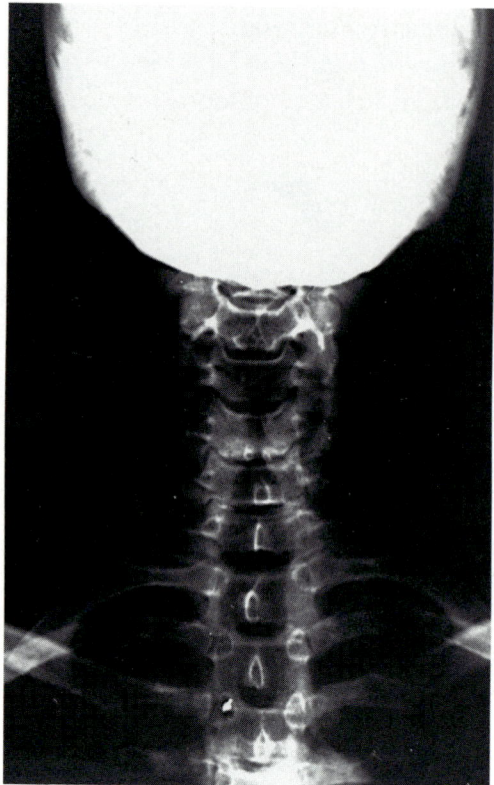

Figure 114. Frontal view of cervical spine with hyperextension of the head. This can place the occipital bone over C3, as almost occurs here.

the head is *extended* too much, the occipital bone will descend over C-3 as in Figure 114. *The correct combination of tube angle and head extension will result in the bottom of the chin and the bottom of the occipital bone being directly superimposed over each other,* with the joint spaces of the cervical spine well opened.

Odontoid View

   Rotation. The open-mouth odontoid view is a special case, involving the positioning of the head. With no rotation of the head, the upper and lower molar teeth will appear equidistant from the midline of the odontoid process. If the left molar teeth (either upper molars or lower molars) obscure the atlantoaxial joint (C1-C2) while the right teeth are out of the way, as shown in Figure 115, the head is rotated to the *right.* If the right teeth obscure the joint, the head is rotated to the *left.* If the teeth on *both* sides obscure the joint, the problem is not rotation, but rather flexion/ extension of the skull.

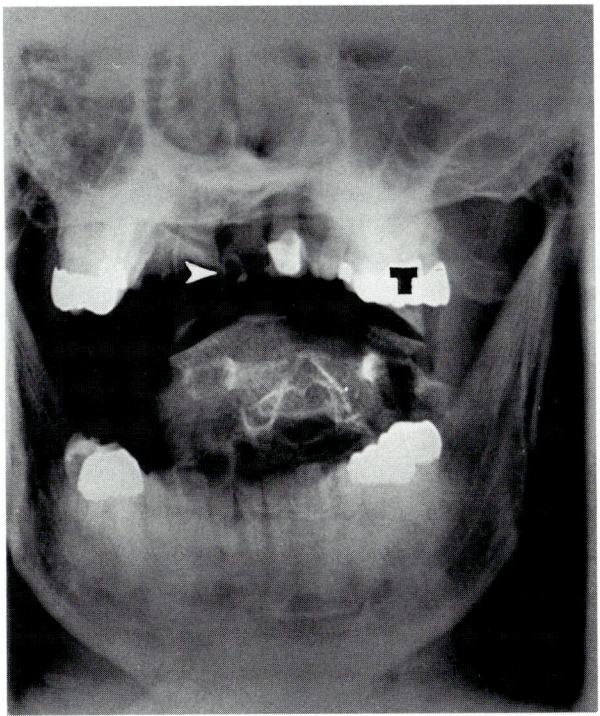

Figure 115. Open-mouth odontoid view with head rotation to the *right* places the *left* upper molar teeth (T) over the atlantoaxial (C1–C2) joint space. Bottom edge of upper incisors (arrow) is below the occipital bone, indicating slight flexion of the head also.

Angulation and Flexion/Extension. Proper flexion/extension of the head will place the bottom edges of the upper central incisor teeth directly over the bottom edge of the occipital bone, as in Figure 116. This normally desuperimposes skull anatomy from all but the very tip of the odontoid process. If the position meets these criteria and yet the odontoid process is still substantially obscured, a repeated exposure using the Fuchs or Judd method is recommended.

Remember that in frontal projections, cephalic or caudal angulation of the x-ray beam is equivalent in its objectives to flexion or extension of the body part. This means, for example, that if a patient was unable to adequately extend his head to get the upper teeth off of the odontoid process, a slight *cephalic angle* of the x-ray beam can accomplish the same thing by projecting these teeth up above the process.

The upper teeth may be properly superimposed over the occipital bone, yet if the lower (mandibular) molar teeth obscure the body of C-2 as in Figure 116, then *the mouth was not opened wide enough.* Hyperextension of the head, however, also can result in the lower teeth obscuring this joint.

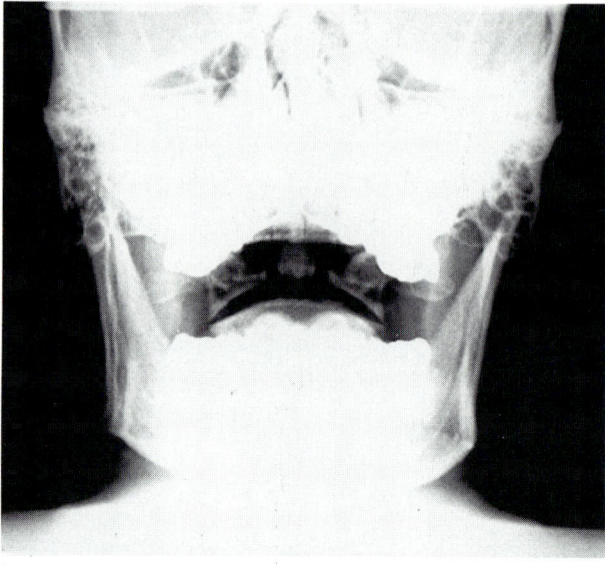

Figure 116. Open-mouth odontoid view with exact flexion/extension of the head (upper incisors superimposed on occipital bone). But, mouth was not opened adequately, leaving lower teeth superimposed over second cervical vertebra.

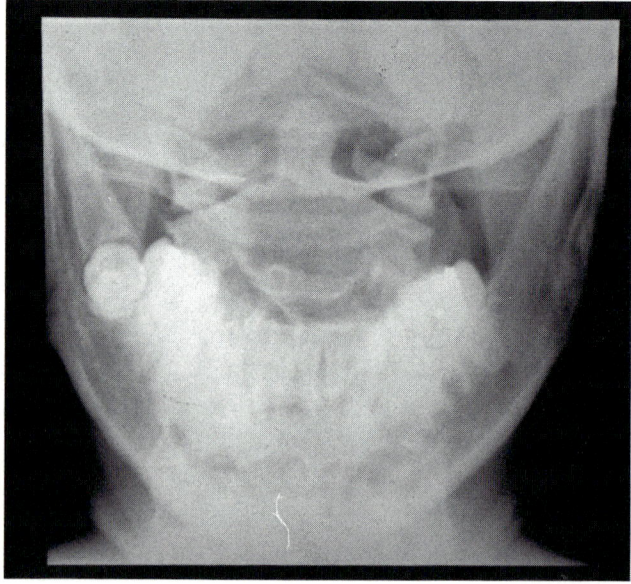

Figure 117. Open-mouth odontoid view with hyperextension of head, placing occipital bone over odontoid process.

Superimposition of the *occipital bone* over the odontoid process, shown in Figure 117, indicates *hyperextension* of the head.

Oblique Views

Rotation. On obliques of the cervical spine, the intervertebral foramina will open and appear as oval holes that are nearly round as shown in Figure 118. If these holes appear narrow, part rotation is either too steep or too shallow from the proper 45 degrees, Figure 119. If the position is much too steep, greater than 45 degrees, the anterior halves of the vertebral bodies will begin to appear "clear" of superimposed neural arch structures. In a full lateral view, the vertebral bodies will be completely clear of such neural arch structures. When the position is much too

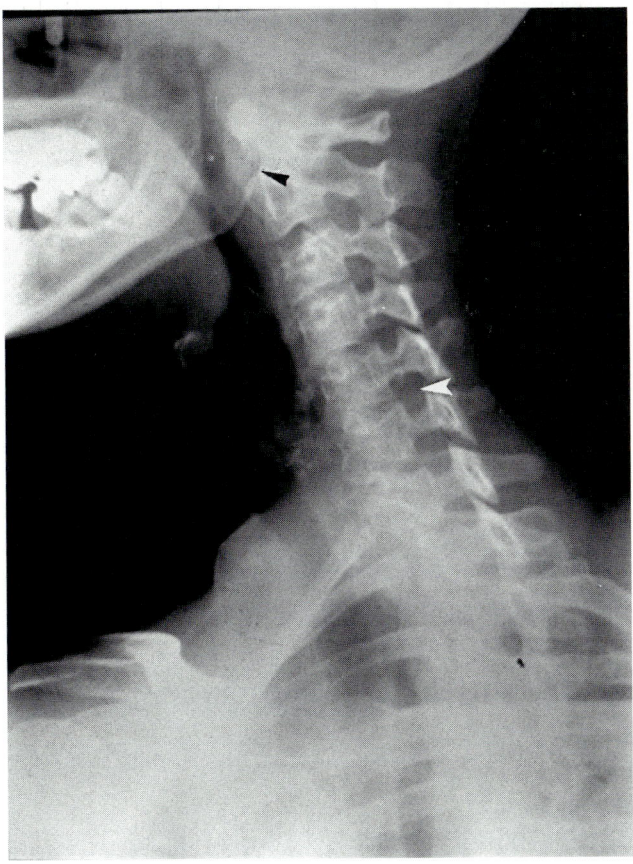

Figure 118. Oblique cervical spine view with good 45-degree rotation opens intervertebral foramina (white arrow). Because head is not fully lateral, upside ramus of mandible overlaps top of C2 (black arrow).

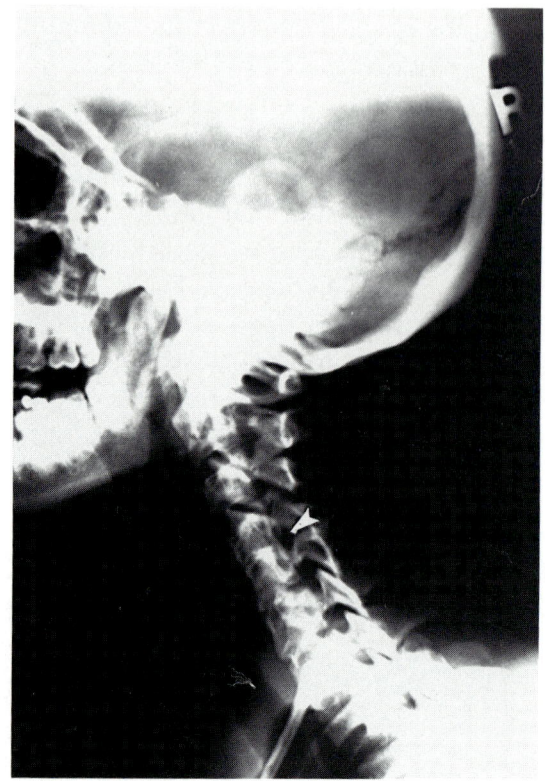

Figure 119. Oblique cervical spine view with body rotation too steep results in narrowing of the intervertebral foramina (arrow).

shallow, less than 45 degrees, one set of pedicles will be seen in the middle of the vertebral bodies.

Rotation of the *head* on oblique cervical spine projections is a controversial issue. Although positioning atlases recommend that the head be in line with the rest of the body (at 45 degrees), this can result in the ramus of the mandible superimposing C-2 as in Figure 118. The author prefers the popular method of turning the head into nearly a lateral position to avoid this superimposition. In addition, the intervertebral foramina of the upper cervical spine open more laterally than the lower ones, so that turning the head laterally tends to demonstrate these upper foramina better.

Angulation and Flexion/Extension. Obliques of the cervical spine which are adequate for evaluation of trauma can be taken if necessary without the recommended 15–20 degree beam angle, but the intervertebral foramina will not be opened up as well vertically. To fully open these foramina for complete diagnosis, the beam angle should be used whenever possible. In addition, the *chin* must be extended on all oblique views of the C-spine to prevent the rami of the mandible from superimposing the anterior aspects of the upper vertebrae as in Figure 120.

Lateral Views

Rotation. The lateral views of the cervical spine should show the vertebral bodies clear of any superimposing processes. As discussed for the thoracic and lumbar spines, the two posterior surfaces of the vertebral bodies should be superimposed and appear as one feature. When

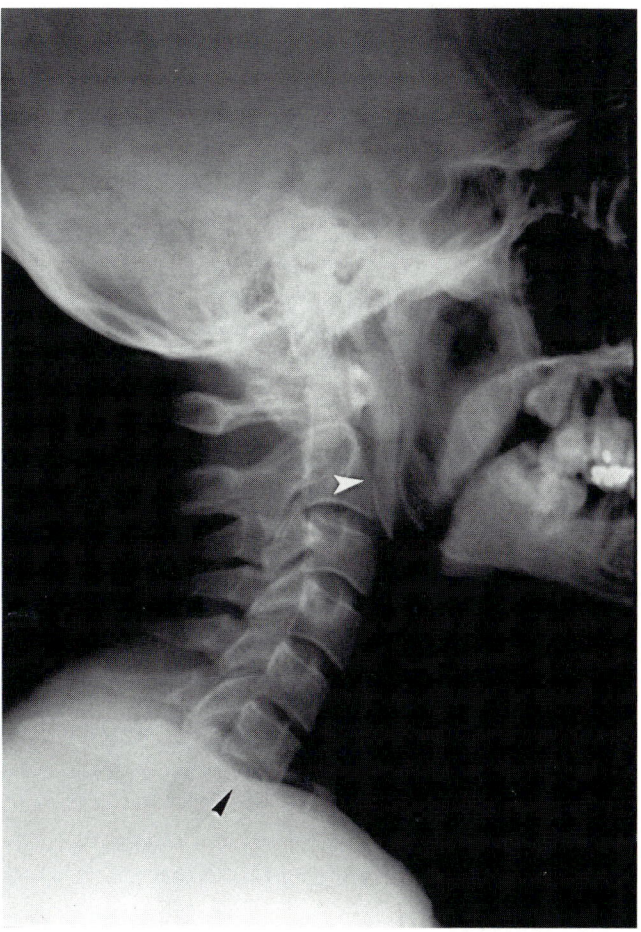

Figure 120. Lateral view of cervical spine with insufficient depression of the shoulders obscures C7 (black arrow). For both lateral and oblique cervical spine projections, slight chin extension would avoid superimposition of mandibular ramus over C2 (white arrow).

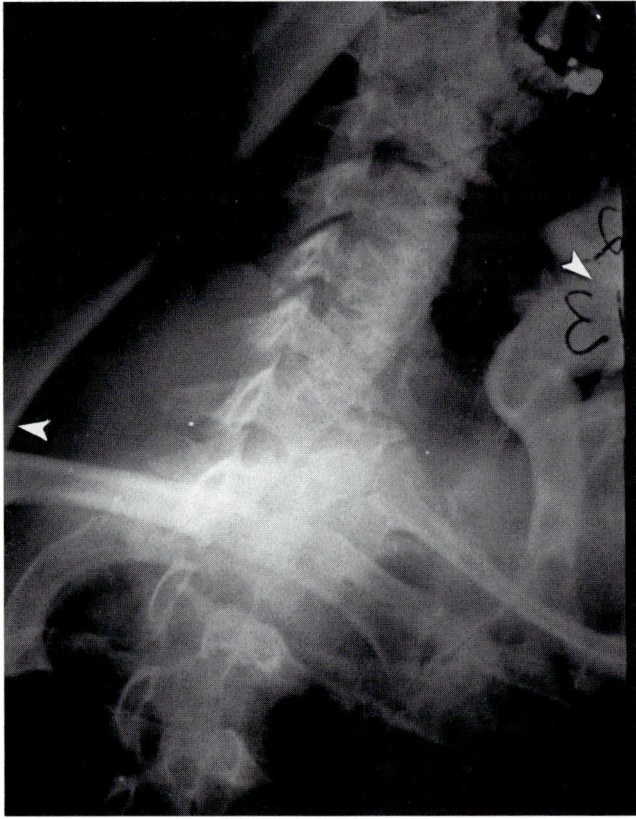

Figure 121. Twining view of cervicothoracic vertebrae with over-rotation of shoulders (arrows). Shoulders (heads of humeri) should be projected just off of spine anteriorly and posteriorly. Opening of cervical intervertebral foramina attest that the spine is in *oblique* rather than near-lateral position.

rotation is present, a double-line will appear along the back of each body as in Figure 104.

Other Considerations. The lateral view of the cervical spine utilizes no tube angle, but both *shoulders* must be depressed enough to desuperimpose the seventh cervical vertebra. If weights do not suffice, stress must be used to pull the shoulders down far enough. Lateral views must include C-1 through C-7, Figure 120. If this cannot be achieved, a Twining view should be taken to demonstrate the seventh cervical vertebra.

Twining View

The Twining view, properly done, should be as near lateral as possible without superimposing either shoulder over the cervicothoracic vertebrae. Radiographers frequently *over*-rotate the patient when adjusting

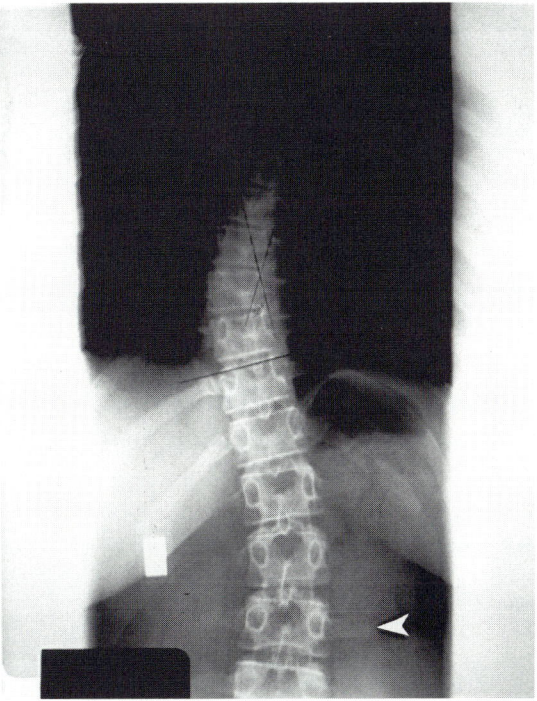

Figure 122. Good technique for spine views should demonstrate the transverse processes as can be seen in the lumbar vertebrae on this view (arrow). But this was an attempted thoracic spine (centered low) and even in lower thoracic vertebrae, the transverse processes are "burned out". Use of a wedge filter would have helped demonstrate the upper thoracic vertebrae.

one shoulder forward and the other backward, as shown in Figure 121. To avoid this error, begin with the patient in true lateral position. *Slide* the downside shoulder forward without moving the torso. Then *roll* the upside shoulder back as far as possible. Very slight body rotation is sometimes necessary, but not as much as shown in Figure 121.

Other Considerations

On all frontal and oblique views of the spines, there should be minimal lateral bending, and if the patient is not placed diagonally on the table, the spine should be aligned vertically down the center of the view. Care must be taken to ensure that the arms are out of the way on lateral thoracic and Twining positions. Reasonable collimation should always be used to prevent the destruction of image contrast from scatter radiation. Generally, the collimated field should not exceed eight inches in width, regardless of the film size used, unless lateral bending or flexion/extension views are being taken.

Technique

A fairly high contrast image is desirable for spine radiography, using kVp levels from 70–80 for adults. In the cervicothoracic views, the shoulder area must be penetrated, and for the L5-S1 "spot" lateral or lateral sacrum, the pelvic ilia must be penetrated so that visibility of the spine itself is maximized. The transverse processes should be visible on frontal and oblique views, and the spinous processes on lateral views. Overexposure (from too much mAs) will obliterate these thin bones from view, as in Figure 122. Use of a wedge filter and the anode heel effect are strongly recommended on the AP thoracic view.

Breathing technique should be used for the lateral thoracic spine, blurring the soft tissue markings in the lung fields so that the spine can be better seen through them, Figure 123.

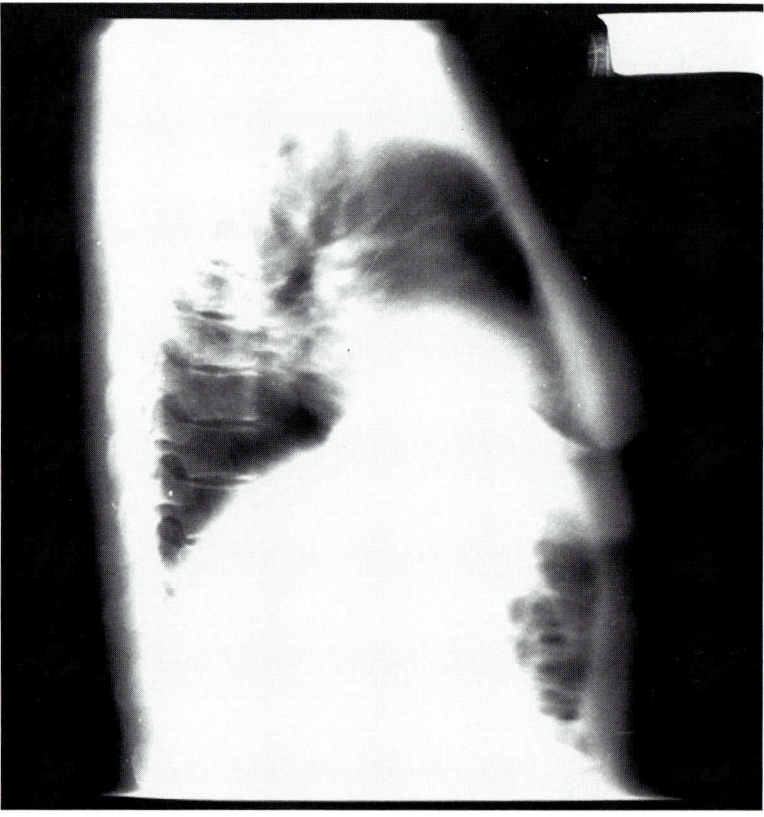

Figure 123. Lateral thoracic spine view using breathing technique. Note clarity of lower thoracic vertebrae with lung markings blurred out.

Chapter 8

EXTREMITY POSITIONS

HAND AND DIGITS

Frontal Views

Rotation. In nonrotated frontal views, the distal phalanx of each finger will appear symmetrical with equal concavity on either side. In true lateral views, the anterior surface of each phalanx will appear more concave than the posterior side, and the distal phalanx will take on a very narrow triangular shape with its base about half as wide as it appears on a frontal view. (Compare the tips of the fingers in Figures 124 and 128.) In rotated or oblique views, the anterior side of each phalanx will appear more concave than the posterior side, but the distal phalanx will still have a broad base, Figure 125. On the PA projection of the entire hand, the four fingers should appear unrotated, while the thumb will naturally lie in an oblique position.

Oblique Views

Rotation. For the oblique hand position, the proper 45 degrees of rotation will separate the *mid-shafts* of all of the metacarpals, even though the bases and heads of these bones will typically overlap as in Figure 125-A. The space between the fourth and fifth metacarpals will be the narrowest, but there should be some space between all of the bones in the mid-shaft area. If the shafts overlap, the hand rotation is *too steep,* greater than 45 degrees, as in Figure 125-B. If none of the *heads* of the metacarpals overlap at all, the position is *too shallow,* less than 45 degrees, as in Figure 126.

Flexion/Extension. If there is diagnostic interest in the digits, oblique hand views must be done with all of the fingers fully extended to place them parallel to the film. With full extension, all of the interphalangeal joint spaces will be open. When the interphalangeal joints are closed as in Figure 126, the fingers were improperly flexed. The best way to ensure that the fingers are parallel to the film is to use a 45-degree "step" sponge

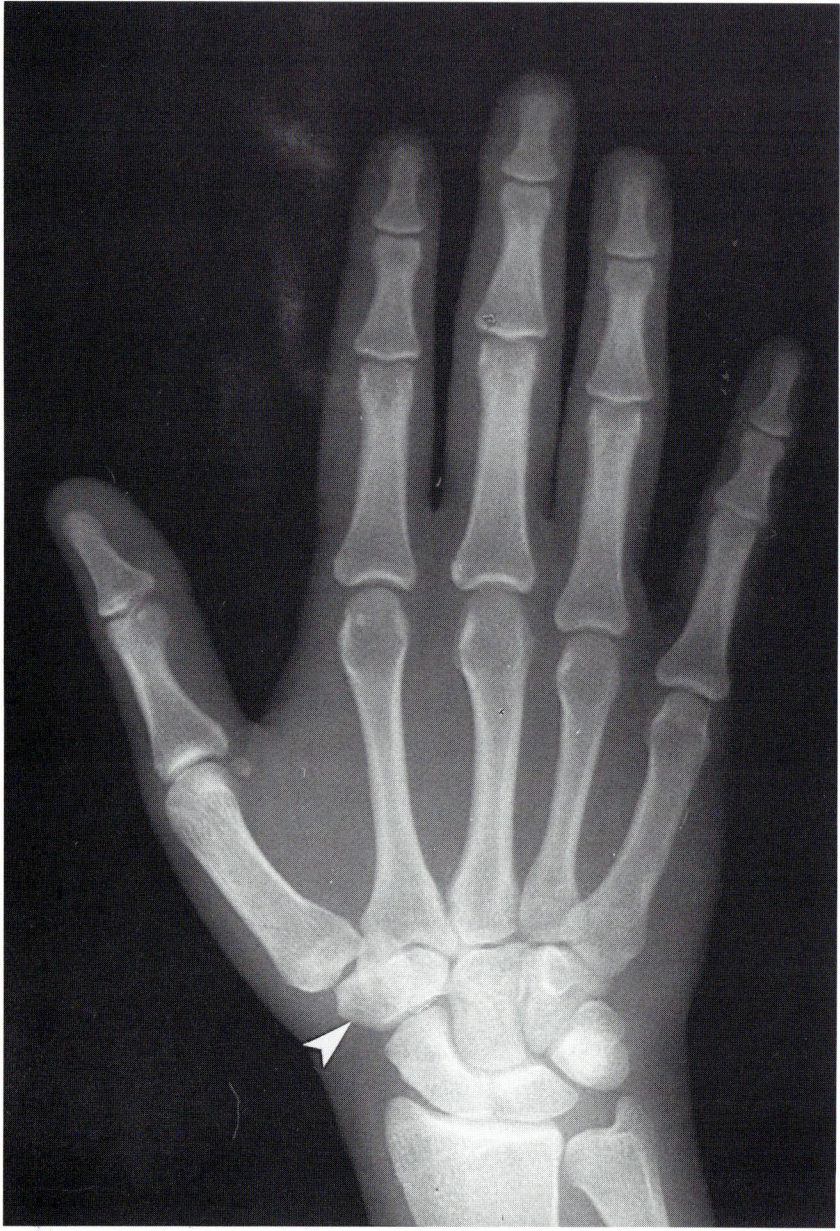

Figure 124. PA view of hand shows symmetrical appearance of distal phalanges on four fingers, (compare with thumb, or with fingers in Figure 125). Greater and lesser multangular bones of wrist (arrow) are superimposed.

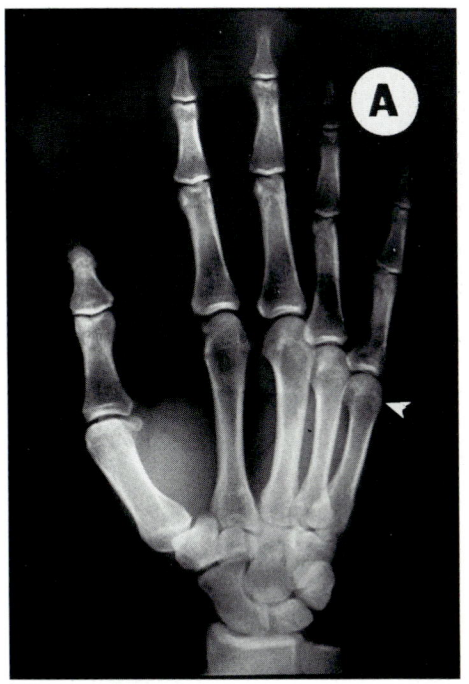 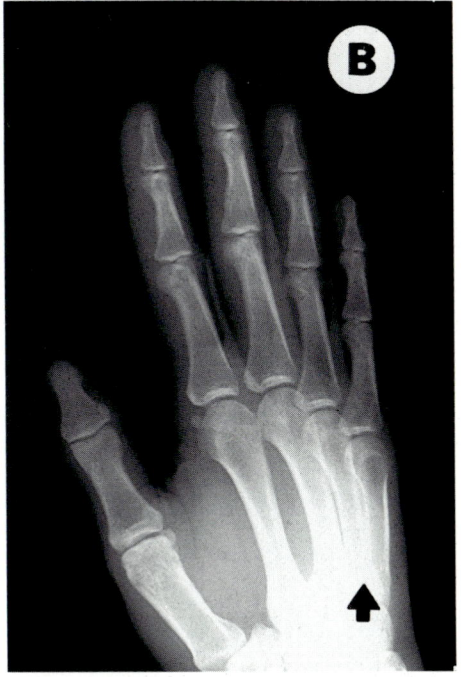

Figure 125. Oblique views of hand. Proper 45 degrees of rotation in *A* shows overlapping of metacarpal heads (arrow), but *not* of shafts. Overlapping of metacarpal shafts in *B* (arrow) indicates too steep rotation.

to support them. It must be noted that some departments allow flexion of the digits for oblique hand views, *provided* there is no direct interest in the digits.

Lateral Views

Rotation. Lateral views of the hand, including the "fanned" lateral, should demonstrate the second, third, fourth, and fifth *metacarpals* superimposed directly upon each other or "stacked". *Pronation* rotation (palm rotated downward) is present when the second digit (index finger) is seen anterior to the other three fingers and shifting toward the thumb, Figure 127. *Supination* rotation shows the fifth digit (small finger) shifting anteriorly toward the thumb, Figure 131.

Flexion/Extension. On the fanned lateral view of the hand, the flexion of the digits should be such that all four fingers are equally spaced, with the second digit (index finger) touching or nearly touching the thumb, Figure 128.

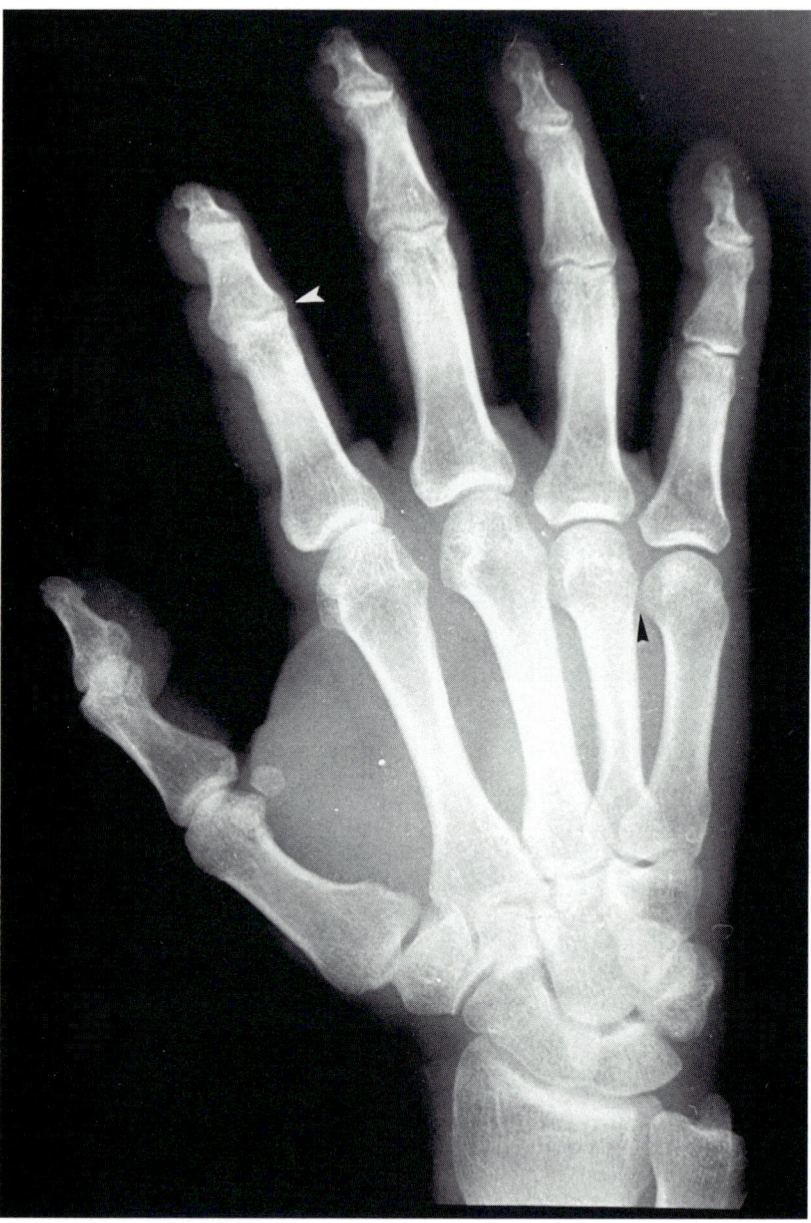

Figure 126. Too shallow rotation for oblique hand view shows no overlapping of *heads* of metacarpals (black arrow). Improper flexion of fingers closes off interphalangeal joints (white arrow) obscuring proximal and distal ends of various phalanges. Use of a "step" sponge is recommended to keep all fingers parallel to film.

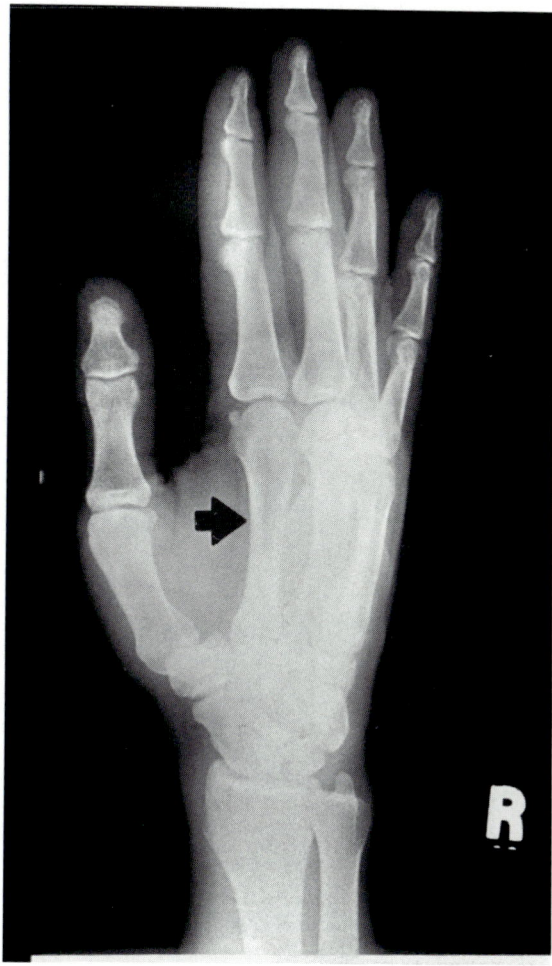

Figure 127. Lateral view of hand with *pronation* rotation, evidenced by shift of second metacarpal (index finger, arrow) toward thumb.

Tilt/Abduction/Adduction. On *any* lateral view of a digit or a fanned lateral of the hand, all interphalangeal joints should be open. Closing of these joints on *lateral* views indicates a lateral tilt to the finger. This is frequently caused by improperly resting the tip of the finger on the film cassette as in Figure 129.

Norgaard Method.

This special "ball catcher's" position to demonstrate arthritis requires that the fingers be left in their natural amount of flexion with the hands

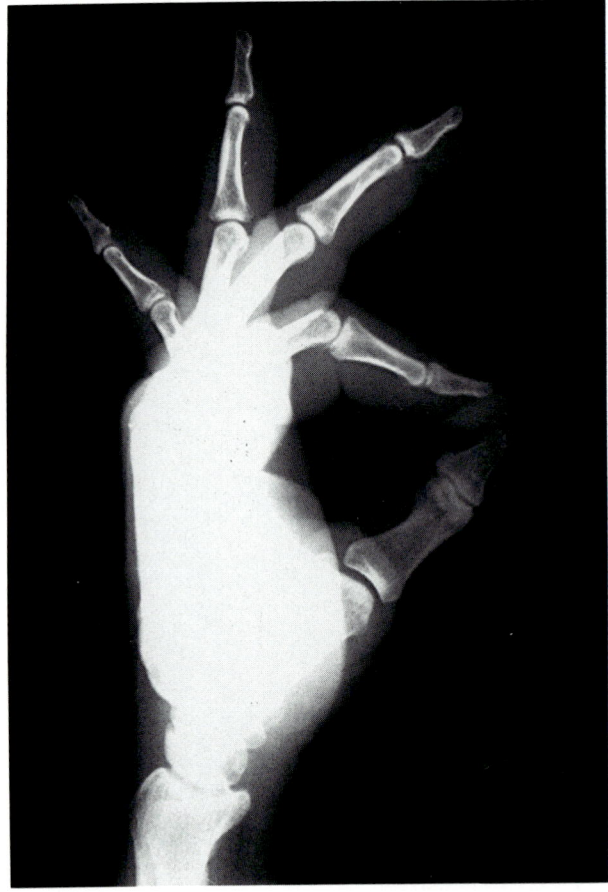

Figure 128. "Fanned" lateral hand with good spacing between all digits.

placed in semisupination. The interphalangeal joints will thus be closed off in appearance, but the *metacarpophalangeal* joints should be open.

WRIST

Frontal View

Rotation. On the nonrotated PA view of the wrist, the distal radioulnar joint space should be open, with no overlapping of the radius and ulna. If any portion of the distal radius and ulna superimpose, rotation is present.

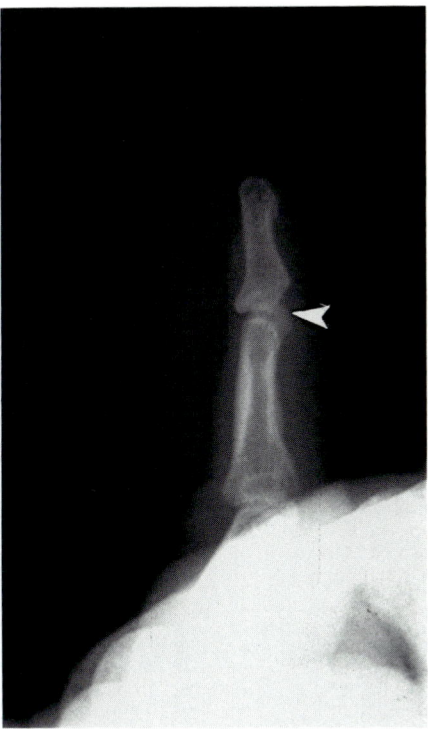

Figure 129. Lateral digit showing closing of interphalangeal joint and overlapping of distal and middle phalanx. This was caused by dropping the finger down to rest on the film, tilting it.

Oblique View

Rotation. A primary purpose of the oblique wrist position is to desuperimpose the *trapezium and trapezoid* (greater and lesser multangulars), which overlap on the frontal view as shown in Figure 124. Proper 45-degree rotation will demonstrate the trapezium and trapezoid free of superimposition from each other as in Figure 130. Approximately one-quarter of the head of the ulna will superimpose the radius. If more than one-quarter of the ulnar head overlaps the radius, or if the mid-shafts of the metacarpals in the hand overlap as in Figure 125-B, the position is too *steep,* more than 45 degrees. If the trapezium and trapezoid overlap as in Figure 124, then the position is too *shallow,* less than 45 degrees.

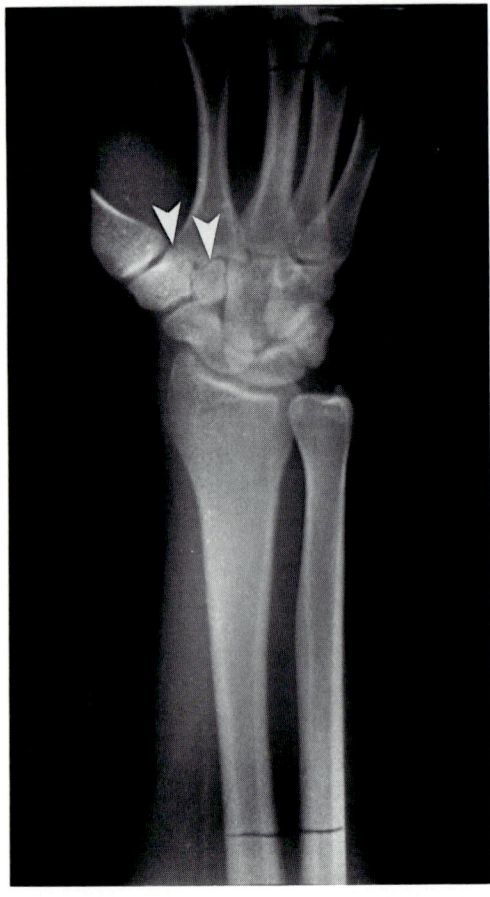

Figure 130. Proper 45-degree oblique view of wrist desuperimposes greater and lesser multangulars (arrows) and overlaps approximately one-quarter of head of ulna over radius.

Lateral View

Rotation. With normal anatomy, a true lateral view of the wrist will place the smaller head of the ulna in the middle of the broader base of the radius. Note that you can palpate the head of the ulna on the posterior surface of your wrist, demonstrating that *the head of the ulna lies slightly posterior to the radius. The plane of the lateral wrist is not exactly aligned with the plane of the lateral hand.* Therefore, to produce a perfect lateral wrist position on most patients, *the palm of the hand should be supinated 5 degrees from lateral,* as demonstrated in Figure 131. This slight rotation will roll the radius back slightly, placing the ulna in mid-shaft for a true lateral position. (Stacking of the metacarpals of the hand, recommended in some positioning manuals, is actually a poor indicator of wrist position.)

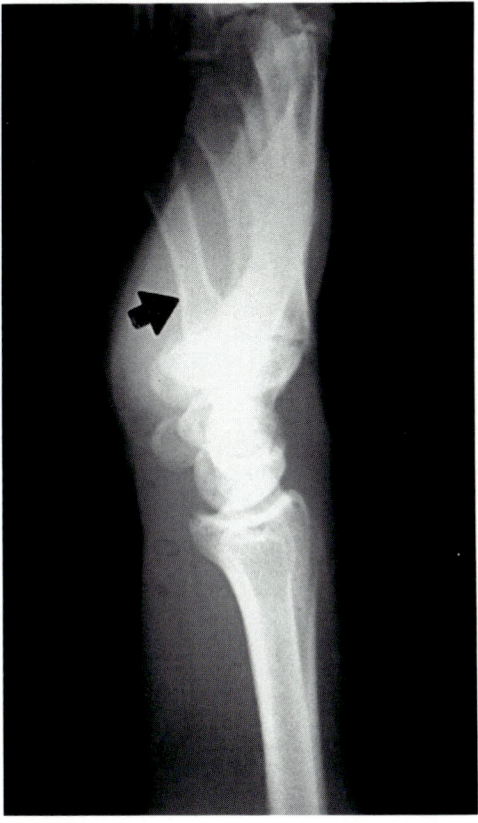

Figure 131. True lateral wrist view with head of ulna centered over radius. Note that the hand is slightly supinated, with the fifth metacarpal (arrow) anterior to the other fingers.

If the head of the ulna is seen lying *posteriorly* in relation to the radius, the wrist is rotated toward *pronation*, Figure 132. If the head of the ulna lies anteriorly against the radius, the wrist is rotated toward *supination*.

Special Views

Navicular. Adequate ulnar flexion (adduction) of the hand will open the joint space between the navicular (scaphoid) and the captitate and lunate to the side. The Stecher method recommends 15–20 degrees of hyperextension, or of a 15–20 degree proximal angulation of the x-ray

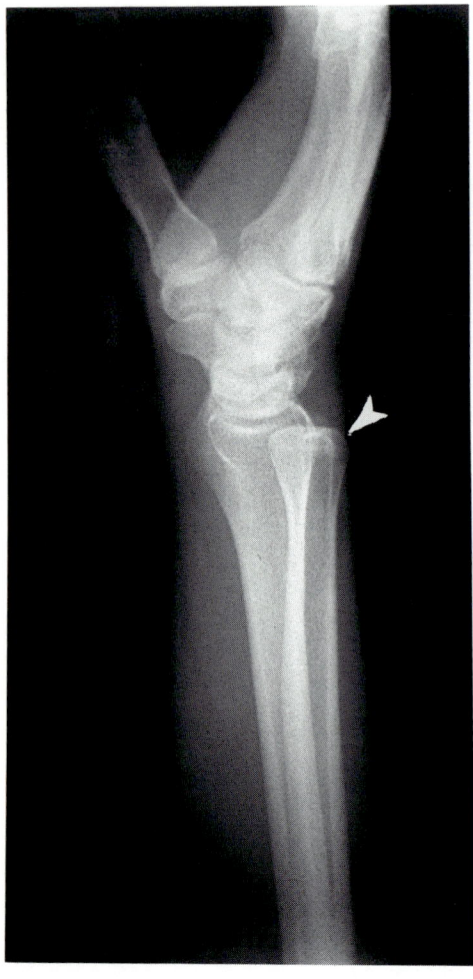

Figure 132. Lateral view of wrist showing *pronation* rotation, projecting head of ulna (arrow) slightly posterior to radius. Note that hand is in true lateral position with metacarpals directly superimposed.

beam. This will open the joint space between the navicular and the trapezium (greater multangular) for an optimal view, as shown in Figure 133.

Carpal Tunnel. With sufficient hyperextension (dorsiflexion) of the wrist, the pisiform will not superimpose the triquetrum and the carpals will be demonstrated in an arch formation.

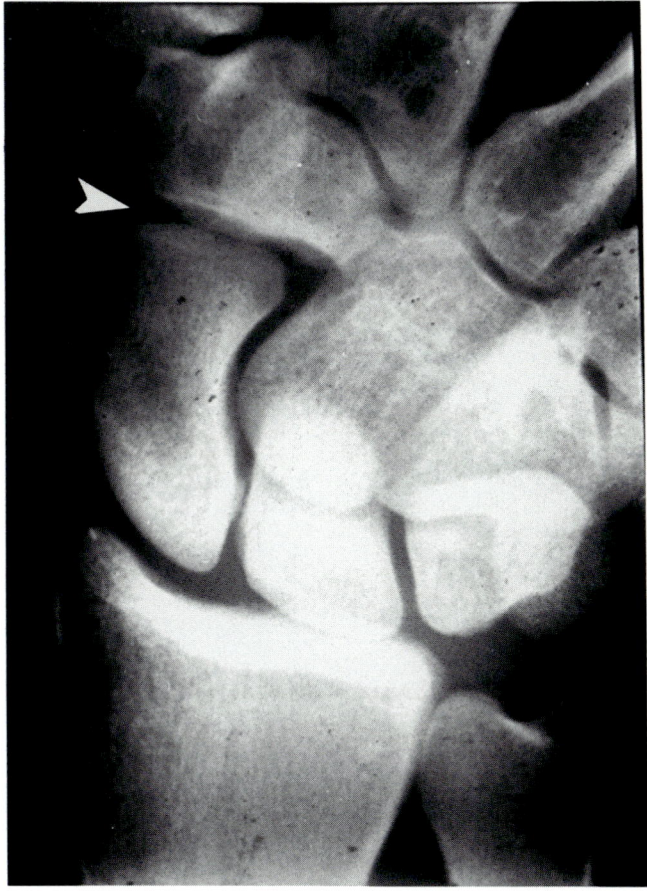

Figure 133. Stecher method for navicular bone using a 15 degree proximal beam angle which opens the intercarpal joint between the greater and lesser multangulars and the navicular (arrow). *Both* the tube angle and ulnar flexion should be used.

ELBOW AND LONG BONES

Frontal Views

Rotation. The elbow area has no symmetrical anatomy and therefore lacks criteria for simple explanations. Figure 134 demonstrates a nonrotated frontal view. The epicondylar area of the humerus is *fairly* symmetrical and broad. The olecranon process of the ulna is *roughly* centered within the distal humerus. The medial one-third of the head and neck of the radius and the radial tuberosity superimpose the ulna. When the elbow

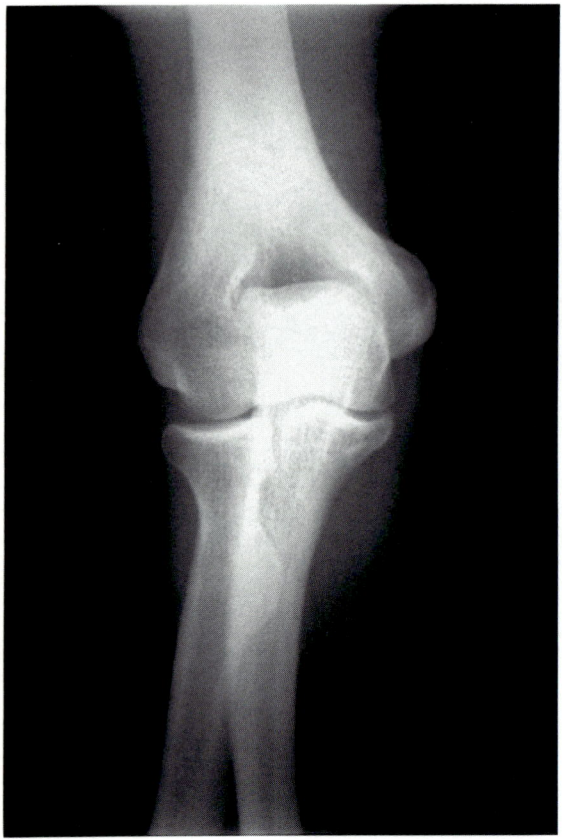

Figure 134. Non-rotated frontal view of elbow demonstrates overlapping of about one-third of the proximal radius over the proximal ulna.

is rotated medially (internally), overlapping of the radial head and the ulna will *increase*. With lateral (external) rotation, this overlap will *decrease* toward complete desuperimposition.

For the frontal view of the forearm, the wrist should also be checked against the criteria described in the previous section. The hand and wrist should be supine. If the proximal radius crosses over the ulna, the hand was improperly pronated.

For the humerus, the positions of the greater and lesser tuberosities should also be checked: In the nonrotated frontal view, the *greater* tuberosity will be placed in profile laterally to the anatomical neck. Also, there will be a distinct internal curvature only on the *medial* surface of the neck as it "turns" toward the scapula, Figure 135. Combining these criteria with the appearance of the elbow, one can make a good judgment of the presence and degree of rotation.

Flexion/Extension. Flexion of the elbow joint will close the joint space

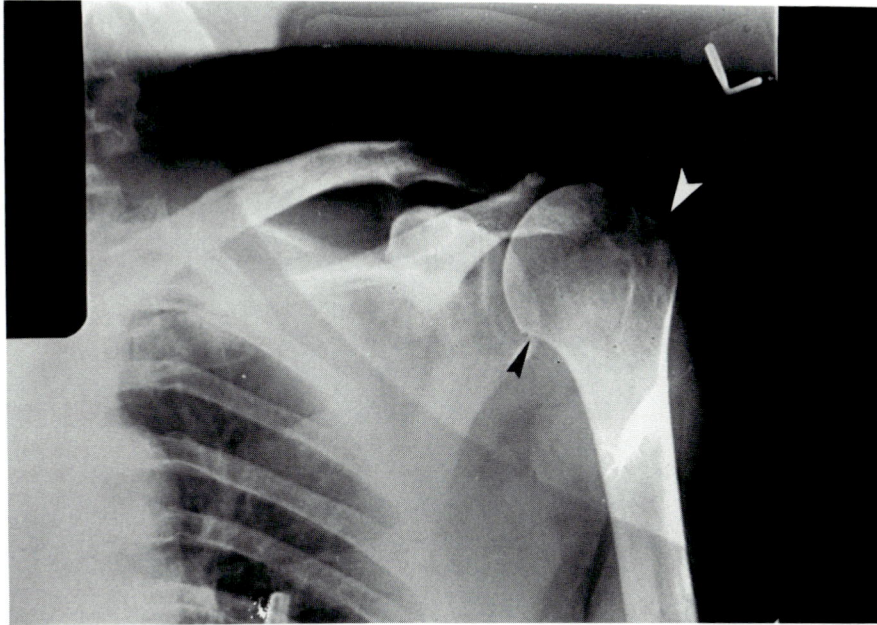

Figure 135. External rotation frontal view of humerus places greater tuberosity in profile (white arrow) and shows disinct medial curvature (black arrow).

between the radius and the humerus off, with the head of the radius superimposing the capitellum of the humerus as in Figure 136.

Lateral Views

Rotation vs Tilt. True lateral views of the elbow, forearm or humerus are all characterized by direct *superimposition of the two condyles of the humerus* as in Figure 137. The line diagram in Figure 138 shows the expected appearance of these two condyles when rotation or tilt are present. Tilt or improper abduction of the humerus occurs when the patient's shoulder is not lowered to the level of the film. This is necessary for all lateral views of the forearm, elbow and humerus. If tilt is present in the humerus, the elbow and proximal forearm will automatically be *rotated* as shown in Figure 139.

When the lateral view of the humerus is improperly rotated, neither tuberosity will appear distinctly in profile, and on the distal end the condyles will shift off of each other side-to-side as diagrammed in Figure 138 and demonstrated in Figure 140.

For the lateral view of the forearm, the *wrist* should also be in true lateral as described in the previous section. For the lateral view of the *humerus,* the *lesser* tuberosity will be placed in profile on the *medial*

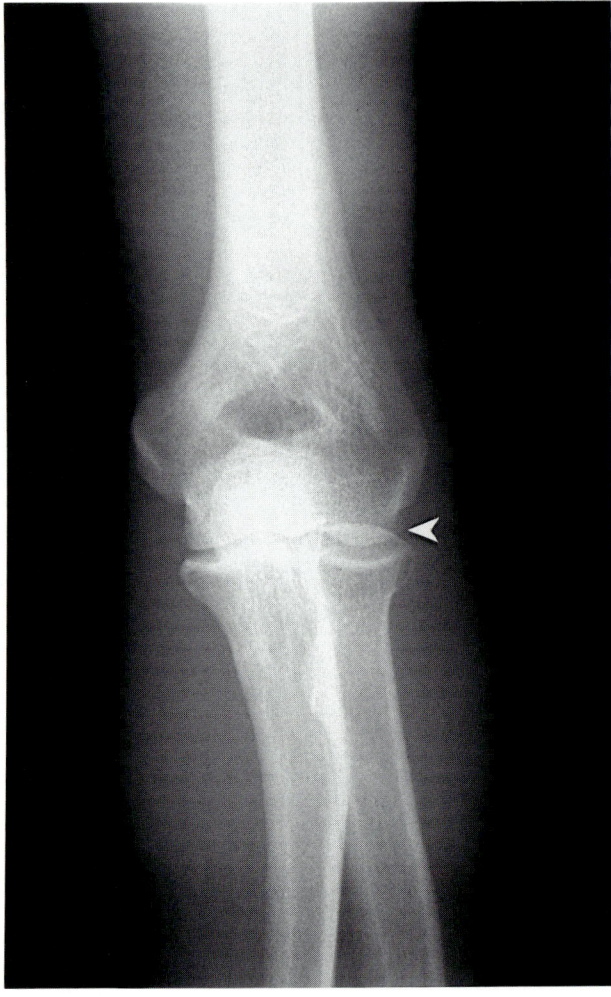

Figure 136. Frontal elbow view with improper flexion of elbow, overlapping head of radius (arrow) with capitellum of humerus, (compare with Figure 134).

surface of the humeral neck, and the general broadening of the neck area will appear symmetrical with the head centered upon it like ice cream on a cone, Figure 141.

Flexion/Extension. On the lateral elbow view, the elbow should be flexed at 90 degrees.

Tilt/Abduction/Adduction. Tilt of the humerus is a common problem with lateral projections of the humerus, elbow and forearm. It is detected by a vertical, superior-to-inferior shifting of the humeral condyles as diagrammed in Figure 138 and demonstrated in Figure 139. Tilt is

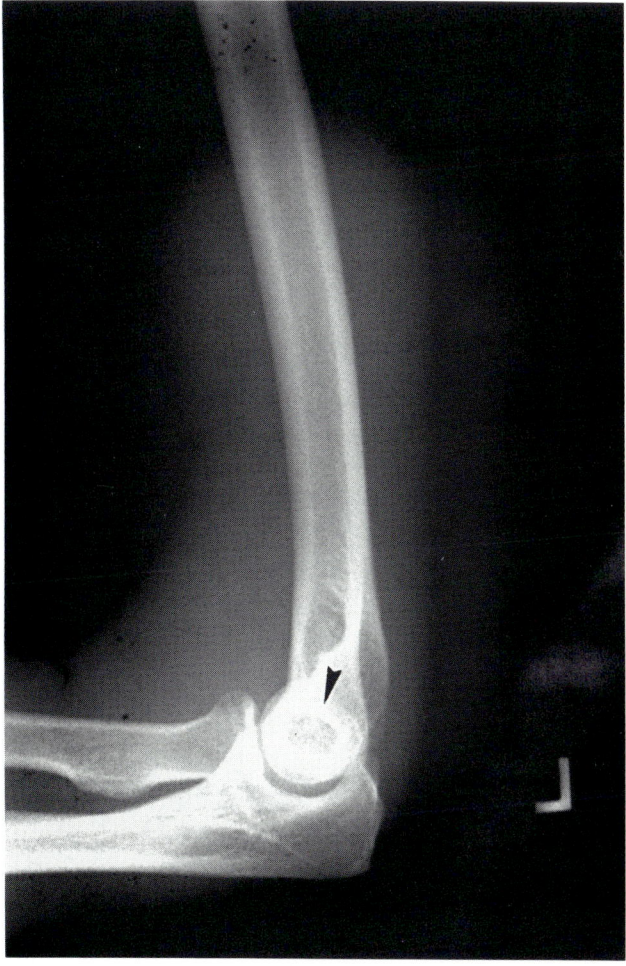

Figure 137. Proper lateral view of elbow superimposes humeral condyles (arrow).

usually due to insufficient *abduction* of the humerus, caused by not lowering the patient's shoulder to the level of the film. To bring the shoulder down to the level of the table, the patient must frequently bend at the waist in seated position.

Transthoracic Lateral View

Rotation. Note that these rules also apply to the *transthoracic* lateral view of the humerus. When possible, the hand should *supinated* as the patient stands against the film (not in "neutral" position, as some positioning manuals suggest). With the hand in near or full supina-

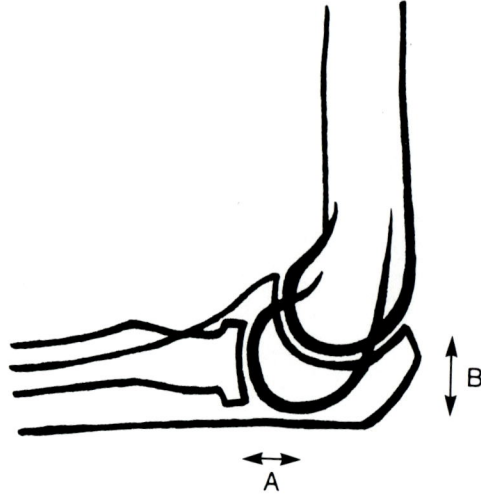

Figure 138. Diagram illustrating expected shift of humeral condyles when humerus is both rotated and tilted during positioning of forearm, elbow or humerus. Side-to-side shift, *A,* indicates rotation in the humerus. Vertical shift, *B,* indicates *tilt* in the humerus or *rotation* in the forearm, either case being caused by insufficient abduction of the shoulder joint to 90 degrees. See Figure 139.

tion, the humeral condyles can be placed in true lateral position against the film. The radiologist should be provided with a true transthoracic lateral view, not a transthoracic oblique! With the humerus in true lateral position, the lesser tuberosity will be in profile anteriorly, and the neck will show a symmetrical broadening with the head in the middle.

Oblique Views

Rotation. With the proper 45-degree rotation, the internal oblique of the elbow places the coronoid process of the ulna in profile, with nearly all of the radial head superimposed over the ulna, Figure 140. Proper rotation on the external oblique opens the proximal radioulnar joint with no superimposition of the radial head and ulna.

SHOULDER GIRDLE

Shoulder Joint

Rotation. The evaluation of shoulder joint views follows precisely the same rules described for the humerus in the foregoing section. The

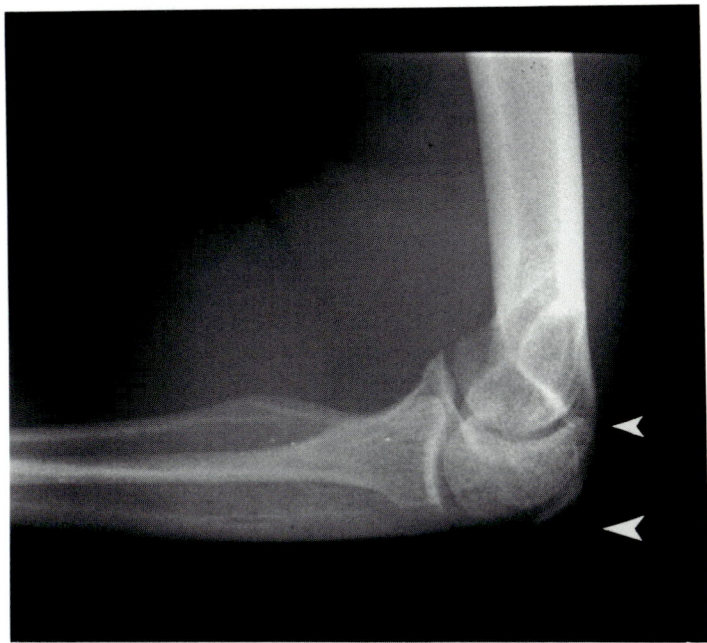

Figure 139. Lateral elbow view showing no rotation, but improper tilt shifting the humeral condyles (arrows) vertically. This tilt was caused by not bringing the shoulder down to the level of the film at the tabletop to achieve a full 90 degrees of shoulder abduction.

frontal view of the shoulder with the humerus in *external* rotation is essentially identical to the AP humerus, and should demonstrate the greater tuberosity in profile with a distinct internal curvature to the medial surface of the neck. The frontal view with *internal* rotation is essentially a lateral view, and should demonstrate the lesser tuberosity in profile with a symmetrical broadening of the neck area. See Figures 135 and 141.

The transthoracic lateral shoulder should be done with the hand supinated enough to place the intercondylar line perpendicular to the film. The *transaxillary* view of the shoulder also requires that the hand be laid in supine position against the tabletop so that the intercondylar line is placed perpendicular to the vertical film. The humerus must also be abducted 90 degrees to open the shoulder joint space. Correctly positioned, both the transthoracic view and the transaxillary view in Figure 142 will demonstrate the lesser tuberosity in profile anteriorly, and the humeral neck will appear to broaden symmetrically with the head in the middle.

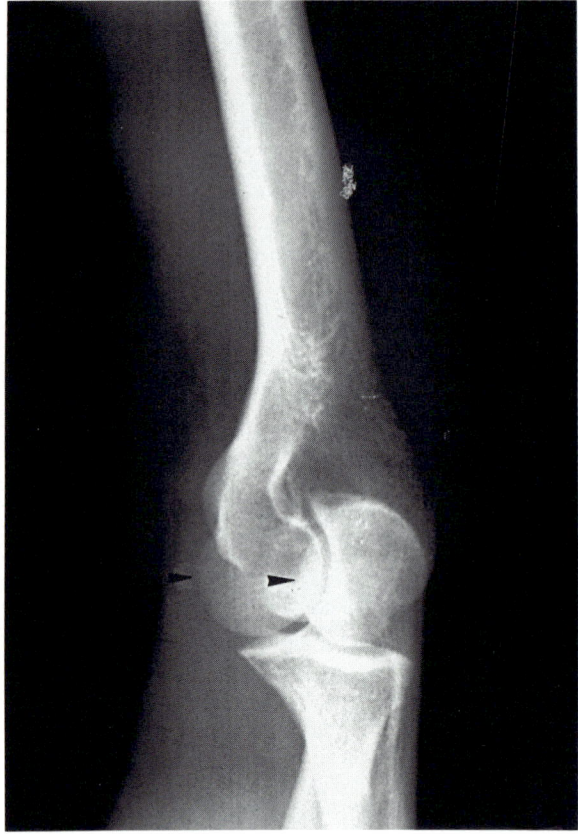

Figure 140. Oblique view of elbow showing side-to-side shift of humeral condyles (arrow). For any lateral humerus view, *including the transthoracic lateral,* such shift would indicate improper rotation.

Scapula and Clavicle

Rotation. Rotation is rarely a problem on frontal views of the scapula and clavicle. With rotation of the body *away* from the affected side, the sternal extremity of the clavicle will superimpose more than one-quarter of the spine, (slight superimposition can be a normal anatomical variation). The scapula should appear flat and parallel to the film in frontal view.

The true lateral view of the scapula will place it on end and leave a clear space between the scapula and the lateral ribs along its entire length as in Figure 143. A very common error is to place the patient's body in *too steep* obliquity, which rotates the scapula *past* lateral into an oblique position superimposing the lateral border over the ribs. Note in Figure 144 that the lateral border can be distinguished because it is

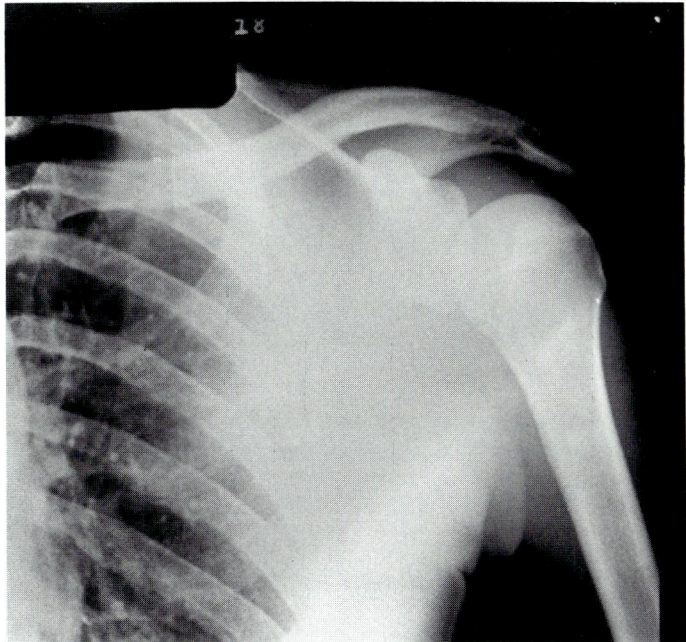

Figure 141. Internal rotation lateral view of humerus shows symmetrical broadening of humeral neck. Compare with Figure 135.

contiguous with glenoid fossa, rising to articulate with the head of the humerus. If the *medial* border of the scapula superimposes the ribs as in Figure 145, the body position was too *shallow*, or the arm was not pulled enough across the chest. The arm should be raised or pulled across the chest on all lateral scapula views so that the *shaft* of the humerus does not superimpose the body of the scapula.

The scapular "Y" position may be critiqued identically to the lateral scapula, with the exception that the humerus will superimpose the lower portion of the scapula. There should be no superimposition of the scapula over the *ribs.*

Angulation, Flexion and Extension. Routine clavicle series typically require one view desuperimposing the clavicle from the upper ribs and scapula as much as possible. This may be accomplished using a prone position with a 25 to 30 degree *caudal* angle, using a supine position with a 25 to 30 degree *cephalic* angle, or with the patient in a *lordotic* position combined with a 10 to 15 degree cephalic angle. With adequate angulation, all of the superior border of the scapula will be projected below the

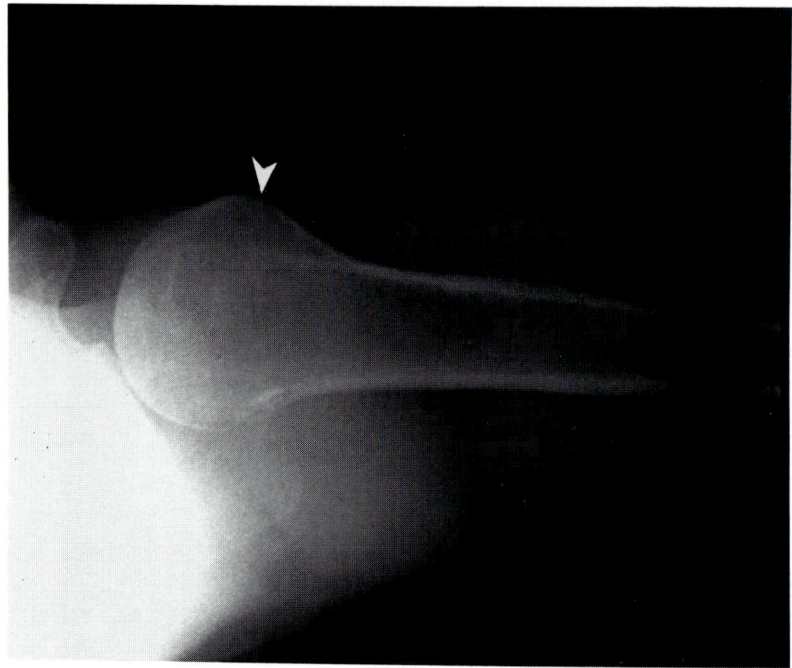

Figure 142. Transaxillary lateral view of shoulder, with care taken to position humeral condyles perpendicular to vertically placed film, should also show symmetrical broadening of humeral neck as in Figure 141, with lesser tuberosity (arrow) in profile anteriorly.

clavicle, and only the *first* rib will cross over the shaft of the clavicle as in Figure 146. The second rib may be seen over the sternal end of the clavicle, but if it crosses the *shaft* of the clavicle, insufficient angle was used. (On the frontal view with no angulation, typically the first three ribs cross over the clavicular shaft.)

FOOT AND TOES

Frontal Views

Rotation. For frontal views of the foot, the *heads* of the metatarsals should not be superimposed at all. If so, rotation is present. Criteria for the toes are identical to those in the previous discussion of the digits of the hand.

Angulation, Flexion and Extension. The interphalangeal joint spaces of the toes are quite difficult to open up due to dorsal curvature, and a 15-degree cephalic angle or use of a 15-degree angled sponge to force

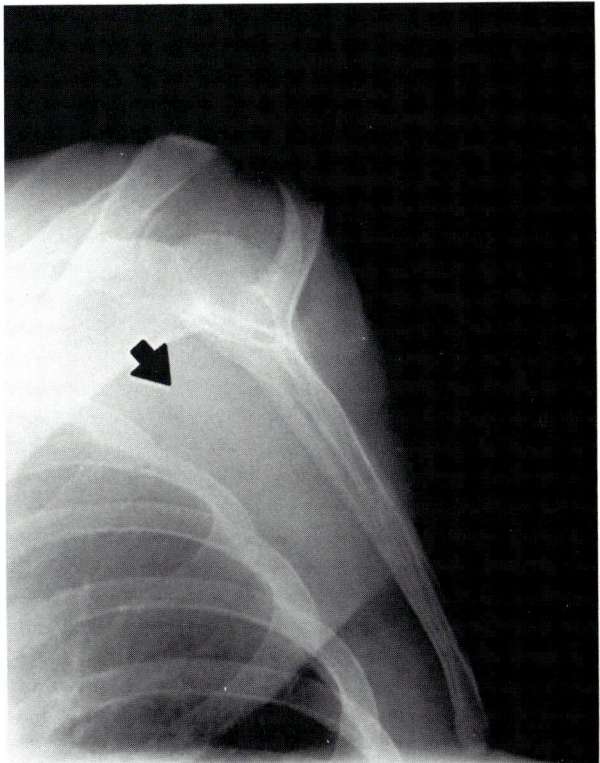

Figure 143. True lateral position of scapula, or scapular "Y" position, leaves clear space between ribs and scapula (arrow) along entire length of the bone.

extension (dorsiflexion) of the foot is recommended. Superimposition of the phalanges and closing of these joint spaces on the *first three toes* indicates that insufficient tube angle, or insufficient dorsiflexion, was used, Figure 147. The prone plantodorsal projection may facilitate demonstrating these phalanges and joints.

A 10-degree cephalic beam angle for the AP projection of the foot is strongly recommended in order to better desuperimpose the bases of the metatarsals and the distal tarsal bones off of each other. This angle will open the tarsometatarsal joints and those distal intertarsal joints which are oriented transversely (across the foot). Failure to open the tarsometatarsal joints, as in Figure 147-A, indicates that insufficient angle or no angle was used.

For patients with *fallen plantar arches* (flat foot), the usual cephalic angle must be decreased to compensate.

On the plantodorsal view of the *calcaneus,* the proper 40-degree cephalic

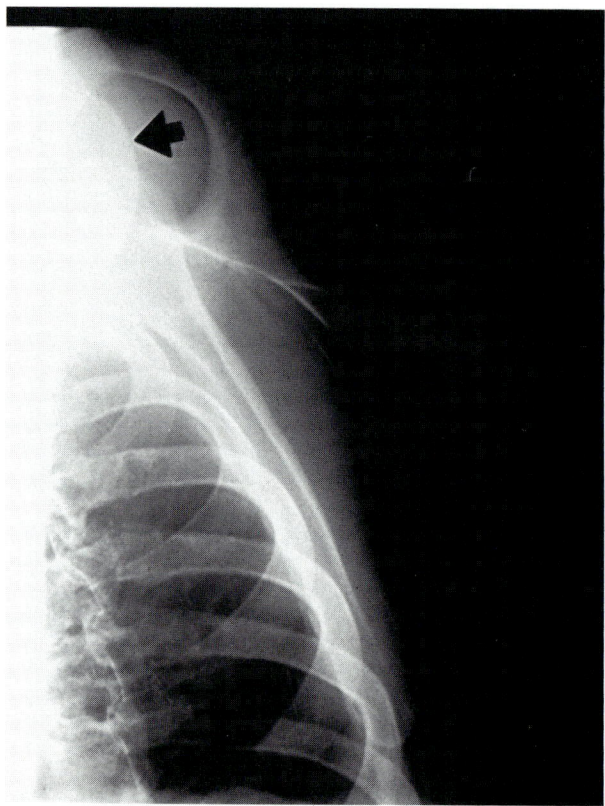

Figure 144. Lateral scapula view positioned with too steep rotation. Note that *lateral* border of scapula, contiguous with head of humerus (arrow) overlaps ribs.

tube angulation will open the subtalar joint, provided that the technique used is penetrating enough to demonstrate this joint.

Technique. The use of a wedge filter and the anode heel effect are recommended for the AP projection of the foot, which is typically light in tarsal bones and dark in the toes, Figure 147.

Oblique Views

Rotation. For the medial (internal) oblique position of the foot, the proper 30 degrees of rotation will begin to slightly overlap the *heads* of the metatarsals, with substantial overlapping of the entire first and second metatarsals. But, clear spaces should exist between the *shafts* of the 2nd through the 5th metatarsal bones. If none of the metatarsal *heads* overlap, rotation is too *shallow*, less than 30 degrees. If the any of the

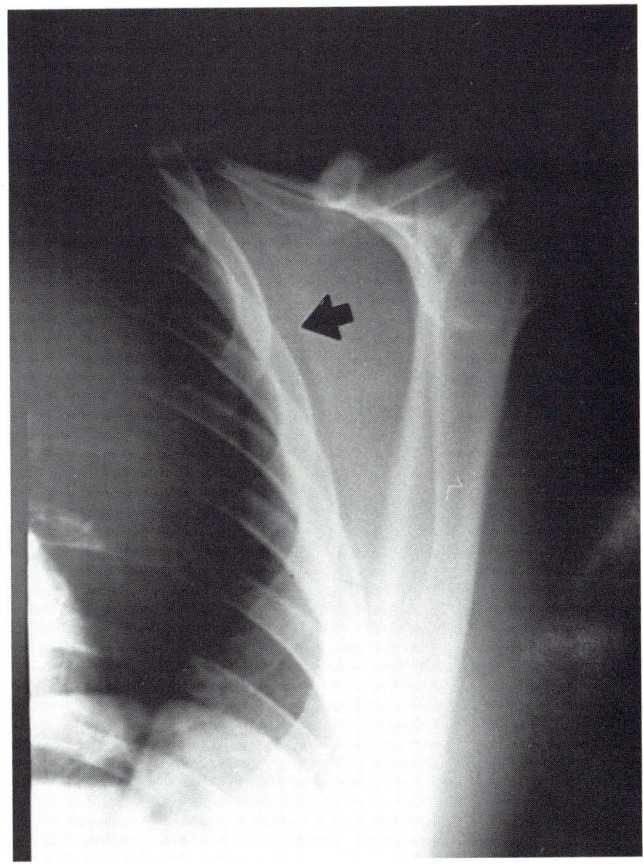

Figure 145. Lateral scapula view positioned with too shallow rotation. *Medial* border of scapula (arrow) overlaps lower ribs.

second through the fifth metatarsal *shafts* overlap, rotation is too *steep,* greater than 30 degrees.

The 30-degree oblique is designed to demonstrate the lateral cuneiform and cuboid bones free of superimposition. Note that on the AP projection the second and third cuneiforms and cuboid overlap each other substantially, Figure 147-A.

Lateral Views

Rotation. The normal transverse arch of the foot makes it impossible to directly superimpose the metatarsal bases or tarsal bones. The *only* reliable criterion for evaluating rotation on the lateral view of the foot is the superimposition of the *heads* of the five metatarsals, Figure 148-A.

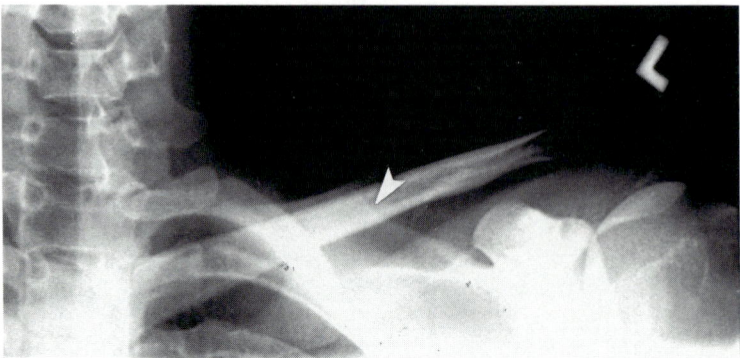

Figure 146. Adequate beam angulation for the frontal view of the clavicle must project all of the superior border of the scapula (arrow) below the clavicle. Only the first rib should cross the mid-shaft of the clavicle. On this thin patient, 25 degrees of beam angle should have been used instead of 15 degrees to project the scapula lower.

When the leg has not been rolled out to the side and down toward the table enough, leaving the foot in a steep oblique position that is not yet fully lateral, the head of the large *first* metatarsal will appear on the radiograph inferior to the other bones, as in Figure 148-B. The first metatarsal can be recognized by its unusual thickness and by its articulation with the great toe.

A much more common error is to *overrotate* the foot past the lateral position so that the plantar surface begins to face up. To prevent this, a support is usually required beneath the *knee* so that the knee is not rolled down all the way onto the table. In the overrotated view of the lateral foot, the head of the *fifth* metatarsal will appear beneath the other bones, as in Figure 149. The fifth metatarsal can be recognized by the pointed process that extends like a hook laterally off of its base.

Flexion and Extension. On lateral views of the foot, dorsiflexion (extension) of the foot so that it lies roughly at right angles to the lower leg is needed because it helps prevent rotation of the part.

Digits are always better desuperimposed from each other by *flexing,* rather than by extending, the fingers or toes that are in the way. Figure 150 shows the unacceptable obscuring of the proximal phalanx when the overlapping toes were improperly hyperextended instead of flexed.

CALCANEUS

For the plantodorsal projection of the calcaneus, dorsiflexion of the foot to place it 90 degrees from the leg, and the proper 40 degrees of

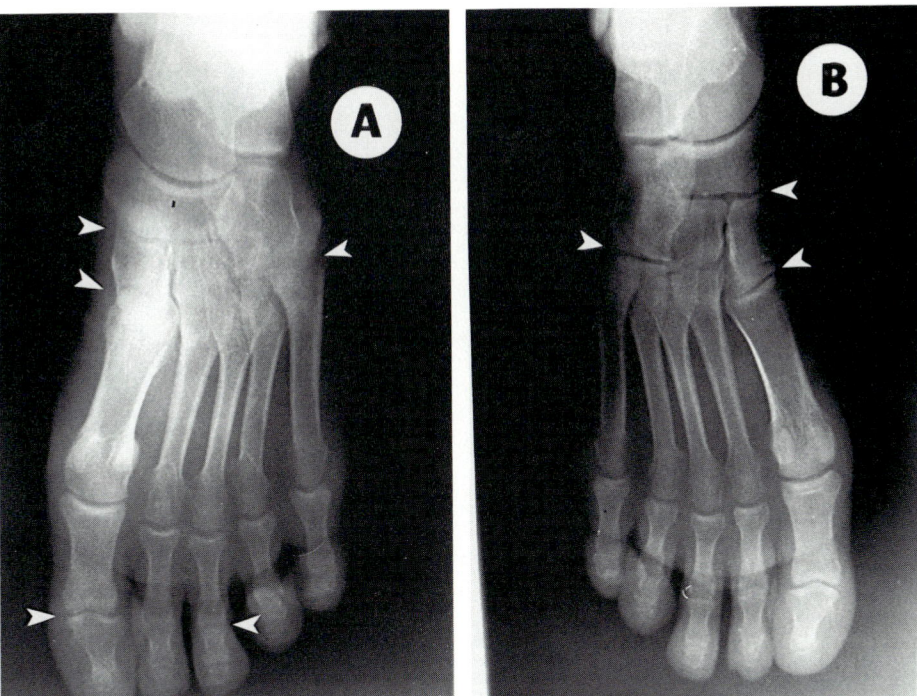

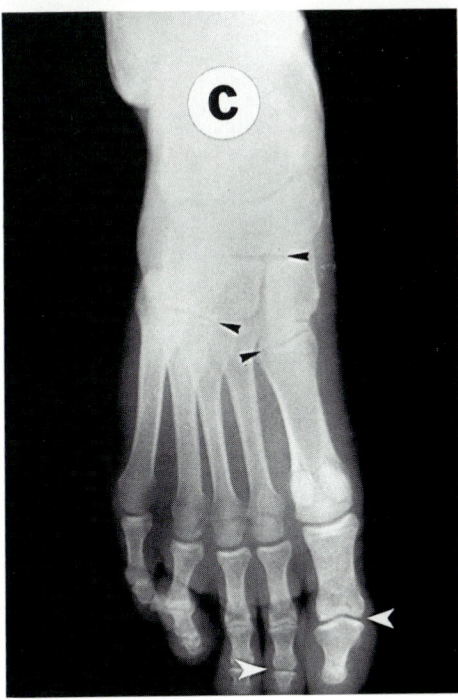

Figure 147. Importance of cephalic angulation on frontal views for both foot (compare A and B) and toes (compare A and C). A, with no angle, shows closing of toe joints as well as tarsometatarsal and transverse intertarsal joints (arrows). Radiographs B and C both utilized a 10-degree cephalic angle. Note that a wedge filter was used for radiographs A and B, but not for C in which the tarsal area is underexposed. The best view is B, using a wedge filter and the proper cephalic beam angle.

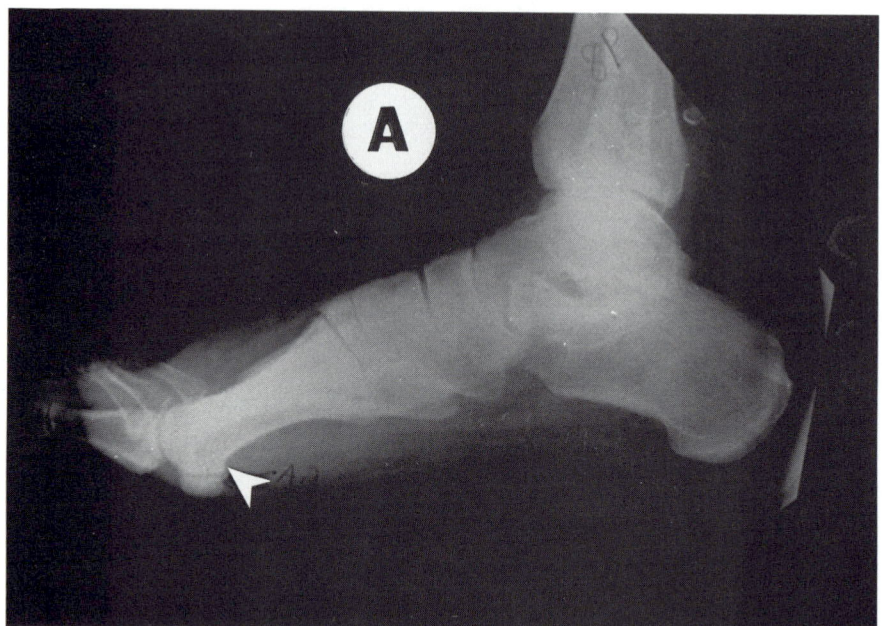

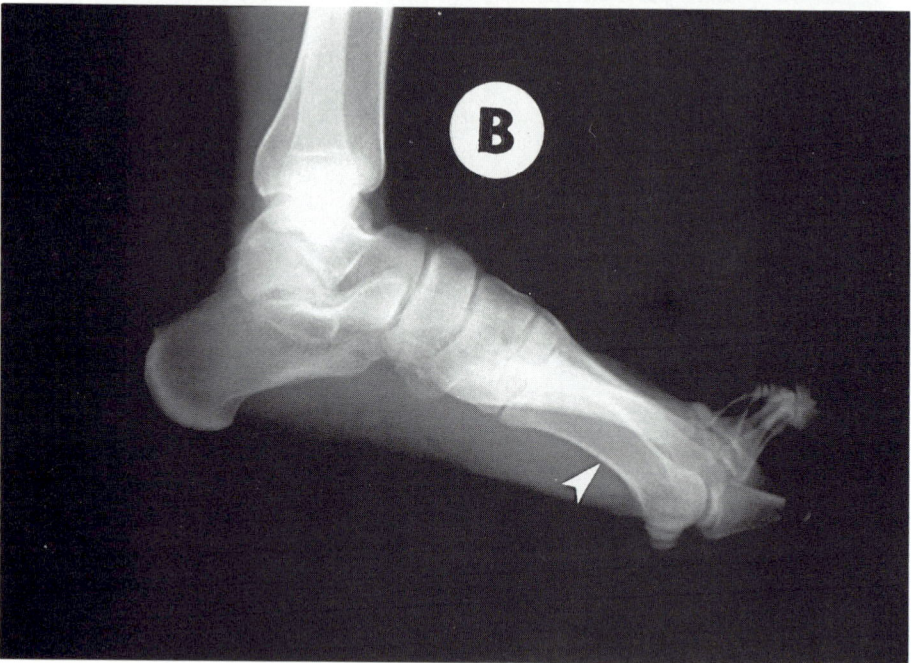

Figure 148. Lateral views of foot. *A* shows a non-rotated view with heads of metatarsals (arrow) directly superimposed. *B* shows *pronation* rotation with thick first metatarsal bone (arrow) projected inferior to other metatarsals, caused by not rolling knee down enough. Note, however, that this same position of the knee (not rolling it all the way down) resulted in a perfect lateral view of the *ankle,* showing the distal fibula centered within the shadow of the tibia.

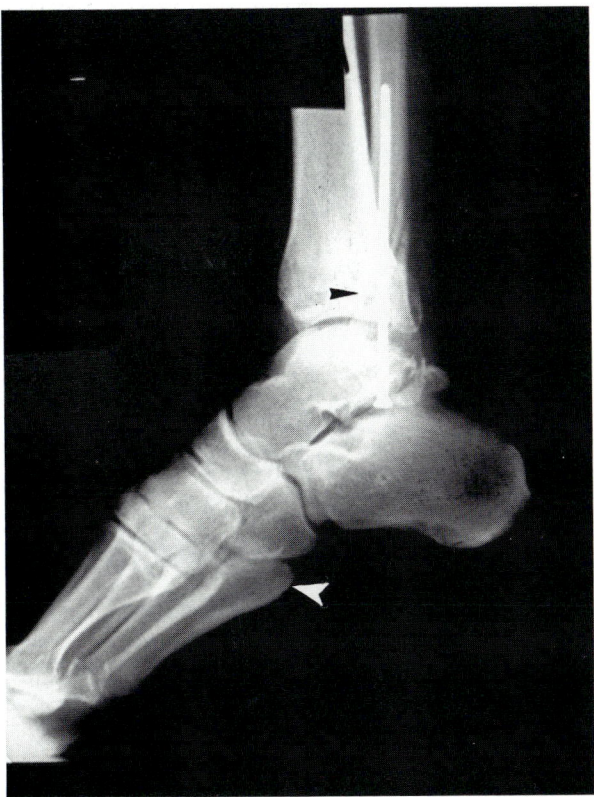

Figure 149. Lateral ankle view showing that *supination* rotation (over-rotation) of the foot places the hook-shaped fifth metatarsal (white arrow) inferior to the other metatarsals. This view also shows how dropping the knee all the way down onto the table usually results in an over-rotated ankle view, placing the fibula (black arrow) posterior in relation to the tibia.

cephalic angulation of the x-ray beam, will show the entire calcaneus including the subtalar joint, Figure 151. This view is typically light at the proximal end and dark at the distal end of the bone. Use of a wedge filter and the anode heel effect are recommended.

The lateral view follows the same basic rotation guidelines as the lateral ankle. The distal fibula should be seen in the mid-shaft of the distal tibia.

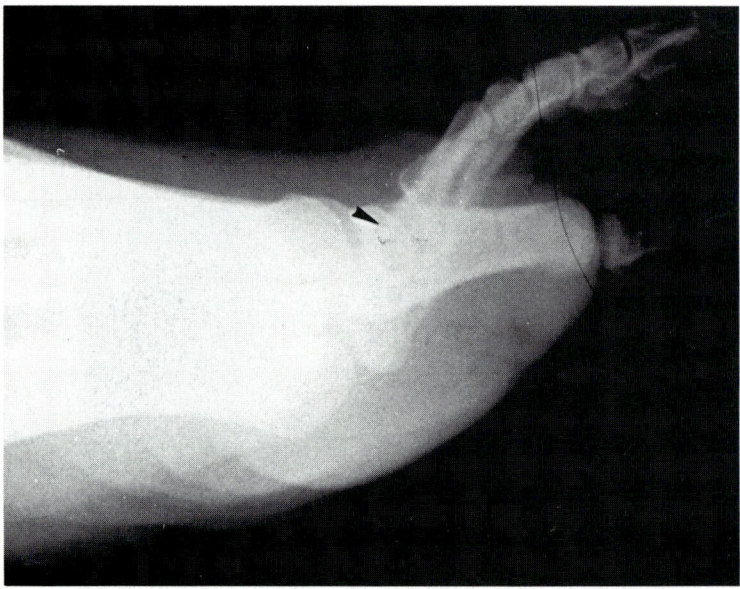

Figure 150. Lateral hallux (great toe) with improper extension of remaining toes causing excessive superimposition of proximal phalanges (arrow). Remaining toes should be *flexed*, not extended.

ANKLE

Frontal View

Rotation. On the non-rotated frontal view of the ankle, there is normally slight overlapping of the distal fibula and tibia, as well as the fibula and talus. However, the joint space between the *medial malleolus of the tibia* and the *medial surface of the talus*, Figure 152, should be opened clearly. If it is not, rotation is present. Slight lateral (external) rotation will be characterized by increasing superimposition of the fibula over the tibia, while medial (internal) rotation tends to desuperimpose these bones and begin to open the distal tibiofibular joint and the talofibular joint space, Figure 154-A.

Angulation, Flexion and Extension. On the frontal view of the ankle, dorsiflexion (extension) of the foot so that it lies roughly at right angles to the lower leg is recommended. It is not essential, however, that this dorsiflexion be exactly at 90 degrees. On a radiograph, when the foot is not thus dorsiflexed, the toes will be seen pointing downward from the ankle as in Figure 152. Properly positioned, the toe area of

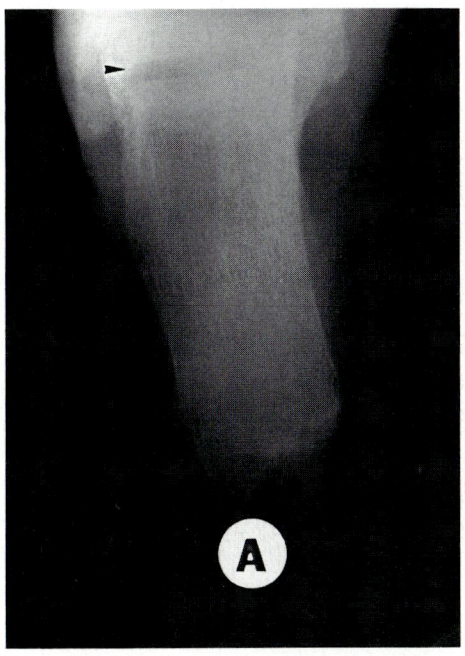 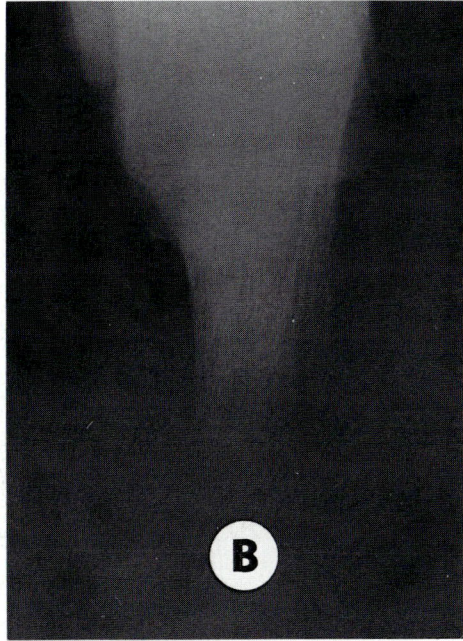

Figure 151. Plantodorsal view of calcaneus should be centered and collimated to include subtalar joint (arrow in A). Note that a wedge filter was used in A to balance densities. Radiograph B, taken without a wedge filter, is both too dark at the distal tip of the calcaneus and too light in the area of the subtalar joint.

the foot will be seen on end and will be underexposed because of its thickness.

Lateral View

Rotation. In the lateral ankle view, the fibula will be projected over the posterior half of the tibia, Figure 153. Some radiographers prefer to use slight internal rotation of the leg, pointing the toes of the foot slightly upward, in order to center the fibula over the tibia as in Figure 148-B. If the fibula appears over the *anterior* half of the tibia, the ankle was not rolled down enough, and medial rotation is present. If the *malleolus* of the fibula extends posteriorly behind the tibia to any degree, as in Figure 149, then the ankle was overrotated past lateral.

Angulation, Flexion and Extension. On lateral views of the ankle, dorsiflexion (extension) of the foot so that it lies roughly at right angles to the lower leg is needed because it helps prevent rotation of the part.

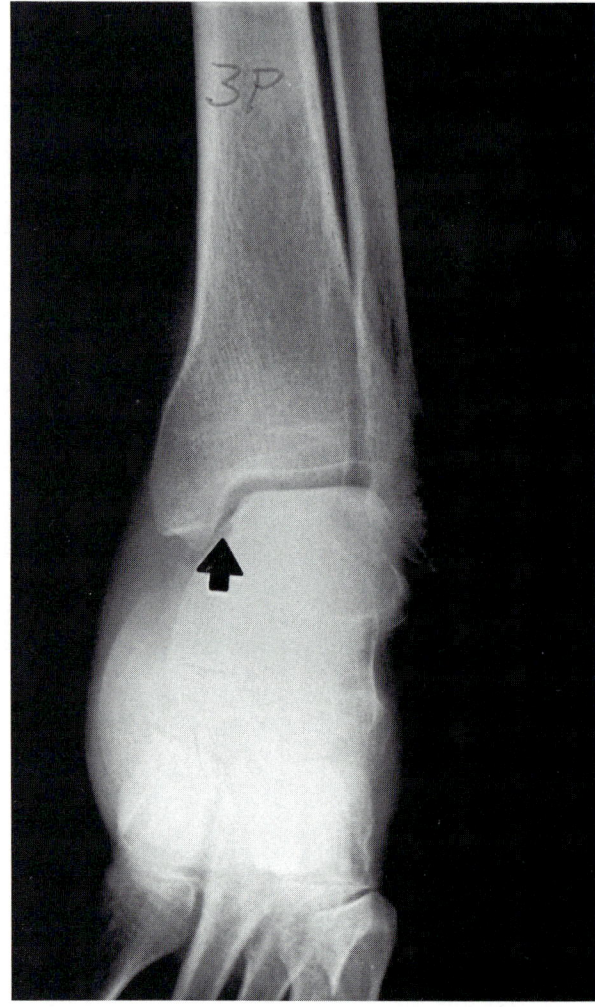

Figure 152. Nonrotated frontal view of ankle shows open joint space between talus and medial malleolus of tibia (arrow). However, on this view the foot was improperly dropped into an extended position.

Oblique Views

Rotation. To best desuperimpose the distal fibula from *both* the tibia and the talus, opening the distal tibiofibular joint and the talofibular joint spaces, 15–20 degrees of internal rotation is recommended as shown in Figure 154-A. Figure 154-B is a true 45-degree medial oblique of the ankle, a routine view in many radiology departments. Note that 45

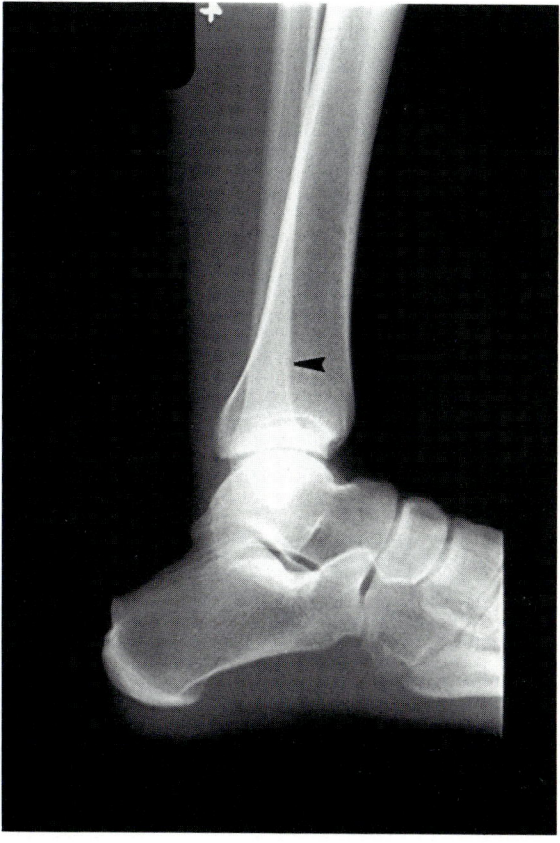

Figure 153. Proper lateral ankle view may show distal fibula over posterior half of tibia (arrow), but *no portion of the distal fibula should extend posteriorly off of the tibia.* If so, lateral over-rotation is present.

degrees of rotation does *not* demonstrate the distal fibula, the distal tibiofibular joint, or the talofibular joint as well as the 15–20 degree view in *A*. The 45-degree view *does* demonstrate the sinus tarsi, a large foramen between the talus and the calcaneus. For trauma cases and ankle series in general, the shallower 15–20 degrees of rotation is the suggested routine for the oblique view.

KNEE AND LONG BONES

Frontal Views

Rotation. On the nonrotated frontal view of the knee, the normal patella will be seen in the middle of the femur, and the two tibial spines

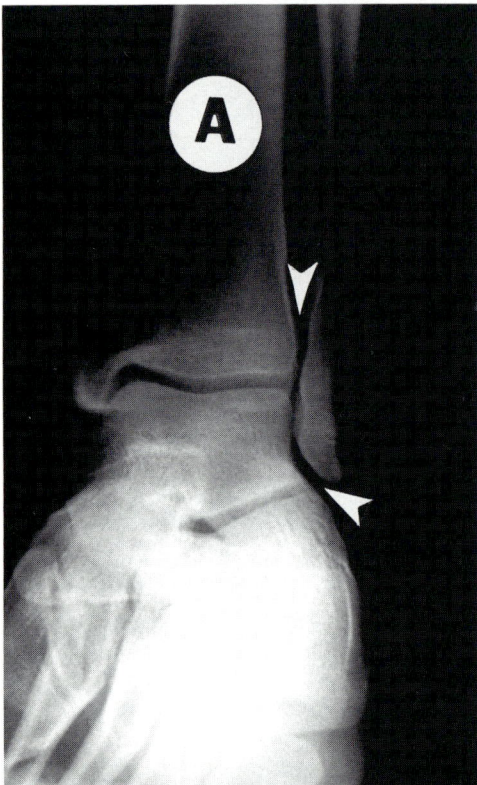 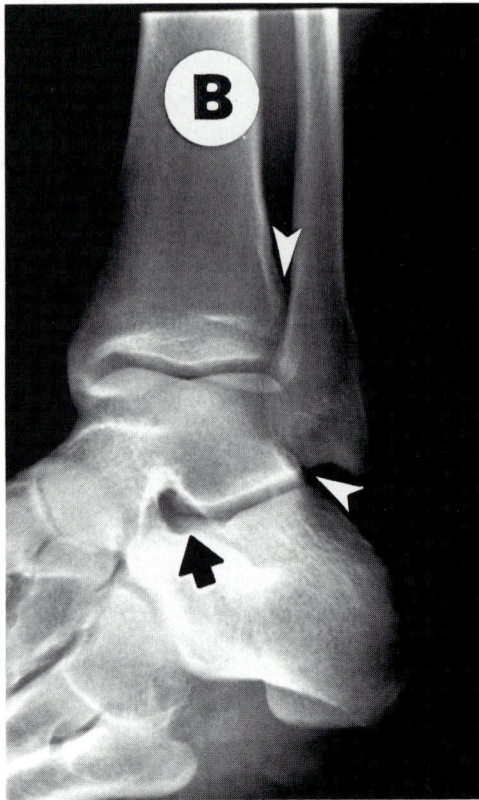

Figure 154. Comparison of routines for medial oblique ankle view. In *A*, 15–20 degrees of medial rotation opens *both* the distal tibiofibular joint and the talofibular joint (white arrows), and provides maximum visibility of the distal fibula. In *B*, 45 degrees of rotation shows the sinus tarsi (black arrow), but is a poor view for the distal fibula and its associated joints (white arrows).

will be centered in the opened joint space as in Figure 155. With lateral (external) rotation, the patella will shift off-center toward the fibula side, and the tibial spines will be assymetrical with one side almost touching the femoral condyle, while the other side shows an open space. With medial (internal) rotation, the patella will shift away from the fibula side, and the tibial spines will again be assymetrical in relation to the femoral condyles as in Figure 156.

For the frontal view of the lower leg, the appearance of the ankle should conform to those criteria described in the previous section.

For the frontal view of the femur, one must choose whether to demonstrate the distal or the proximal portion in true frontal projection,

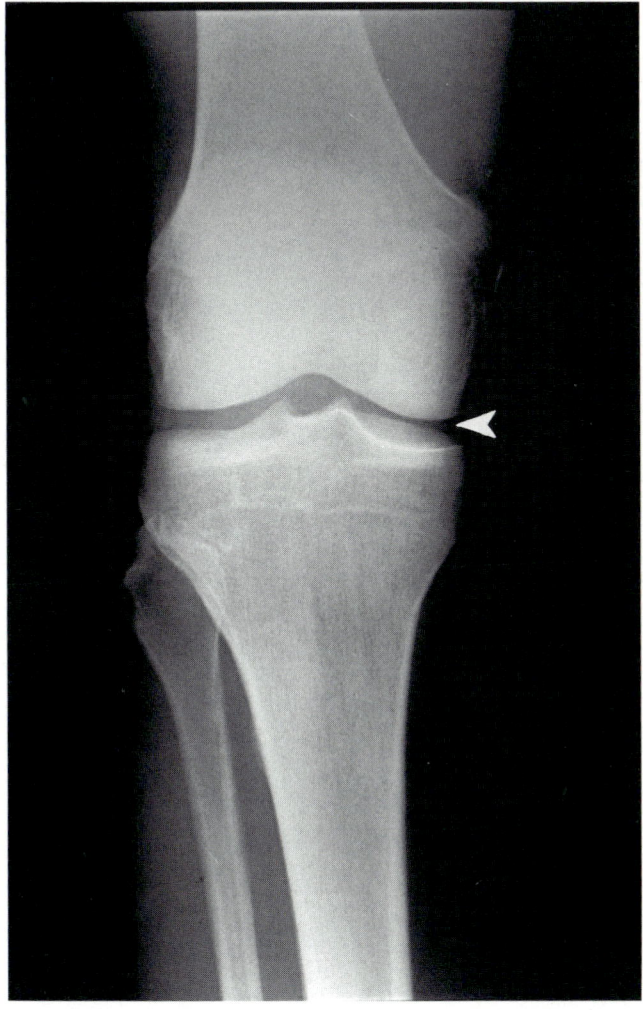

Figure 155. Nonrotated frontal knee view demonstrates open joint (arrow) throughout.

because they do not lie in the same planes. Generally, *if the entire femur is included or only the distal portion, the knee should be straight,* placed according to the criteria in the previous section. *If only the proximal femur is included, then a 15-degree internal rotation of the knee and leg is necessary in order to place the neck of the femur parallel to the film.* This is fully described in the following section on hip views.

Routines for Femur Views. Since the entire femur can often not be fit on a 17-inch long film, *and since the axis of the neck and axis of the condyles*

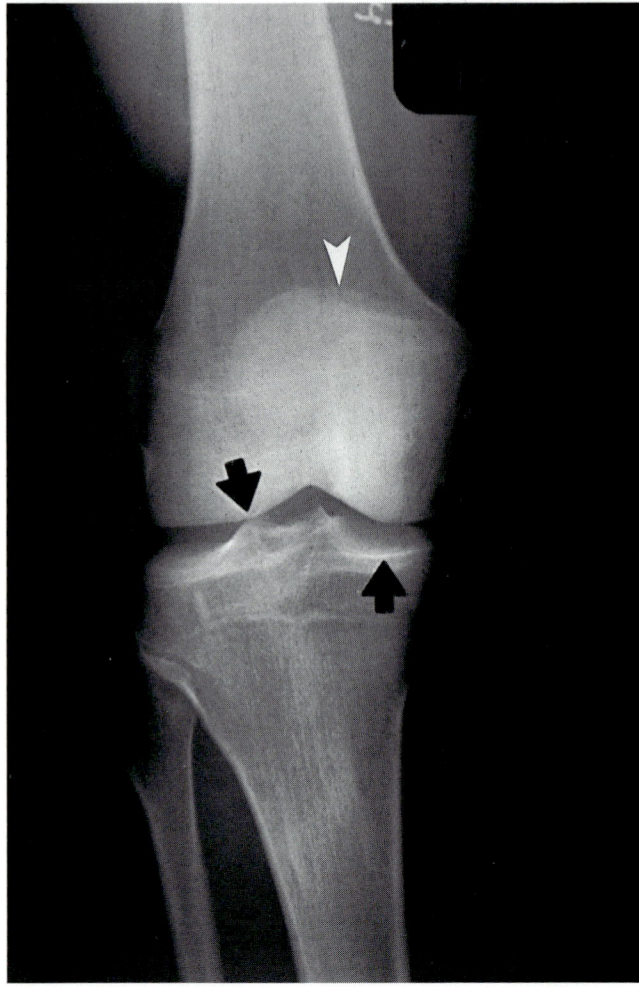

Figure 156. Slight medial rotation on the frontal knee view shifts patella (white arrow) medially over femur shadow and begins to superimpose tibial spines and tibial plateaus (black arrows) over distal femur. Note that *flexion* of the knee will also cause superimposition of the tibial plateaus over the femur as shown here, but the patella would be centered.

are not in the same plane, it is recommended that the routine views for a femur series include the following:

1. AP distal femur on 17-inch film to include the knee with no rotation of the leg
2. LAT distal femur on 17-inch film to include the knee with the knee in true lateral
3. AP proximal femur on 12-inch film to include the hip joint, *with*

15 degrees of internal leg rotation if possible to place the femoral neck in true frontal view

4. LAT proximal femur on 12-inch film to include the hip joint, *with* 15 degrees of internal leg rotation if possible to place the femoral neck in true lateral view

Angulation and Flexion/Extension. Ideally, there should be no flexion of the knee to best open the joint for the frontal view. Flexion will result in the posterior edges of the tibial plateaus rising up and covering the joint space, as in Figure 156. Most often, however, with the patient supine, slight flexion of the knee cannot be helped, and the knee will be up off of the table. In these cases, a 5-degree cephalic angle is required to open the joint space.

Oblique View of the Knee

Rotation. The medial or internal oblique view of the knee is designed to open the proximal tibiofibular joint space and completely desuperimpose the proximal fibula and tibia, Figure 157. Any superimposition of these bones indicates improper rotation. If the knee is *steeper* than the recommended 45 degrees (not rolled down enough), nearly all of the patella will still overlie the distal femur as in Figure 156. If the position is *shallower* than 45 degrees, or too laterally rotated, more than one-half of the patella will be seen off of the distal femur.

Lateral Views

Rotation. The nonrotated lateral view of the knee will demonstrate the normal patella in lateral profile, with the subpatellar joint opened throughout. The posterior aspects of the two femoral condyles will be nearly superimposed as in Figure 158-A. If the subpatellar space is closed and there is substantial side-to-side shifting of the femoral condyles, the position is rotated. It can be difficult on the rotated knee view to determine *which way* the knee was rotated, internally or externally. Remember that the larger of the two femoral condyles is the *medial condyle.* If the posterior surface of this larger condyle lies behind the other condyle, as in Figure 158-B, the knee was rotated medially. That is, the knee was not rotated down enough toward the table. If the smaller condyle lies posterior, the knee was overrotated laterally toward the table.

For a lateral view of the *distal femur,* these same rules for side-to-side

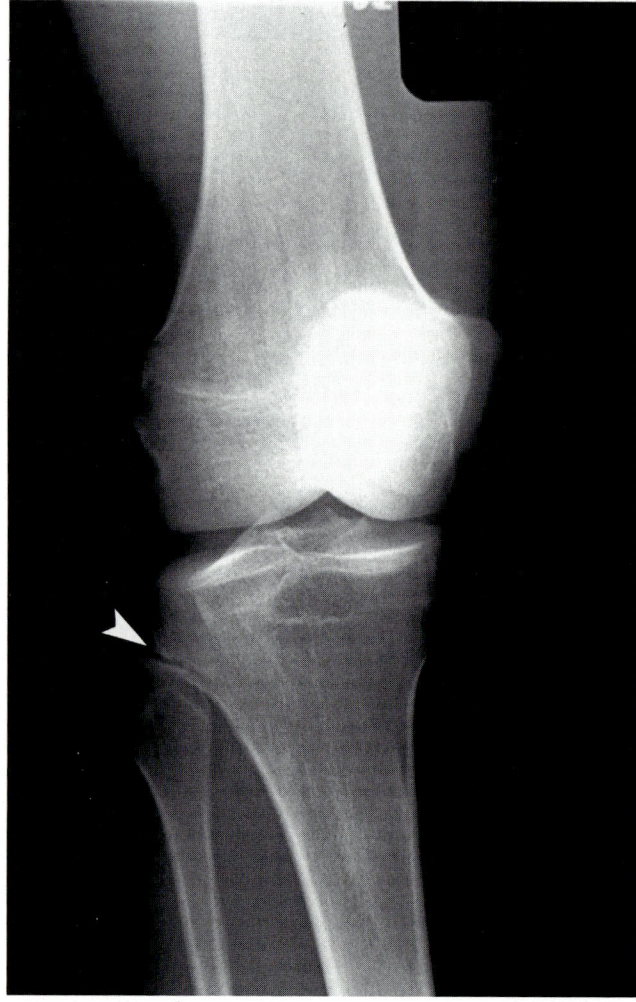

Figure 157. Proper 45-degree rotation for the medial oblique knee view opens the proximal tibiofibular joint (arrow) completely desuperimposing the proximal fibula from the tibia. Compare to Figures 155 and 156.

shift of the condyles hold true, except one will expect substantial superior-to-inferior shift of the condyles because the location of the central ray is far above the knee area. The same criteria can be used for lateral views of the *leg*.

Angulation and Flexion/Extension. The medial condyle of the femur is larger and extends lower than the lateral condyle, as can be seen on any AP knee radiograph (see Figure 155) or on a skeleton. When the

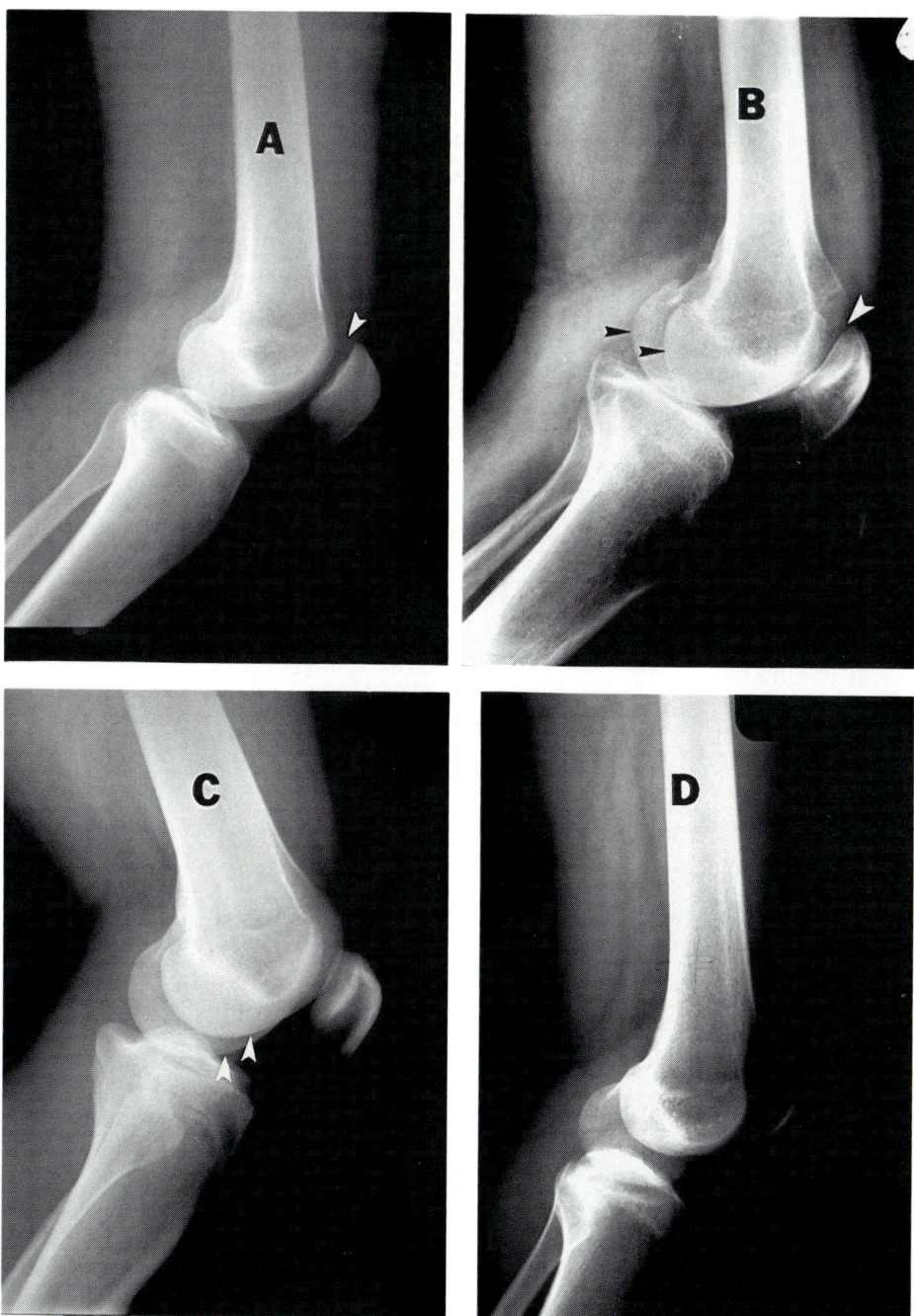

Figure 158. Lateral views of the knee. *A* shows no rotation and uses a five-degree cephalic angle to project the larger medial condyle up onto the lateral condyle, opening both the knee joint proper and the subpatellar space (arrow). *B* utilized the cephalic tube angle, but shows medial rotation, placing the medial condyle posterior to the lateral condyle (black arrows) and closing the subpatellar space (white arrow). In *C*, no cephalic tube angle was used, so the medial condyle is projected inferior to the lateral condyle (arrows). *D* is a view of the distal femur centered above the knee, and the caudally diverging rays at the bottom of the field are *expected* to shift the condyles vertically.

mediolateral view of the knee is taken with a vertical x-ray beam, the larger medial condyle will be projected not only into the knee joint proper, as shown in Figure 158-C, but also into the subpatellar space in many cases. This occurs because the patella is rarely directly anterior to the femur, but rather lies antero-*inferior* to the femoral condyles. This closing of the subpatellar space is frequently mistaken as rotation of the knee, when all that is needed to correct the projection is to utilize the 5-degree cephalic angle recommended in positioning atlases. This cephalic angle should be used on *all* lateral knee projections.

For the lateral view, the knee should also be flexed 20 to 30 degrees. This helps eliminate any rotation and also opens the joint spaces better.

On lateral views of the distal femur, Figure 158-D, the condyles are expected to shift vertically because the diverging rays near the bottom of the field are angled *caudally.*

Axial Patella

Angulation and Flexion/Extension. For the Settegast method, the knee should be flexed until the palpated patella lies parallel to the beam. The subpateller joint should appear open throughout, and the patella itself on end with very little of its undersurface visible. When the undersurface of the patella closes off the joint space, an improper amount of beam angle was used. When there is *too much upward angle* of the beam, the undersurface of the patella will be superimposed by the anterior edge of the *tibial plateaus* curving upward as in Figure 159. The edge of the tibia is recognizable because it is a smooth convex upward curvature *without* two distinct, prominent condyles like the femur has. When there is *not enough upward angle* of the beam (or it is too "horizontal"), the patella will be superimposed by the condyles of the femur, easily recognized with the indentation of the intercondylar fossa between them, Figure 160.

For the prone Hughston method, the leg is flexed approximately 55 degrees to rest the pointed toes atop the 45-degree angled collimator. Closing of the subpatellar space on this projection is usually due to a failure to point the toes so that the lower leg is within 10 degrees of the 45-degree angled beam.

Tunnel View

Angulation and Flexion/Extension. With 70 degrees of knee flexion and a beam that is perpendicular to the tibia, the intercondylar fossa of

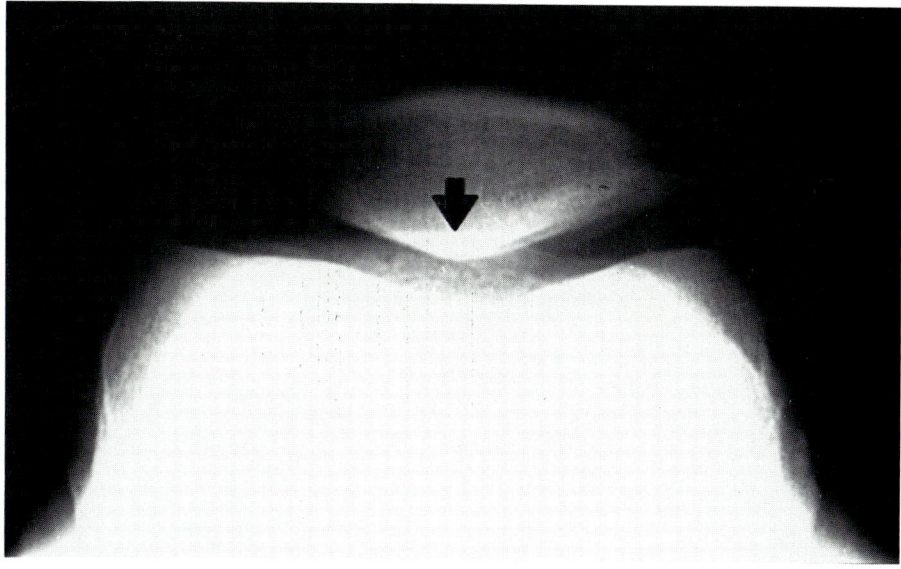

Figure 159. Too much upward beam angle on this "sunrise" axial patella view projected the rim of the *tibia* (arrow) over the patella.

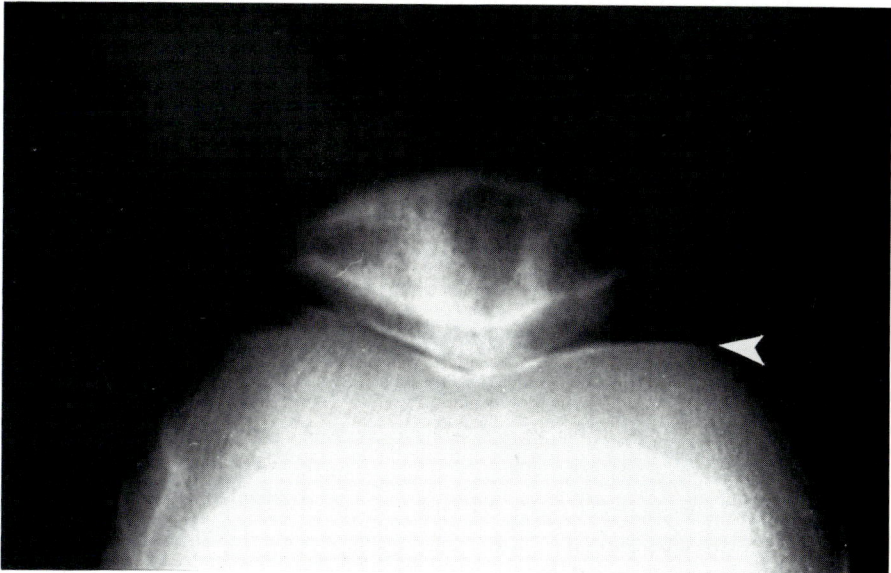

Figure 160. Insufficient upward beam angle on this "sunrise" patella view caused the patella to be projected over the femoral condyles (arrow).

the femur will be opened best. The *entrance* and *exit* arches of this deep fossa will be superimposed so that there is little or no "ceiling" seen within the "tunnel" as in Figure 161. A common positioning error is to rotate the patient's hips too far forward so the femur is less than 70 degrees from the table. This error and other legitimate methods which require less flexion can be distinguished by a sense of looking up at the "ceiling surface" of the arch, as in Figure 162, with a double edge cause by the its entrance and exit, and will usually also show a vertical foreshortening of the fossa space.

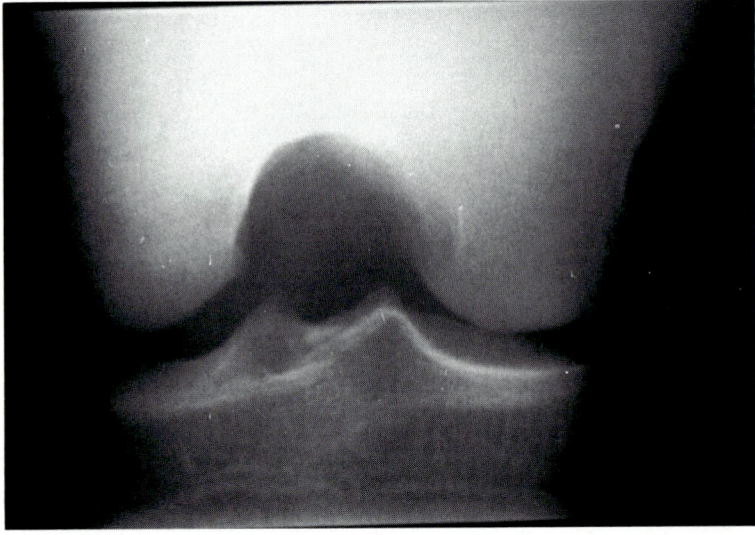

Figure 161. Good "tunnel" view of the intercondylar fossa (Holmblad method) with thigh at steep 70-degree angle to the tabletop.

HIPS

Frontal Views

Rotation. The *bilateral* view of the hips is essentially identical to the frontal view of the pelvis. The non-rotated view will demonstrate the symphysis pubis aligned with the midline of the sacrum and spine, the obturator foramina symmetrical, and the iliac crests symmetrical. Rotation will foreshorten the upside iliac crest and open the upside obturator

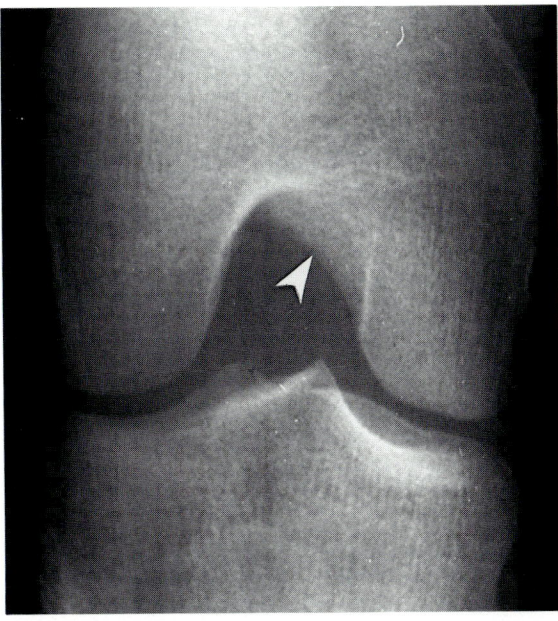

Figure 162. "Tunnel" view of intercondylar fossa (Holmblad method) with thigh improperly placed at 50–55 degree angle from tabletop shows "ceiling" of tunnel, not fully opened.

foramen. Full discussion and radiographs illustrating these criteria are found in Chapter Seven under "Abdominal and Pelvic Views."

On any frontal view, bilateral or unilateral, if the legs are properly rotated internally 15 to 20 degrees (touching the toes together), the femoral neck will be seen in its entirety with no superimposition of the greater trochanter. The greater trochanter will lie in profile laterally to the neck, and the lesser trochanter will be mostly or completely hidden *behind* the upper femoral shaft as in Figure 163. Insufficient internal rotation of the legs leaves the greater trochanter superimposing the lateral end of the neck, with the lesser trochanter arising from the medial surface of the upper shaft as in Figure 164.

Lateral Views

Rotation. Any true lateral view of the hip, whether using unilateral or bilateral Cleaves method, Lauenstein method, or the cross-table "groin lateral" (Danellius-Miller method), will ideally demonstrate the greater trochanter directly superimposed upon the femoral neck with a very straight appearance to the entire proximal femur with the shaft, neck and head in line, as in Figure 165-A. (If some internal rotation of the

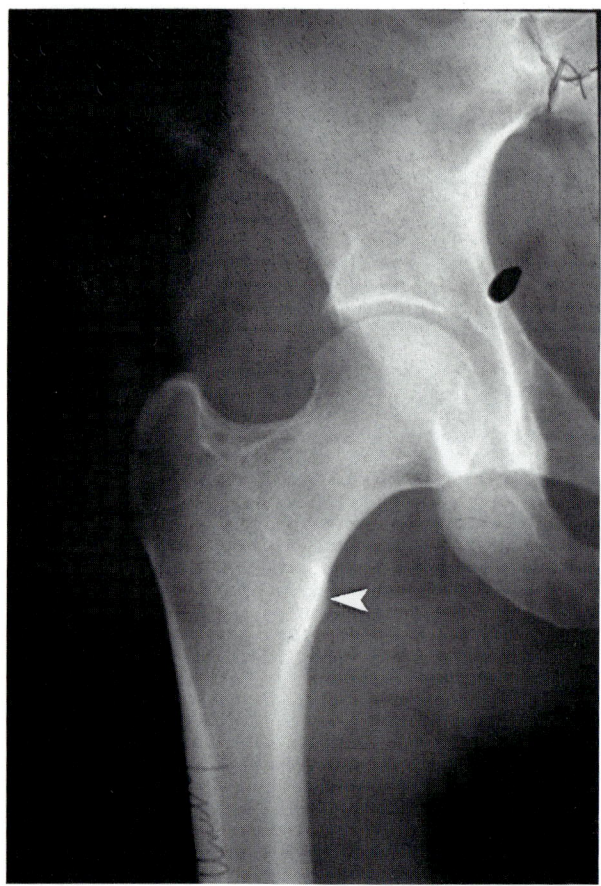

Figure 163. Proper frontal view of hip with 15 degrees of internal leg rotation places lesser trochanter (arrow) nearly behind shaft of bone and lays neck and greater trochanter out parallel to film.

affected leg can be accomplished on the cross-table groin lateral method, this places the femoral neck in more true lateral position.) When hip pins are present, they will also appear straightened on a true lateral view, with little or no angle of the pin visible, Figure 166.

The *Cleaves* method is often improperly used on adult patients to try to procure a bilateral projection of both hips in lateral position. This method is designed primarily for *congenital* hip deformities and is therefore primarily a *pediatric* positioning method. Small children can abduct their thighs enough while lying flat on their backs to obtain good lateral hip views with the Cleaves method. Adults, however, are typically not able to bring both thighs very near the tabletop in hyper-abduction. This

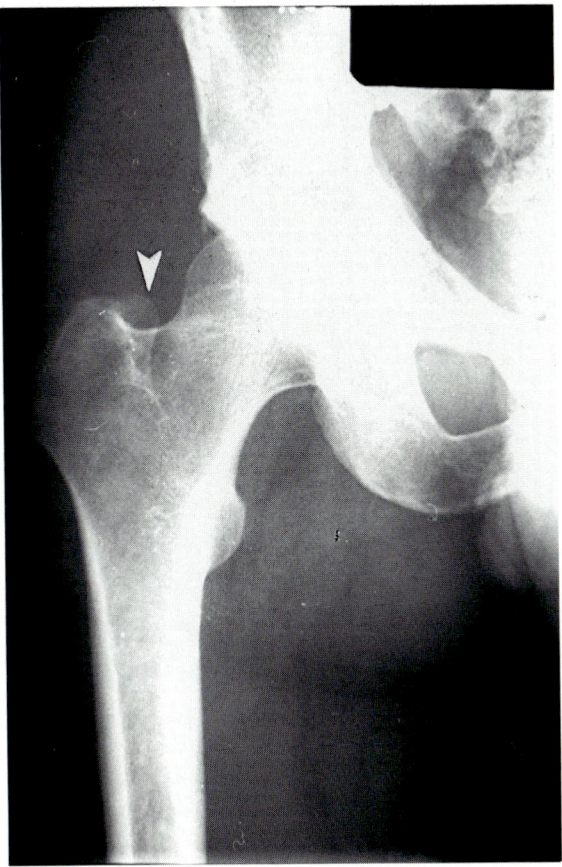

Figure 164. Failure to rotate leg medially on frontal hip view shows superimposition of greater trochanter (arrow) behind neck of femur, and lesser trochanter in profile.

effectively results in bilateral *oblique* views of the hips, and should not be used. For adults, the *Lauenstein* method is highly recommended.

In the Lauenstein position, shown in Figure 165-A, the pelvis is intentionally rotated toward the affected side until the femur can be laid flat on the table in true lateral position. Since hip routines universally include a preliminary AP view of the pelvis, there is no reason to assume that the *pelvis* must be unrotated for the lateral hip views. It is the *neck of the femur*, not the pelvis, which must be placed into a true position. Figure 165-B shows an attempt at a lateral hip leaving the pelvis in a non-rotated supine position and placing the thigh in "frog-leg" position. Note that the femur is rotated, as evidenced by the prominence of the lesser trochanter (compared to *A*).

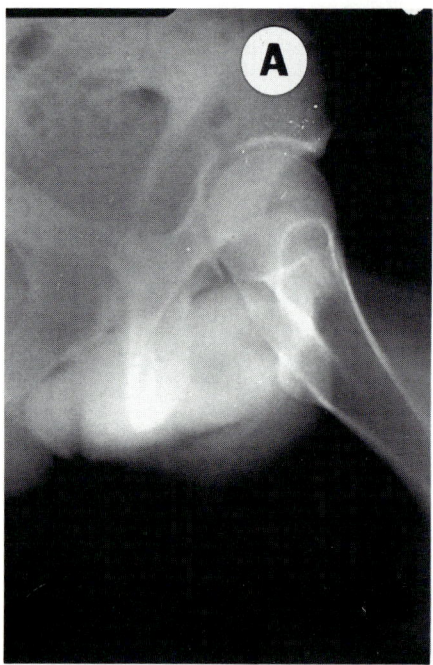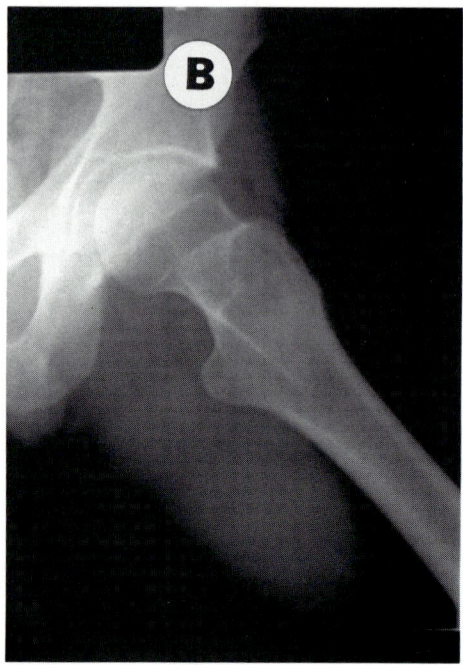

Figure 165. Lateral views of one hip. In *A*, the Lauenstein method uses rotation of pelvis in order to bring femur all the way down onto table into true lateral position. Note linearity of bone, with greater trochanter directly superimposed over neck of femur. In *B*, improper attempt at unilateral "frog-leg" position leaving pelvis supine resulted in rotated lateral view of femur compared to *A*.

Of course, if a fracture to the proximal femur is suspected, the groin lateral Danellius-Miller method is recommended, and some rotation may be expected, but the same basic criteria apply.

Groin Lateral Hip

Tilt/Abduction/Adduction. For the groin lateral view of the hip, proper *abduction* and flexion of the unaffected side is crucial. Many radiographers flex the unaffected thigh up well, but only slightly abduct it to the side. On larger patients, this leaves a substantial amount of soft tissue from the buttock on the unaffected side still superimposing the affected hip. The view appears light in density, and frequently the repeated view is done with an increased technique rather than recognizing the improper position. Figure 167 shows how much difference proper abduction of the unaffected side can make. Both views were taken with identical techniques.

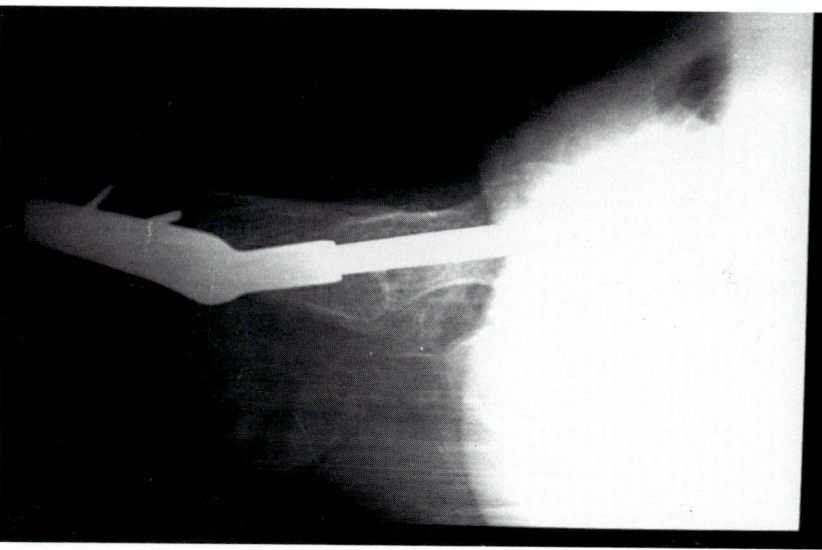

Figure 166. Groin lateral projection of pinned hip. Internal rotation of leg results in straightened appearance of pin. Here the pin shows a slight angle, indicating the femur is almost in true lateral position.

Technique

Radiographic technique for all extremities should provide adequate penetration (kVp) to see details *through* the bones of interest, with relatively high contrast and medium density.

194

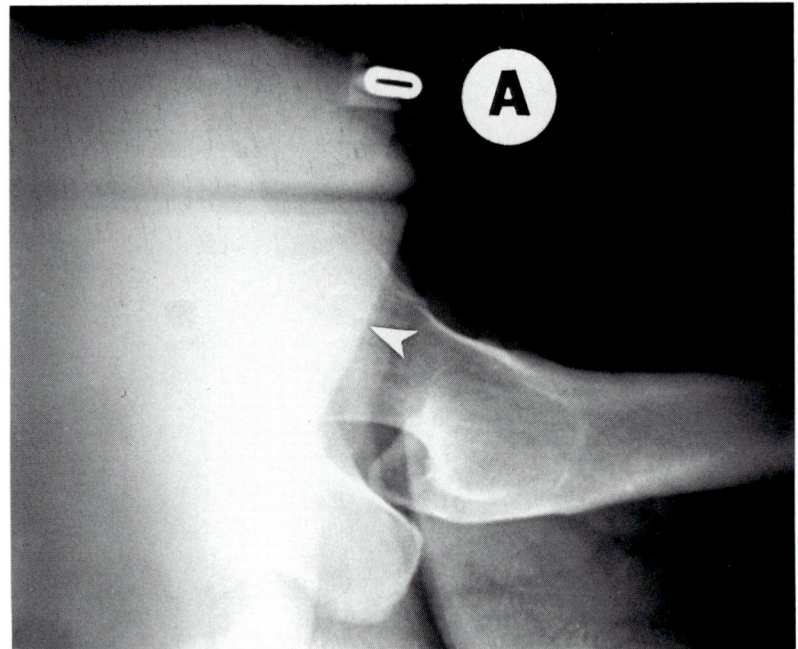

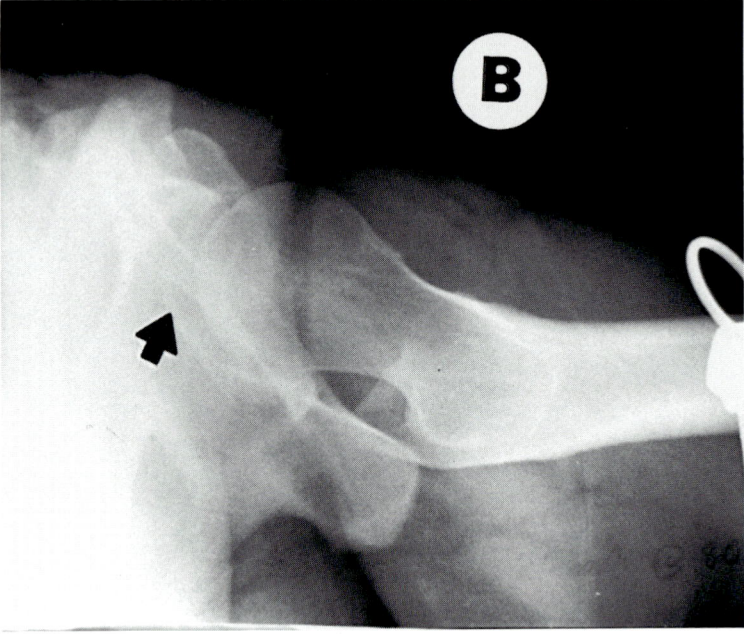

Figure 167. Importance of abduction of the unaffected leg for groin lateral hip view. Both views were taken with *identical technique* and with *the same amount of hip flexion* on the unaffected side. In *A,* failure to abduct the unaffected leg to the side results in the soft tissue of this thigh (arrow) superimposing the acetabulum and head of the femur of interest. In *B,* the unaffected thigh is abducted to the side with the foot resting on the collimator, demonstrating the acetabulum (arrow) and head of the femur.

Chapter 9

HEAD POSITIONS

SKULL

Frontal Views

Rotation. For the PA, Caldwell, and Waters projections of the skull, the same criteria can be used to evaluate head rotation. One of the most reliable criteria, when the sides of the skull are included within the view, is the symmetry of the distances between the lateral rims of the orbits and the sides of the skull. When the face is rotated toward the right, this distance will foreshorten on the patient's right and elongate on the left as in Figure 168-B. The *foreshortened* side is the direction of rotation.

For coned-down views which do not include the sides of the skull, such as Figure 171, the symmetry between the lateral rims of the orbits and the *sides of the greater wings of the sphenoid* bone can be used. (The lateral surfaces of the greater wings form the "temple" areas on the side of the head just behind the orbital rims.) On a frontal skull view, these surfaces appear as a straight white line running vertically at a slight diagonal through the lateral quarter of each orbit, Figures 168-A and 171. When the face is rotated toward the patient's right, the space between the greater wing and the orbital rim on the right side will be broadened, while this space on the left side will foreshorten and become narrower, as in Figure 168-B.

Other good criteria for rotation on frontal skull views include the symmetry of the orbital rims, greater wings of the sphenoid, or rami of the mandible from the midline of the skull. The "straightness" or thickness of the bony nasal septum should *not* be used because there is too much normal deviation in the thickness and linearity of this structure. Nor should any of the sinuses be used—even the maxillary sinuses are not reliably symmetrical.

The Waters views in Figure 174 is rotated to the patient's right. Note that more of the left side of the skull can be seen lateral to the orbit and

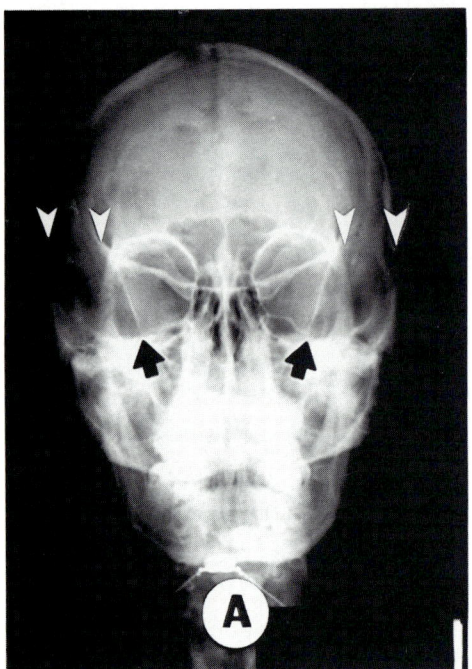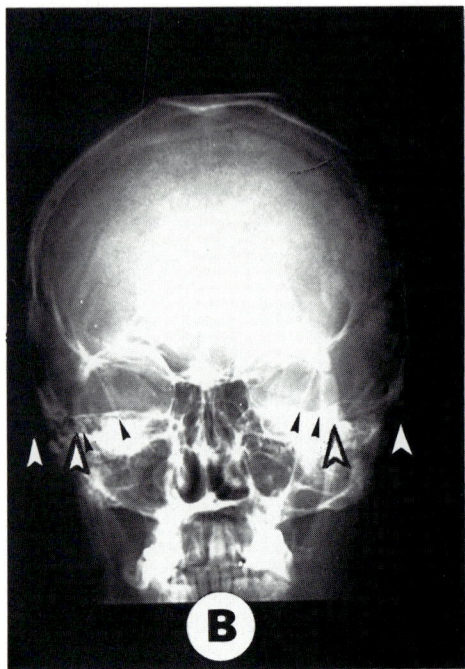

Figure 168. Rotation on frontal skull views. *A* shows a non-rotated view with equal distance from the lateral orbital rims to the sides of the cranium (white arrows) and symmetrical greater wings of the sphenoid bone (black arrows). *B* shows rotation to the right, with the distance from the orbital rim to the cranial wall lessening on the patient's right (white arrows) and the distance from the greater wing to the lateral orbital rim increasing on the patient's right (black arrows). However, note that *B* demonstrates proper flexion/extension for a Caldwell view with the petrous ridges in the lower one-third of the orbits.

ramus of the mandible. The bony septum dividing the sphenoid sinus, seen within the mouth, is also off-centered to the arch of the upper teeth, indicating rotation.

Angulation and Flexion/Extension. For the nonangled PA or AP view of the skull, the petrous pyramids should almost "fill the orbits," so that the petrous ridge lies just under the superior rim of the orbits as in Figure 169-A. When the petrous ridges lie *above* the superior orbital rim as in Figure 169-B, the most likely cause is *hyperflexion* of the head whereby the chin was depressed too much. The same appearance may be created, however, when a cephalic tube angle was present with the patient in prone position, or when a caudal tube angle was present with the patient in supine position.

For the Caldwell method with a 15-degree beam angle, the petrous

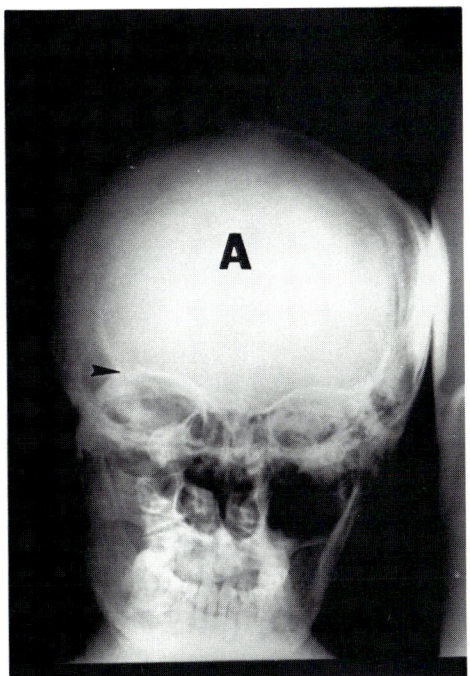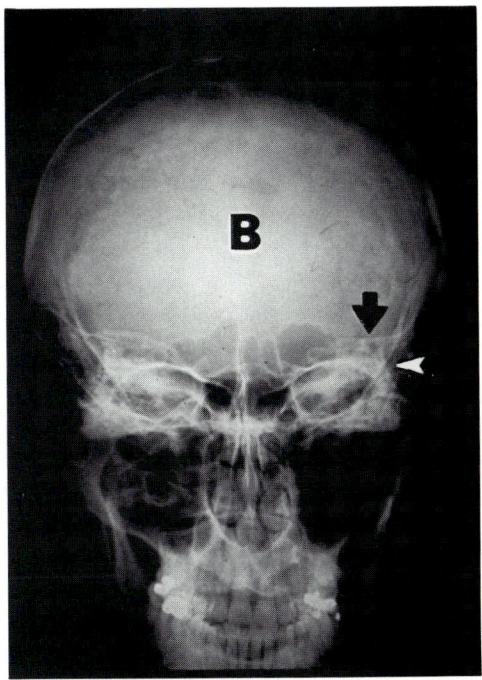

Figure 169. PA skull projections showing (*A*) correct flexion/extension placing the petrous ridges (arrow) just below the upper rim of the orbits, and (*B*) with *hyperflexion,* placing the petrous ridges (black arrow) above the orbits (white arrow). Note that in *A* the combination of head tilt and poor centering and collimation resulted in clipping off the left side of the cranium.

pyramids should "fill" the lower one-third of the orbits as in Figure 168-B. The angle of the x-ray beam should be caudal with the patient in prone position, or cephalic with the patient in supine position. Assuming that the orbitomeatal line of the skull is maintained perpendicular to the film, if the petrous ridges are seen in mid-orbit, Figure 170, then the tube angle was about 5 degrees *too little* (it was approximately 10 degrees instead of 15). If the ridges lie at the upper one-third of the orbit, only 5 degrees of angle was used. Conversely, when the ridges are seen at or near the inferior rim of the orbits, as in Figures 168-A and 171, 5 to 7 degrees *too much* tube angle was used.

Each of the problems just described can *also* be caused by improper flexion or extension of the head. In prone position, with the tube properly angled at 15 degrees caudal, *flexion* of the head will "cancel out" the tube angle, placing the petrous ridges too high within the orbits as in Figure 170. *Extension* of the head will place the ridges too low within the

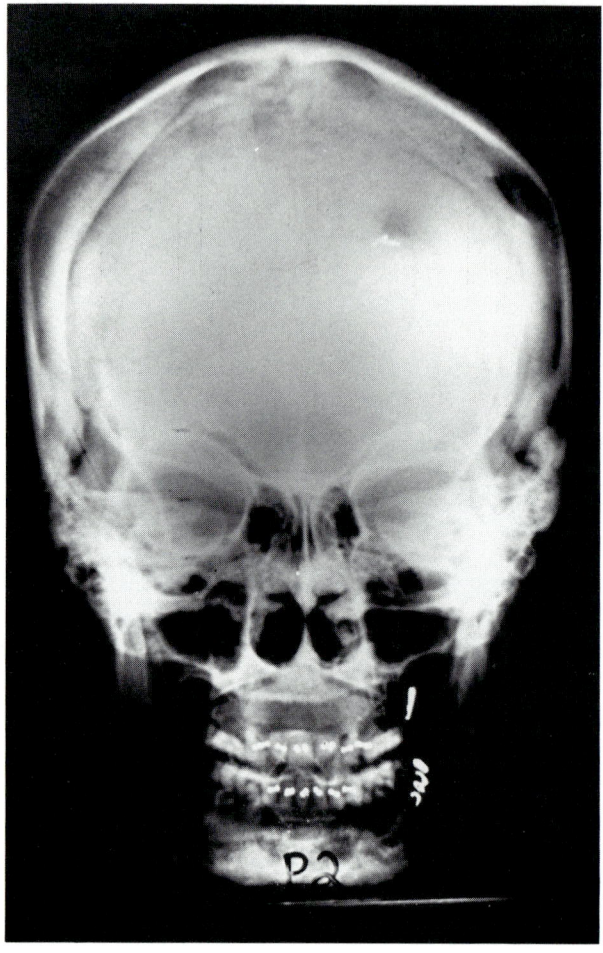

Figure 170. Caldwell view showing petrous ridges in mid-orbit. This indicates either A) 10 degrees of caudal beam angle, 5 degrees short of the needed 15, or B) 5 degrees flexion of the chin, cancelling out part of the caudal beam angle.

orbits as in Figures 168-A and 171. These effects of flexion and extension are identical for both prone and supine positions.

The *Waters* projection for sinuses or facial bones should place the petrous ridges just below the floors of the maxillary sinuses as in Figure 172. Given that this view uses 37 degrees of head extension, and knowing where the Caldwell view places the petrous ridges, we can closely determine the *amount* of inadequate head extension when it occurs: We know that a 20-degree tube angle or 20 degrees of head extension places the ridges at the lower margin of the orbits as in Figure 171, and that 37

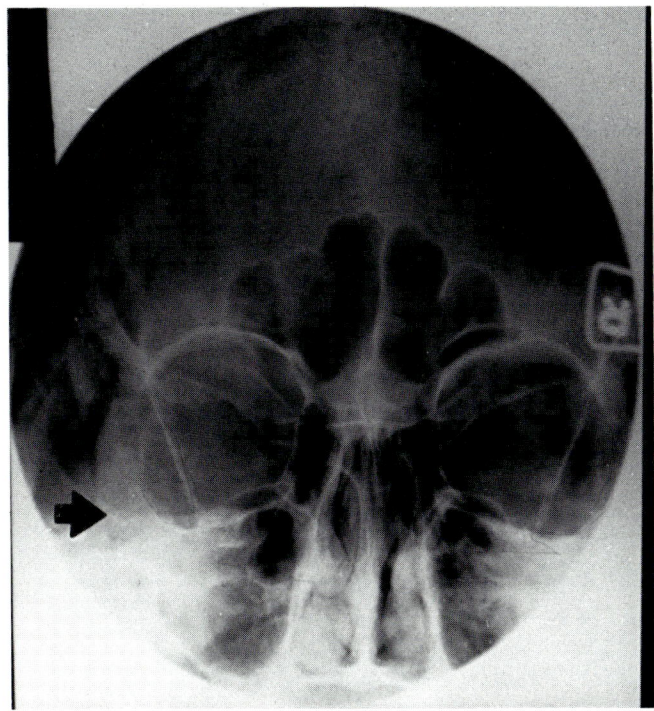

Figure 171. Coned Caldwell view for sinuses showing petrous ridges at lower orbital rims (arrow). This indicates either A) 20 degrees of caudal beam angle, 5 degrees too much, or B) 5 degrees of chin extension with a 15-degree caudal beam angle. *Note that since the sides of the cranium are not included, one must use the symmetry of the greater wings of the sphenoid bone within the orbits to assess rotation: This view is NOT rotated judging by these criteria, but the coned field is off-centered, which is often mistaken for rotation on coned-down views.*

degrees places them at the lower margin of the sinuses. There are approximately 17 degrees difference. It can therefore be deduced that 25 degrees of head extension places the ridges at the upper one-third of the maxillary sinuses, while 30 degrees places them at the lower third of the sinuses as in Figure 173.

When the petrous ridges are seen more than one-quarter inch below the floors of the maxillary sinuses, they will begin to overlap the chin. This appearance indicates that *too much* head extension was used, *or* that the tube was improperly angled caudal.

The placement of the petrous ridges on the Waters view is also dependent upon tube angulation. Any time that the x-ray beam is angled caudal for a prone position, or cephalic for a supine position, the petrous ridges will be projected *lower* than they should be. When the beam is angled

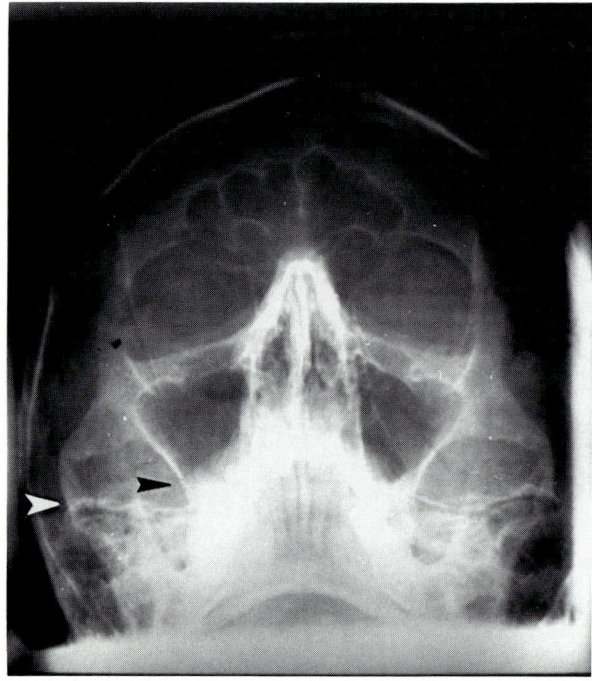

Figure 172. Proper Waters view for sinuses, showing petrous ridges (white arrow) projected just inferior to the floors of the maxillary antra (black arrow). Like Figure 171, this view is *not* rotated, but the coned field is off-centered, clipping the left side of the cranium more than the right side.

cephalic for a prone position or caudal for a supine position, the ridges will be projected *higher* than they should be. Of course, improper placement of the petrous ridges can be the result of any combination of improper head extension and improper tube angle.

For the *open-mouth Waters view*, inadequate extension of the head leaves the top teeth over the sphenoid sinuses as in Figure 174, while hyperextension of the head places the lower teeth over the sphenoid sinuses, Figure 175. Hyperextension is common on open-mouth Waters views because opening the mouth *after* resting the chin against the table forces the head back further still. With the mouth opened wide and the proper 37-degrees of extension at the orbitomeatal line, the rounded pair of sphenoid sinuses with a thin bony septum between them will be seen in the middle of the open mouth.

Tilt. Slight tilt of the head is not normally a crucial element for frontal projections. As a matter of professionalism, one should try to

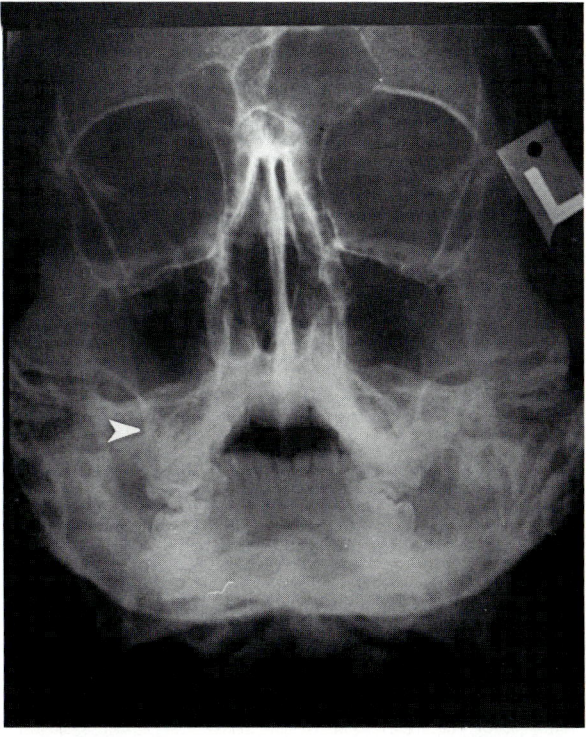

Figure 173. Waters view for sinuses showing inadequate head extension (about 30 degrees), placing the petrous ridges in the lower third of the maxillary sinuses. Note that improper angling of the beam could also cause this appearance. If this patient cannot extend his head further, a 7-degree caudal angle of the central ray will combine with the 30 degrees of head extension to produce an adequate view.

keep the film aligned with the head. But a frontal radiograph is not repeatable for small amounts of tilt—a slight rotation of the film while viewing it, hanging it by its corner, is all it takes to "correct" this minor error. However, note that in Figure 169-A a combination of head tilt, collimation and centering errors resulted in clipping off the side of the cranium, requiring a repeat.

Semi-Axial (Townes) View

Rotation. On the nonrotated semi-axial view of the skull, the distance from the lateral margin of the foramen magnum to the side of the skull on either side should be equal and the petrous pyramids should appear symmetrical. Also, the mid-point of the junction of the two petrous ridges should be in line with the opisthion (the mid-point of the poste-

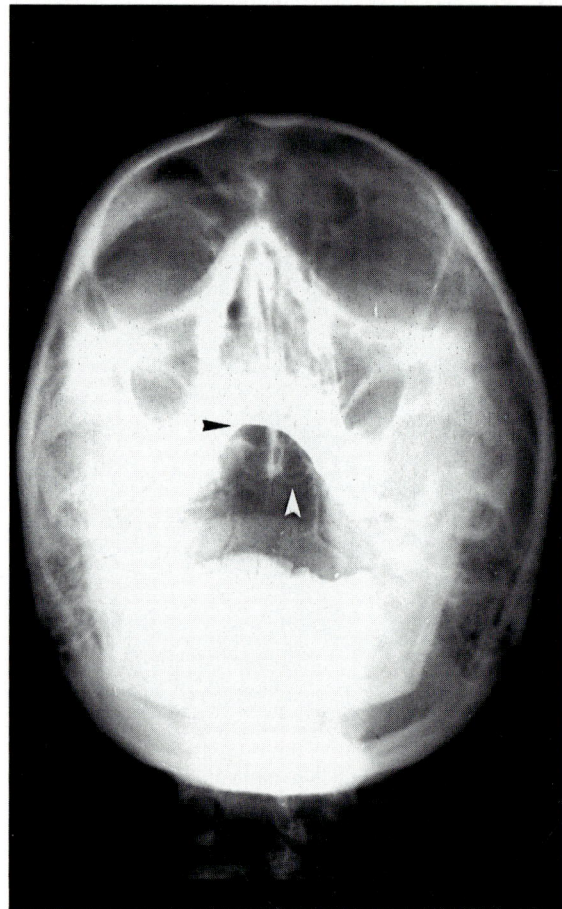

Figure 174. Open-mouth Waters view for sphenoid sinuses (white arrow), showing inadequate head extension and placing the upper teeth (black arrow) over the anterior sphenoid sinuses.

rior arch of the foramen magnum) and the ridge of bone that extends from the opisthion to the inion, as in Figure 176.

When the head is rotated, the petrous pyramids appear asymmetrical. Since the foramen magnum (and the opisthion) lies behind the petrous pyramids anatomically, it will appear to shift in the opposite direction of head rotation. For example, with the head rotated to the right the center of the foramen magnum will appear to shift to the patient's *left* in relation to the junction of the petrous pyramids, shown in Figure 177.

Angulation and Flexion/Extension. With the proper head position and a true 30-degree caudal tube angle to the obitomeatal line, *at least* one-half of the foramen magnum will rise above the junction of the petrous

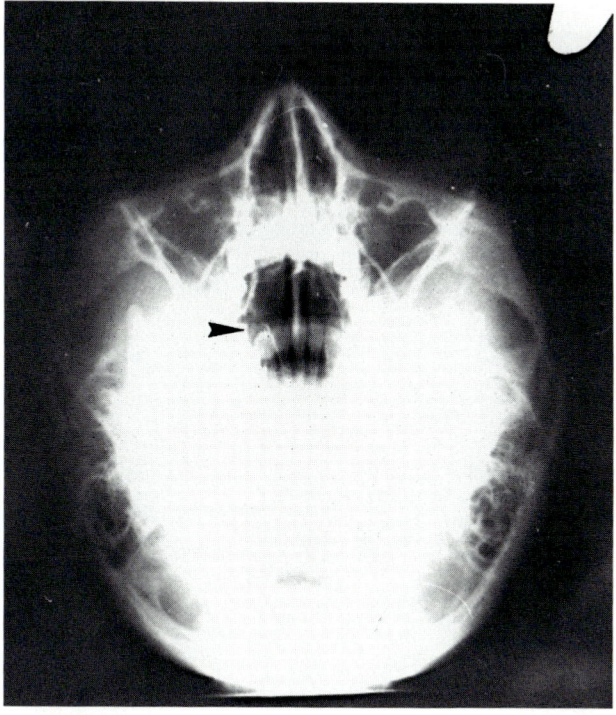

Figure 175. Open-mouth Waters view for sphenoid sinuses showing hyperextension of the head when the mouth was opened *after* placing the patient's chin against the table. This placed lower teeth (arrow) over sphenoid sinus.

ridges, with the dorsum sellae and posterior clinoid processes framed within it. Further, the two petrous ridges will nearly form a perfect right angle to each other, each descending at a 40–45 degree angle from the midline, as in Figure 176.

When improper angulation or flexion/extension are present, the petrous ridges will each appear to descend at a shallower 30-degree angle to form an obtuse angle between each other at the center. When the x-ray beam is *not angled enough* in relation to the orbitomeatal line, one-half or less of the foramen magnum will rise above the junction of the petrous ridges, and the posterior clinoid processes are not seen framed within the foramen as in Figure 178. If the beam is angled *too much,* the dorsum sellae and clinoids are superimposed over the occipital bone and the posterior arch of the first cervical vertebra is framed in the foramen magnum as in Figure 179. The posterior arch of C-1 is distinguished from the dorsum sellae because the arch has an almost continuous rounded curvature to it, usually with two small "bumps" of bone at the middle.

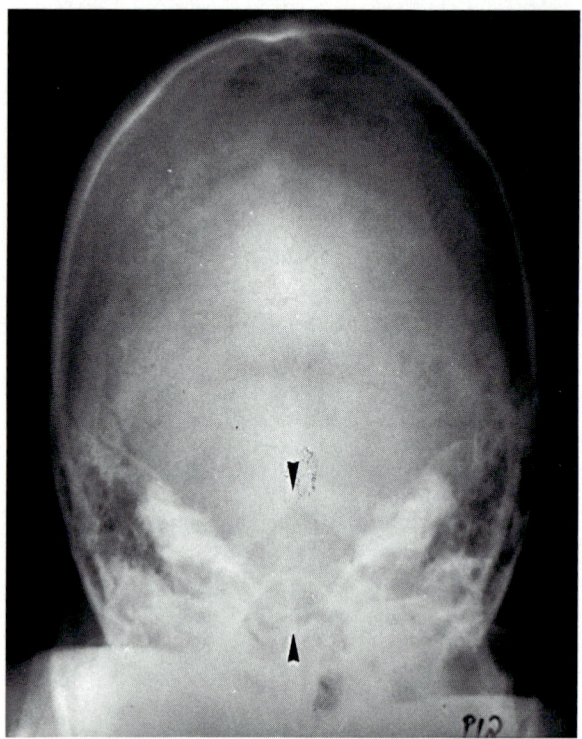

Figure 176. Non-rotated Townes (Grashey) view of skull showing the opisthion (top arrow) and foramen magnum centered to the junction of the petrous pyramids (lower arrow) and symmetry of the ridges. Framing of the dorsum sellae within the foramen magnum, three-fourths of which appears above the petrous ridges, and 45-degree angle of the ridges, indicate proper tube angle and flexion/extension. Note, however, that a collar superimposes the inferior portion of the right petrous pyramid.

For the Townes view, hyperflexion of the head causes a radiographic appearance identical to that of an excess tube angle, while hyperextension of the head produces the same results as inadequate tube angle. In hyperflexion, the posterior arch of C-1 begins to come into view within the foramen magnum.

Hyperextension of the head is a very common problem during supine positioning of the Townes projection. As the patient lies on his back, the head normally drops back into an extended position to rest on the table, and it is difficult for most patients to flex their chins down while lying supine. Typically, 5 to 7 degrees of head extension is present even after attempting to pull down the chin. In practice, a tube angle of *35 degrees from vertical* is strongly recommended for most patients in order to

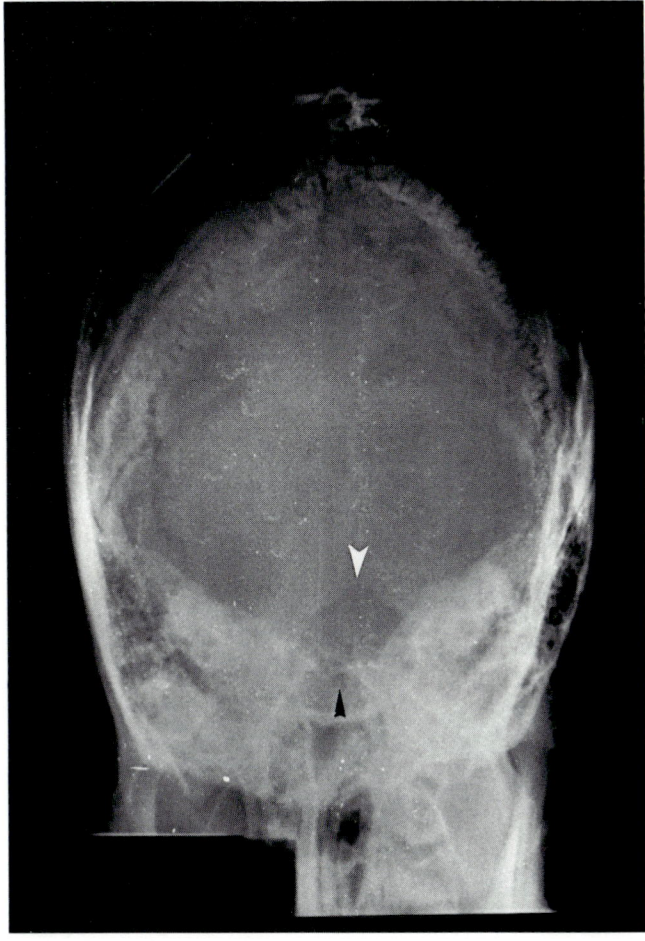

Figure 177. Rotated Townes (Grashey) view showing opisthion (white arrow) and foramen magnum shifted to the patient's left in relation to the junction of the petrous pyramids (black arrow), and asymmetrical appearance of the ridges. Face was rotated toward the *right*.

assure a 30-degree angle between the central ray and the extended orbitomeatal line.

Tilt. For the Townes view, tilt has very similar effects to rotation — it makes the petrous pyramids and occipital anatomy assymetrical. Tilt can be readily distinguished by observing the overall long axis of the head in relation to the film.

Other Considerations. Note that in Figure 176 the collar of a jacket overlaps the lower portions of the petrous pyramids and the occipital

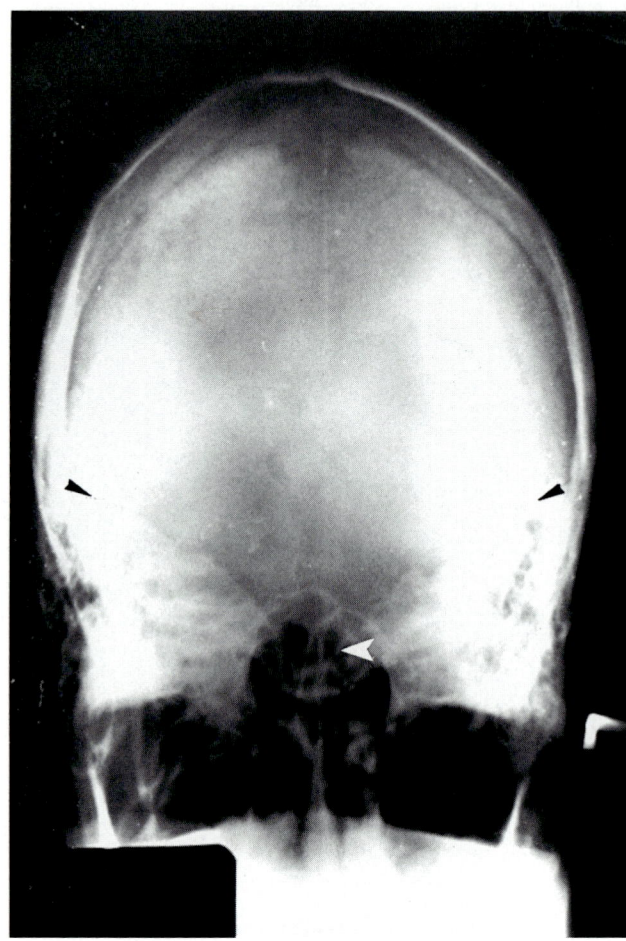

Figure 178. Townes (Grashey) view of skull showing less than one-half of the foramen magnum rising over the junction of the petrous ridges (white arrow), with the ridges (black arrows) at an obtuse angle (less than 45 degrees). This indicates either (A) insufficient caudal angle of the central ray, or (B) extension of the head which cancels out a portion of the caudal beam angle.

bone. With the angle used on the Townes view, even the patient's shoulders can get in the way if they are hunched up. Be sure to take the angle of the projection into account.

Lateral Views

Rotation. In selecting criteria to evaluate rotation on lateral radiographs of the head, it is important to bear in mind the general rules for

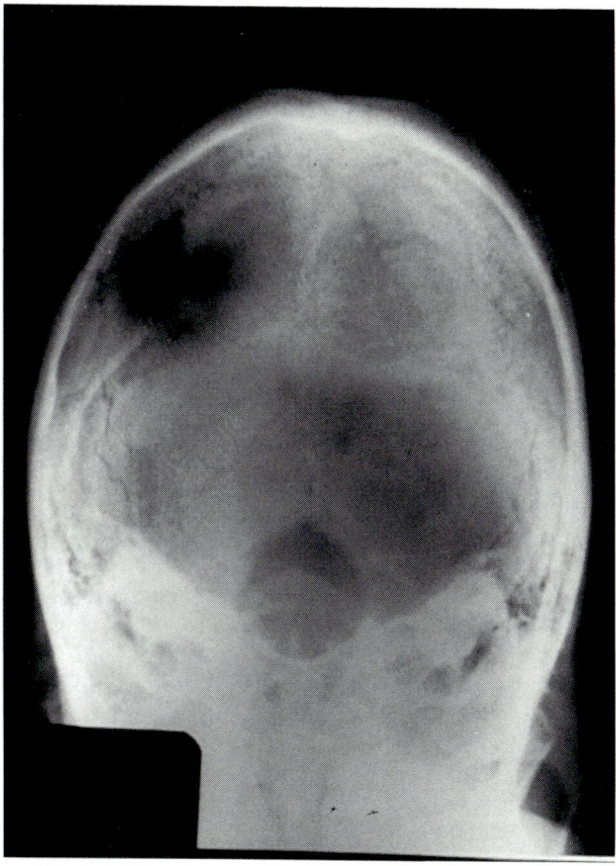

Figure 179. Townes (Grashey) view of skull showing posterior arch of the first cervical vertebra framed within the foramen magnum. This most likely indicates excessive caudal tube angulation, but can be also caused by excessive *flexion* of the head for this view. The blocker impedes the lower petrous pyramid, and should have been placed up.

good criteria discussed in Chapter Six. Foremost is the rule that the anatomical parts observed must be as close as possible to the central ray location. For example, the orbital rims are *very poor* criteria for evaluating rotation on a routine lateral skull, yet they are good criteria for a *lateral sinus or facial bone* view. This is because on the lateral skull, the x-ray beam is centered to the mid-cranium, at least 10 centimeters away from the rims of the orbits. It should therefore be expected that diverging beams will shift the orbital rims off of each other even though the position is in true lateral. This important concept is diagrammatically illustrated in Figure 180 here and in Figure 74, Chapter 6. For the lateral view of the facial bones, sinuses, or nasal bones, the beam is centered to the body of the malar bone, very near the orbital rims, and for *this* view the orbital rims should be superimposed directly on top of each other as in Figure 182.

Superimposition of the two posterior clinoid processes is often suggested for critiquing lateral skull rotation. These are near the central ray indeed, but the two processes are only one-half inch away from each other and close to the midline of the skull. As described in Chapter 6, anatomical parts so close together are reliable indicators only for *extreme* rotation. That is, it takes a lot of rotation to noticeably shift them off of each other.

Two anatomical criteria for skull rotation will be recommended here, each with a single disadvantage. These are the greater wings of the sphenoid bone and the rami of the mandible. The greater wings of the sphenoid are the "C"-shaped bones separating the sphenoid sinuses from the ethmoid sinuses diagrammed and shown in Figures 180 and 182. The *vertical* portion of the wings, or middle of the "C", should not be shifted more than about one-quarter inch off of each other side-to-side, Figure 181. The only disadvantage to using the greater wings is that they are still a couple of inches away from the central ray location, so that slight shift must be expected. For the coned-down lateral view of the sella turcica, the greater wings of the sphenoid bone make *excellent* criteria for rotation, because the central ray is located very near to them.

Alternatively, when they are included in the view, the posterior surfaces of the two mandibular rami may be checked for superimposition, Figures 180 and 181. They should not be more than about one-quarter inch shifted off of each other side-to-side. The disadvantage to using the rami of the mandible is that this is a movable bone and it is possible for the patient to have the jaw cocked to one side. When they are visible, the two mastoid tips also make good criteria for evaluating rotation.

Unfortunately, it can be difficult to distinguish *which way* the skull is rotated, to the right or left. With practice, the *upside* of the skull may be determined by observing which of the two mandibular condyles is more magnified and blurry. Then one can observe whether this magnified side is shifted anteriorly or posteriorly in relation to the opposite condyle.

It may be useful to point out that rotation on lateral skull positions is almost always with the face rotated *toward* the table. It is natural for the patient to drop their head somewhat during positioning or prior to exposure. Furthermore, radiographers often fail to get the patient's upside shoulder far enough off of the table to bring the head up into true lateral, as is discussed in the following section on head tilt. Downward rotation also

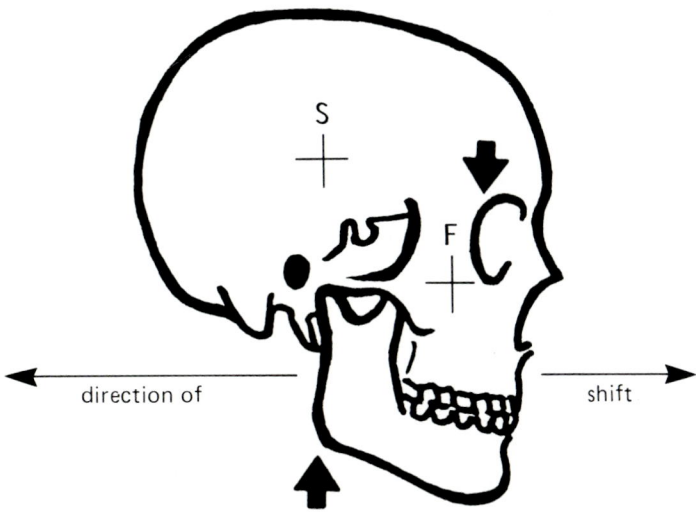

Figure 180. Diagram showing centering points for lateral skull (S) and for lateral facial/sinus views (F), with proper criteria for rotation indicated. Rotational shift is side-to-side, so anatomical criteria selected to evaluate rotation must be close to the central ray location side-to-side. The orbital rims are good for a lateral facial or sinus view, but too far from the central ray for use on a lateral skull position. For the lateral skull, the rami of the mandible (lower arrow) or the greater wings of the sphenoid should be used.

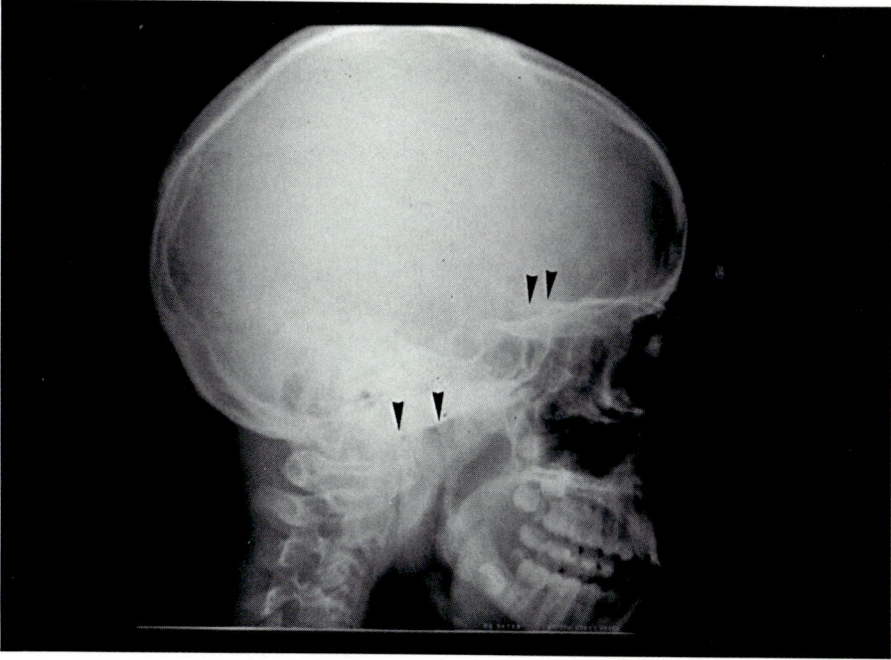

Figure 181. Non-tilted lateral skull showing criteria for rotation. If the rami of the mandible or the greater wings of the sphenoid (arrows) are shifted more than a quarter inch, rotation is unacceptable.

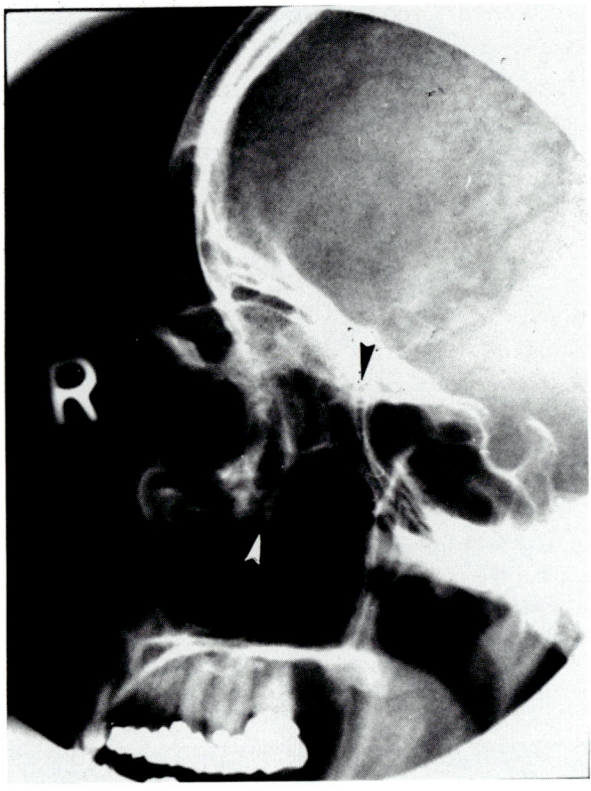

Figure 182. Proper coned lateral view of the sinuses. Both the rims of the orbits (white arrow) and the greater wings of the sphenoid bone (black arrow) are closely superimposed, indicating no rotation is present. Superimposition of the orbital plates of the frontal bone indicates that no tilt is present. Note also that coning and centering include posterior extent of the sphenoid sinuses.

seems less noticeable than upward rotation. Rarely is the skull rotated upward past lateral position without being noticed and corrected.

For coned-down lateral views of the sinuses or facial bones, the lateral rims of the orbits should be superimposed, and the vertical walls of the maxillary sinuses may be observed for confirmation of a rotated position.

Flexion/Extension. Positioning the infraorbitomeatal line transversely perpendicular to the table brings the chin up enough to ensure that the rami of the mandible do not obscure the anterior body of the first cervical vertebra. This is a fine point, and flexion/extension is not a crucial factor in lateral skull views.

Tilt. The most reliable criterion for head tilt on lateral views of facial bones, sinuses or skulls is the *orbital plates of the frontal bone,* or "roofs" of the orbits, as shown in Figure 183. These should not be shifted *vertically* off of each other more than one-quarter inch. The posterior fossae of the occipital bone form horizontal lines, but are far from the plane of the central ray and typically are shifted vertically up to one-half inch. Extreme shift of these bones or the mastoid tips can be used to confirm head tilt.

Avoiding tilt in lateral head positioning is both crucial and challenging. The key to eliminating it is to remember that the head is attached to the shoulders, *and* that the upside shoulder is attached to the upside elbow. The most frequently encountered type of head tilt with the patient in prone position is with the chin lower than the glabella as in Figure 184. To eliminate it, perform the following three steps *in order:*

1. Raise the upside *elbow* off of the table and have the patient support his arm with his hand.
2. Rotate the *shoulder* up as far as needed until the head appears close to being untilted.
3. To eliminate the last bit of tilt, *tuck the chin slightly.*

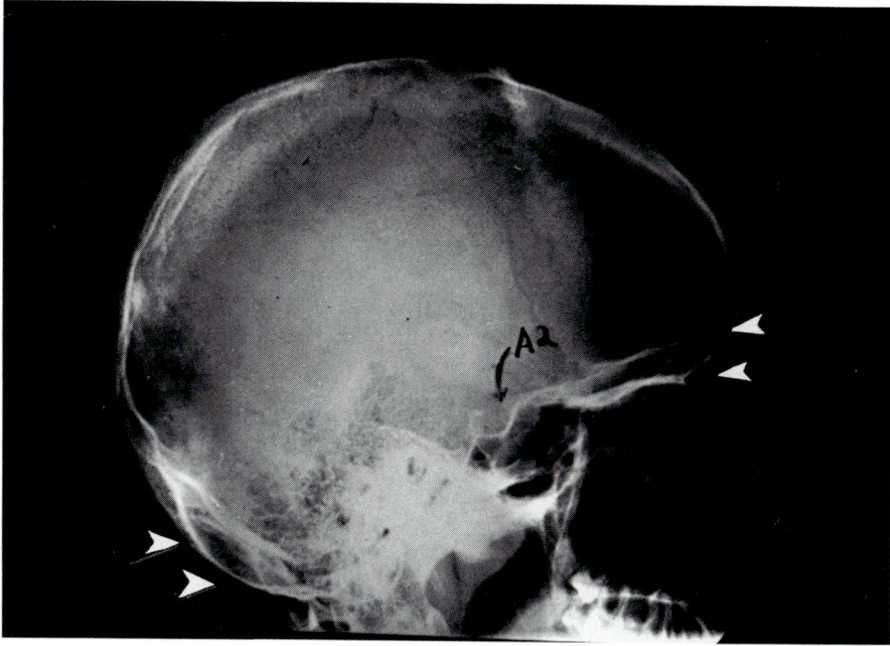

Figure 183. Non-rotated lateral view of the skull showing improper tilt. Tilt is evidenced by vertical desuperimposition of the orbital plates of the frontal bone (roofs of the orbits), as well as of the posterior fossae of the occipital bone (arrows).

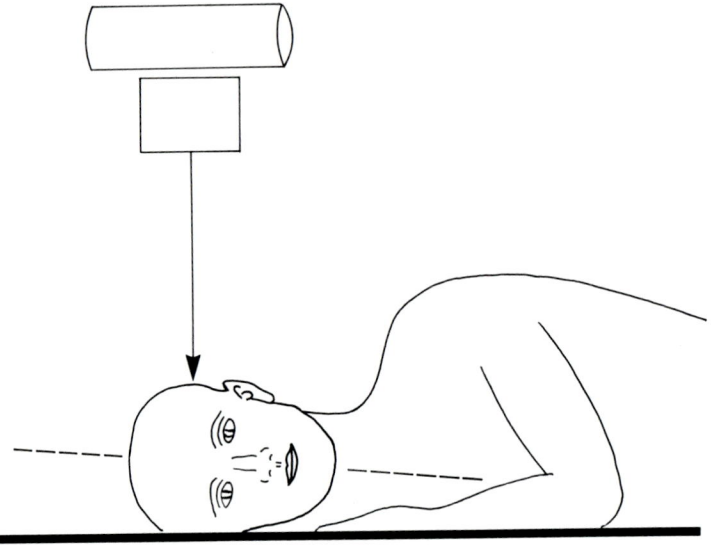

Figure 184. Typical head tilt during lateral skull positioning with chin lower than the glabella, caused when the elbow is rested on the table. Large-shouldered patients can present the opposite kind of tilt with the glabella lower than the chin.

The patient can only pull his shoulder up so far with the elbow still resting on the table.

Occasionally, a patient has such thick shoulders that head tilt results with the glabella lower than the chin. This type of tilt is difficult to eliminate in the prone position. For slight tilt, use a thin sponge under the side of the cranium to raise it. For tough cases, try repositioning the patient *supine* with the head turned laterally.

Axial Basilar View

Tilt. On the basilar view (submentovertex or verticosubmental projection) of the skull, sinuses or mandible, head tilt is often mistakenly called "rotation." (Actually, true head rotation is not crucial on this view, since it would be corrected by simply rotating the film and hanging it by its corner.) In the nonrotated view, the bony nasal septum appears to be exactly centered within the inverted "U"-shaped arch of the mandible, so that the two rami of the mandible are equidistant from the midline septum. Also, an equal amount of the side wall of the cranium will be visible laterally to each mandibular ramus, as in Figure 185.

When the cranium is tilted to the patient's left, more of the side of the cranium will be seen lateral to the mandibular condyle on the left, and

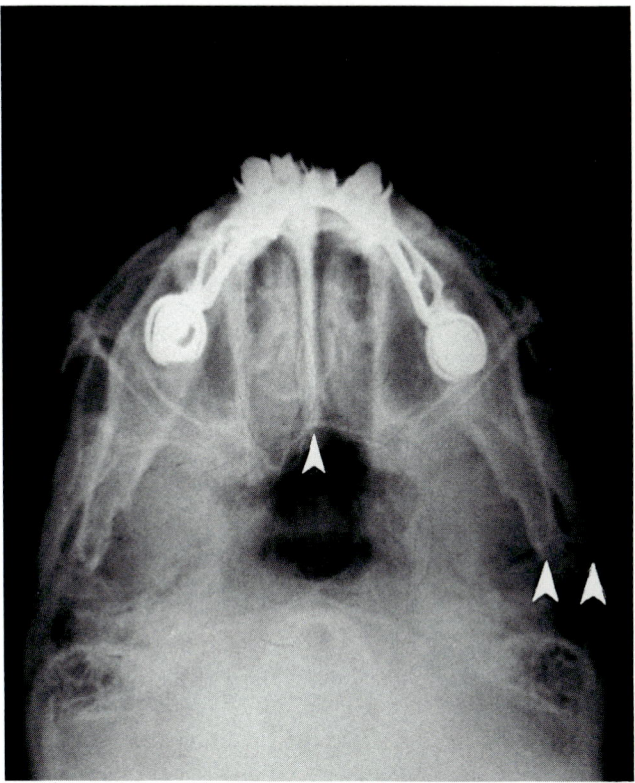

Figure 185. Proper submentovertex view of skull. Distance from mandibular ramus to side of cranium (arrows) is equal on both sides, and bony nasal septum is centered within arch of mandible, indicating no tilt is present. Mentum superimposes the forehead precisely, indicating full and adequate head extension.

less cranial wall will be seen lateral to the condyle on the right as shown in Figure 186. Also, the bony nasal septum will appear to shift off-centered to the left within the arch of the mandible, so that there is less distance from the septum to the left mandibular condyle and more distance from the septum to the right condyle. In other words, in the direction that the head is tilted, *more* cranial wall will be seen and *less* cranial base will be seen on that side.

Angulation and Flexion/Extension. The properly positioned basilar view places the mentum (chin) directly superimposed over the forehead, with no facial bones visible above the chin, as in Figure 185. The entire petrous pyramids should be free of superimposition from the condyles of the mandible. This requires the correct combination of head extension and cephalic beam angulation. Many patients are unable to hyperextend

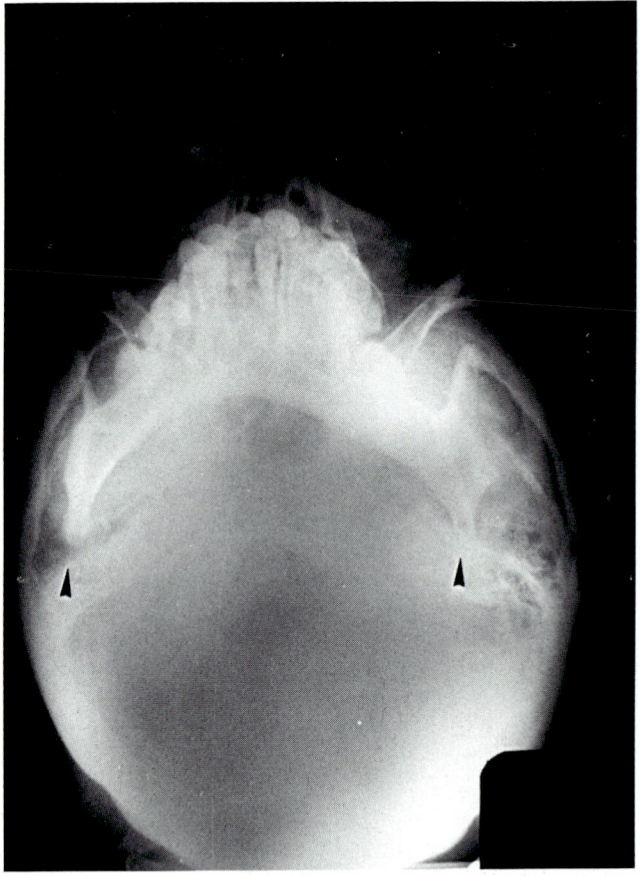

Figure 186. Submentovertex view of skull showing uneven distance from rami of mandibles (arrows) to sides of cranium, indicating improper head tilt. Insufficient head extension is also present, since facial anatomy is visible above the chin.

their heads to the point where the infraorbitomeatal line parallels the film as recommended in most positioning texts. More importantly, the *central ray* should be kept *perpendicular* to the infraorbitomeatal line. If the head is not fully extended, then the beam must be angled cephalic *until the shadow of the chin begins to rise above the shadow of the forehead.* This simple positioning tip will assure an adequate view of the basilar structures free of superimposition from the chin.

If the head is not extended enough, *or* if the x-ray beam is not angled cephalic enough, the orbits and other facial bones will be seen above the chin, as in Figure 186. *There should be no structures projected anterior to the chin.*

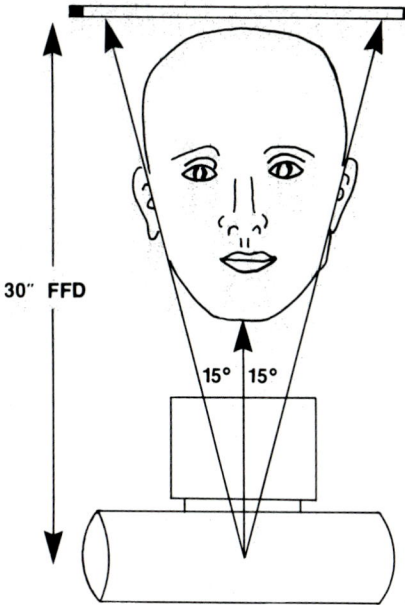

Figure 187. Diagram of reduced-distance submentovertex method for demonstrating the bilateral zygomatic arches. Focus-film distance of 30 inches results in the diverging beams which project the zygomatic arches to each be angled 15 degrees from the central ray. This successfully projects each arch off of the cranial wall, producing the view demonstrated in Figure 188.

Zygomatic Arches

The submentovertex projection just described is also very effective for obtaining a bilateral view of the zygomatic arches, with the following modification: Reduce the focus-film distance to about 30 inches, with an appropriate reduction in technique (use a PA hand technique). Otherwise, the position is like any other SMV, with the central ray centered about two and one-half inches below the chin, perpendicular to the infraorbito-meatal line. With the shortened FFD, the diverging beams form 15 degree angles to either side of the central ray as they pass through the zygomatic arches, as diagrammed in Figure 187. The resulting image shows a magnified mandible just superimposing the front *and* sides of the cranium, with the zygomatic archs in full view, Figure 188. This is an easy way to position zygomatic arches and obtain a bilateral view with one exposure.

Another effective way to desuperimpose the cranium from the zygomatic arches is to use an additional 10 degrees of cephalic beam angle

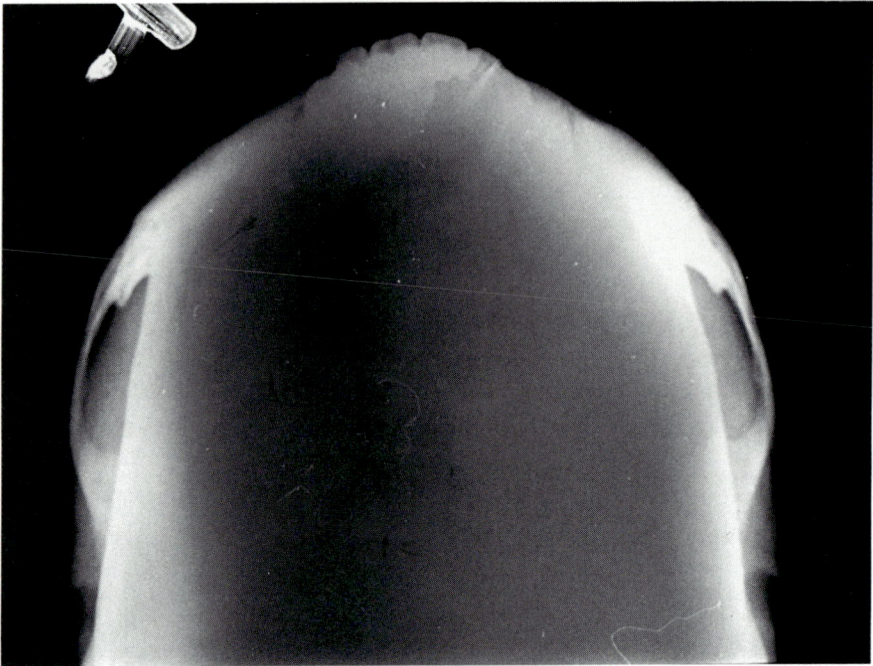

Figure 188. Submentovertex projection for bilateral zygomatic arches taken with reduced 30-inch FFD as diagrammed in Figure 187.

past perpendicular to the infraorbitomeatal line. For a routine submento-vertex view, Figure 189 would be considered as *hyperextended* or with too much cephalic tube angle, because the chin is projected well above (anterior to) the forehead. Note, however, that this method is well-suited for demonstrating the *zygomatic arches.* Since the angle creates slight elongation distortion of the arches, this method should be a second choice to the reduced FFD approach. Some patients have unusually "flat" arches which are very difficult to demonstrate. If the reduced FFD method has been attempted and fails to adequately demonstrate the arches, this extra-angle method may be needed.

The Mays method for each individual arch uses a 15-degree lateral beam angle to produce the same effect as the reduced-FFD submentovertex. On *either* the submentovertex bilateral view or the Mays view, if the straight lateral edge of the mandible or soft tissue of the cheek obscures the zygomatic arch of interest, as in Figure 190, the head was *not tilted enough* or the x-ray beam was *angled too much laterally.* On either view, if the curved edge of the cranium superimposes the arch, as in Figure 191,

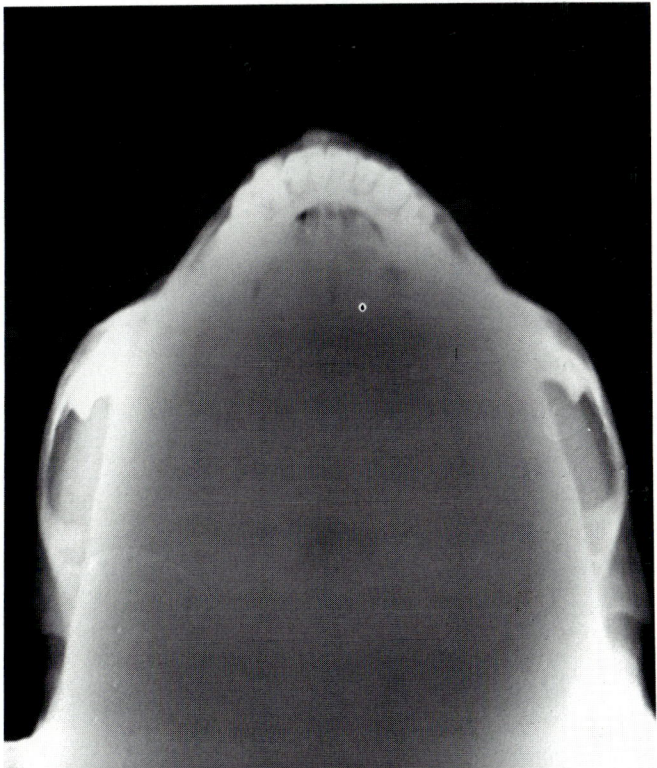

Figure 189. Submentovertex projection for bilateral zygomatic arches taken at 40 inches FFD with *hyperextension* of the head in relation to the central ray. (Note that the chin is projected well above the forehead. Compare to Figure 188.)

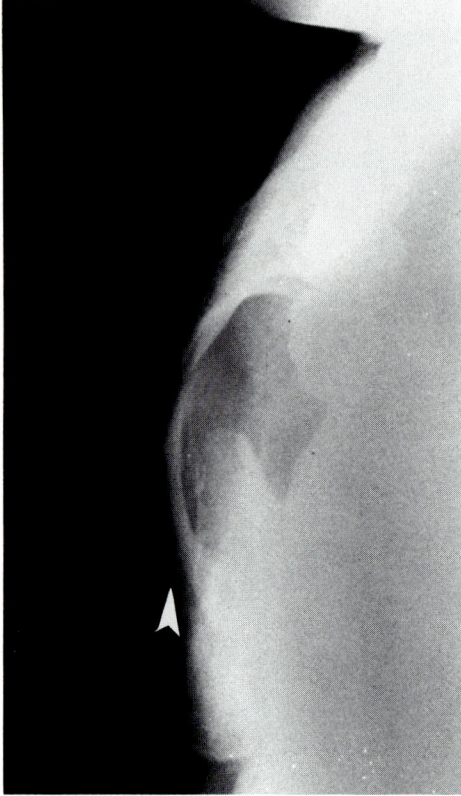

Figure 190. Mays method for zygomatic arch showing superimposition of soft tissue of cheek (arrow) over arch due to *over-tilting* the head away from the affected side.

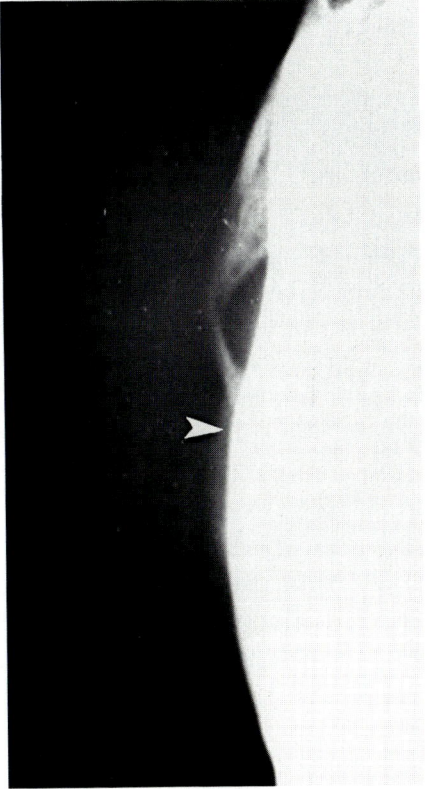

Figure 191. Mays method for zygomatic arch showing superimposition of cranial wall (arrow) over part of the arch due to *insufficient head tilt.*

the head was *tilted too much* or the x-ray beam was *not angled enough laterally.*

Optic Foramina/Orbits

Criteria for the Waters and Caldwell views are presented earlier in this chapter. We will now discuss the specific criteria for the Rheese method to demonstrate the optic foramen and the interior of the orbit.

With the head extended so the acanthiomeatal line is perpendicular to the film, and with the proper 53 degrees of head rotation, the optic foramen is placed in the *middle* of the lower outer quadrant of the orbit as in Figure 192. The optic foramen can be found by following the bony edge of the lesser wing of the sphenoid bone laterally within the orbit until it terminates at the foramen, Figure 192. When the head is rotated *too steep,* greater than 53 degrees, the foramen will lie in the middle of the lower orbit. When the head is rotated *too shallow,* less than 53 degrees, the foramen will lie over or near the lateral rim of the orbit, Figure 193. If the head is not extended enough, the foramen will lie too high, in the middle or upper portion of the orbit as in Figure 194. If the head is overextended, the foramen will lie over the lower rim of the orbit.

Mandible

The frontal view of the mandible is similar to the frontal views for the skull—the rami of the mandible should be equidistant from the bony nasal septum and are indicative of rotation. Most commonly there is no flexion or extension of the head, but some texts recommend extension when there is interest in the mentum, to place the chin against the film.

The axiolateral oblique position is designed to maximize desuperimposition of the body of one side of the mandible. To accomplish this, there are three essential considerations:

1. The head must be tilted enough to desuperimpose the upside mandibular body from the downside,
2. The head should be slightly rotated toward the film to place the body as parallel as possible,

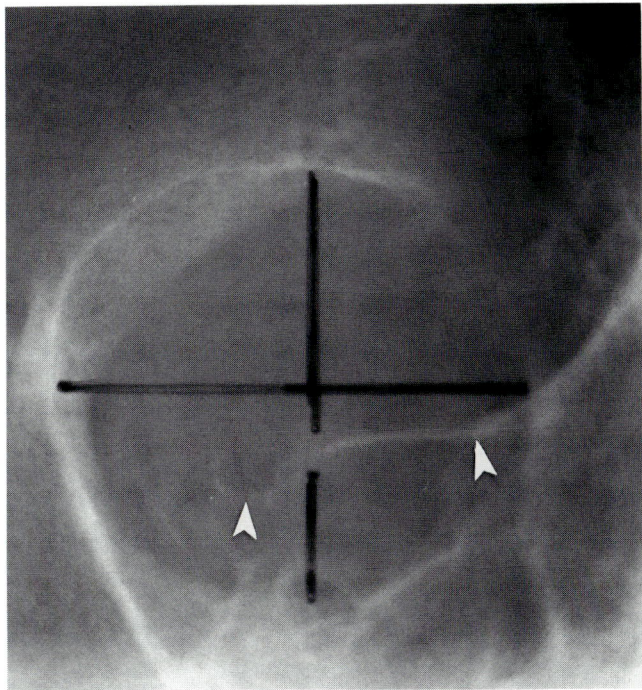

Figure 192. Proper Rheese view projecting the optic foramen (left arrow) into the middle of the lower-outer quadrant of the orbit. Right arrow shows lesser wing of sphenoid bone which can be followed laterally to its termination to help locate the optic foramen.

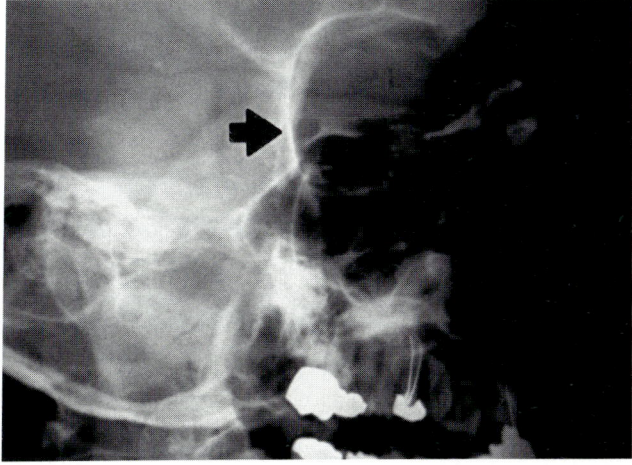

Figure 193. Rheese view showing shallow head rotation (head rotated *too lateral* or less than 53 degrees from tabletop), placing optic foramen at lateral rim of orbit (arrow).

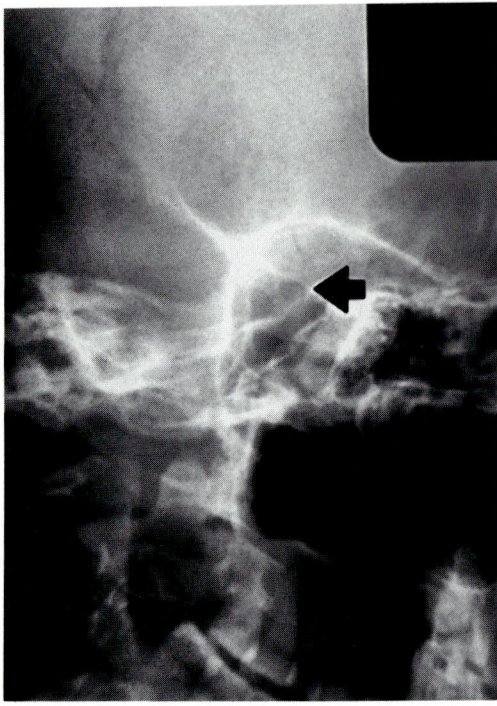

Figure 194. Rheese view showing insufficient head extension, (chin was not brought up enough to place acanthiomeatal line perpendicular to table edge), projecting optic foramen (arrow) into upper half of the orbit.

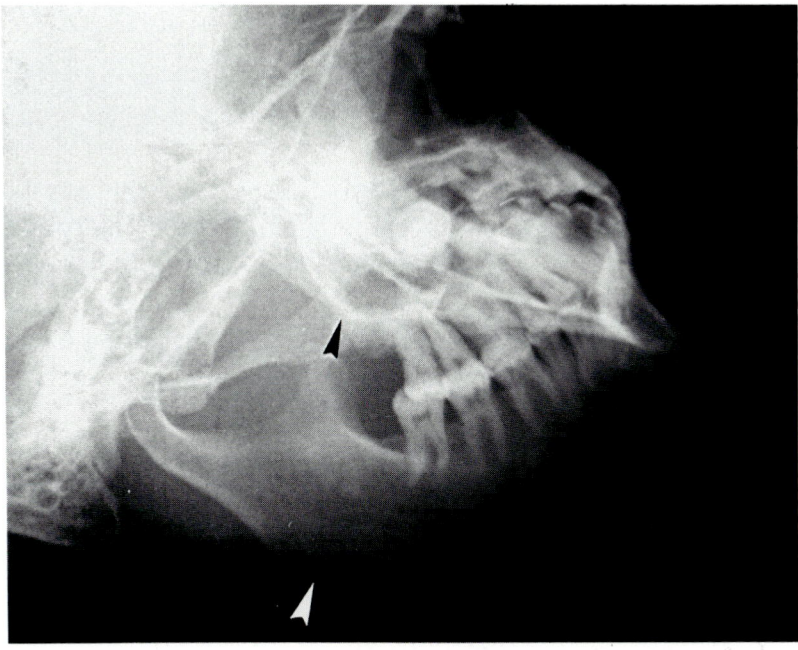

Figure 195. Proper oblique mandible view with gonions (arrows) shifted 3 inches vertically. Note how much of downside mandible is visible, including condylar and coronoid processes.

3. The chin must be extended forward to ensure that the gonion does not superimpose the cervical spine.

Figure 195 demonstrates a good mandible position. The upside gonion is approximately 3 inches above the downside gonion of interest, because a combination of head tilt toward the film and cephalic tube angulation resulted in a *30-degree angle* between the beam and the interpupillary line. The upside gonion is slightly anterior to the downside gonion, indicating slight rotation of the face toward the film. Too much rotation will place the downside gonion of interest over the cervical spine. Finally, the chin is extended also to keep the downside gonion of interest out of the cervical spine.

Figure 196 shows an oblique mandible view with inadequate head tilt or insufficient cephalic angulation. The upside body obscures the downside body. Figure 197 shows what happens when *only* a cephalic tube angle is used—the shoulder may be projected into the mandible. To avoid this, it is recommended that a combination of 15 degrees of head tilt toward the film and 15 degrees of cephalic beam angle be used in combination. (The author prefers to use tilt only by placing the downside shoulder against the film and tilting the head 30 degrees, with *no* angulation of the tube.)

Figure 198 shows the downside gonion superimposed by the cervical spine. This can be caused by either rotating the head too much toward the film or by allowing the chin to drop into a flexed position. Rotation can be distinguished by observing the side-to-side shift of the vertical posterior surfaces of the mandibular rami.

Temporomandibular Joints and Mastoids

The *Law's* method is the most commonly used projection for both temporomandibular joints and mastoid air cells. On a properly positioned Law's view, the magnified and blurred upside condyle of the mandible will appear an inch and a half *below* and an inch and a half *anterior* to the sharp downside condyle. The upside external auditory meatus and the dense petrous bone surrounding it will also be projected *below and in front* of the downside EAM and petrous bone, as in Figure 199. The small, round internal auditory meatus will be projected within the larger, oval external auditory meatus.

Remembering the general rule from Chapter 6 that there is about one inch of anatomical image shift for every 10 degrees of rotation, tilt or angulation, one can accurately analyze the various lateral projections for mastoids and TMJ's. The Law's view in Figure 200 shows the upside TMJ

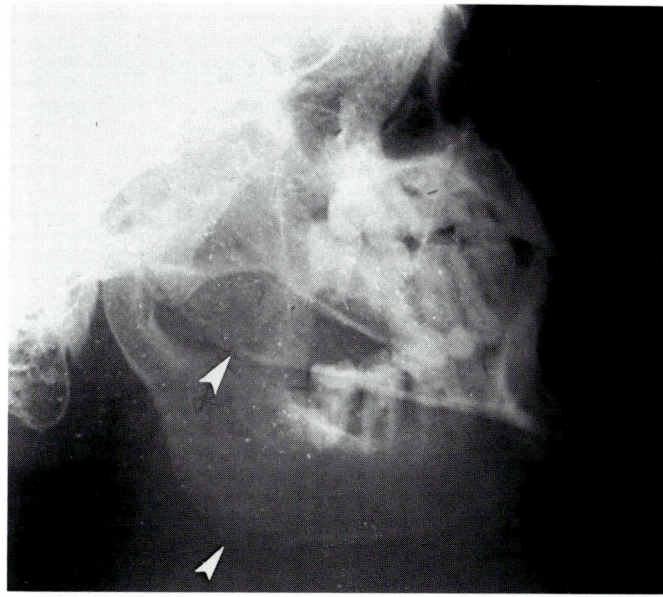

Figure 196. Oblique mandible view showing insufficient head tilt (about 15 degrees, displacing the gonions one and one-half inches), obscuring the coronoid process and mental area on the downside.

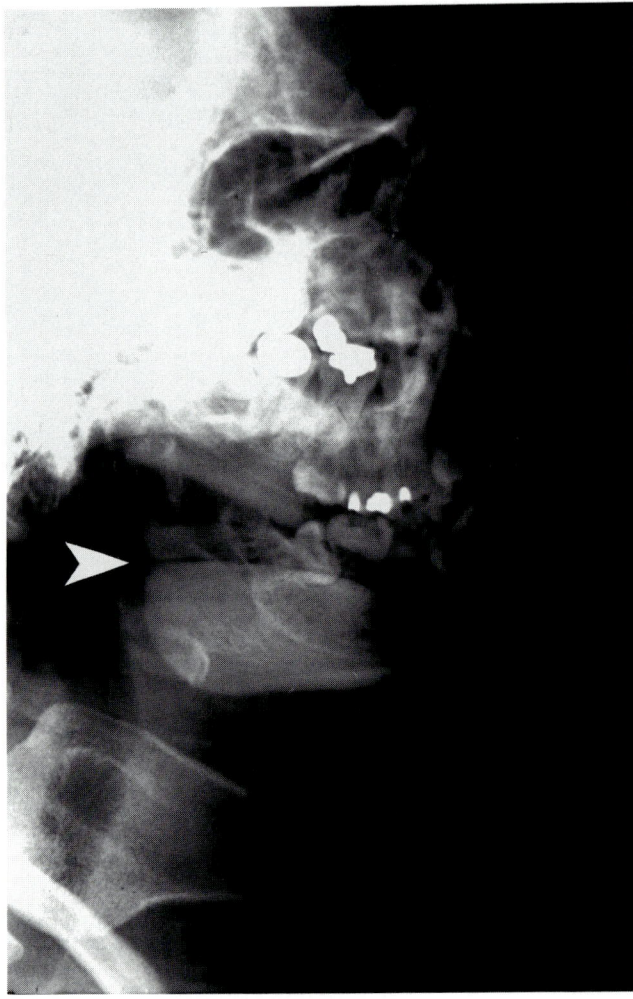

Figure 197. Attempt at an oblique mandible view using a 30-degree cephalic beam angle, projecting the soft tissue of the upper arm (arrow) over the mandible. Head tilt, or a combination of head tilt and a beam angle not to exceed 15 degrees are recommended.

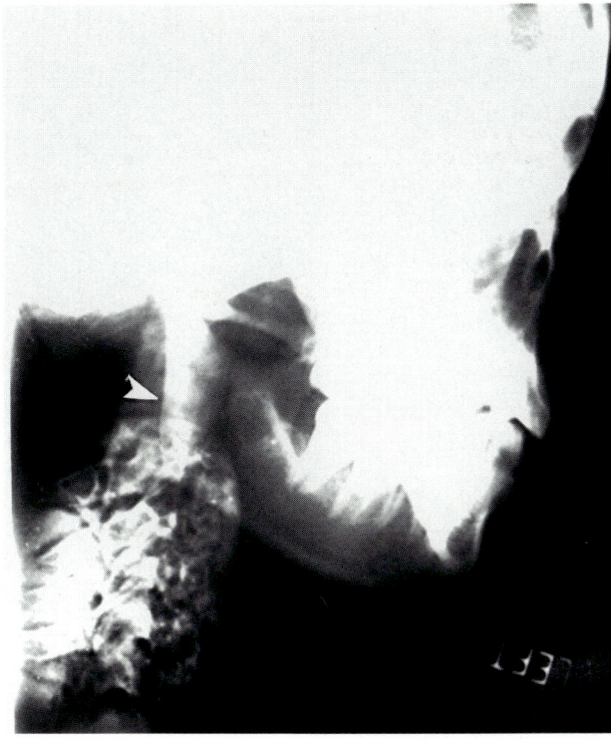

Figure 198. Oblique mandible view showing overrotation of the head toward the film, superimposing the ramus of the mandible over the cervical spine (arrow).

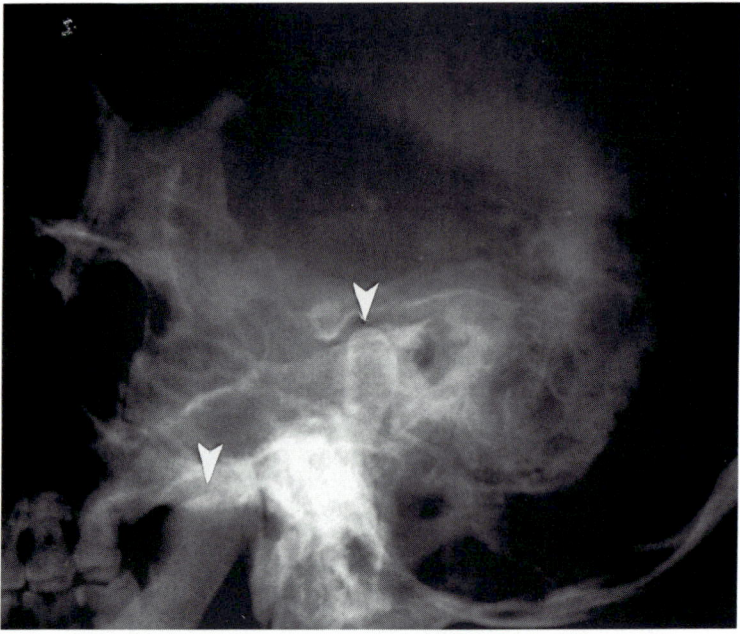

Figure 199. Proper Law's method for temporomandibular joints or mastoids. The double 15-degree method projects the upside TMJ one and one-half inches *below* and one and one-half inches *anterior* to the downside TMJ (arrows). The external auditory meati are visible just posterior to each TMJ and are shifted in identical fashion.

and condyle an inch and a half below, but only one inch in front of, the downside TMJ. This indicates a proper 15-degree caudal tube angle, but only 10 degrees of head rotation. To correct this position, the face should be rotated 5 degrees more toward the film.

Figure 201 illustrates the upside condyle two and a half inches straight below the downside condyle. This indicates 25 degrees of caudal tube angulation with no head rotation (head in true lateral position). This is correct positioning for the lateral Schuller method for mastoids. The Henschen method should place the upside condyle one and one-half inches directly below the downside condyle. The Lysholm method should place it three and one-half inches directly below. The Owen method, which uses a 30-degree caudal angle and a 30-degree head rotation in supine position, places the upside condyle and EAM three inches below and three inches posterior to the downside condyle and EAM.

Petrous Portion of Temporal Bone

The Stenver and Arcelin methods for profiling the petrous pyramids are reverse to each other, sharing the same evaluation criteria with

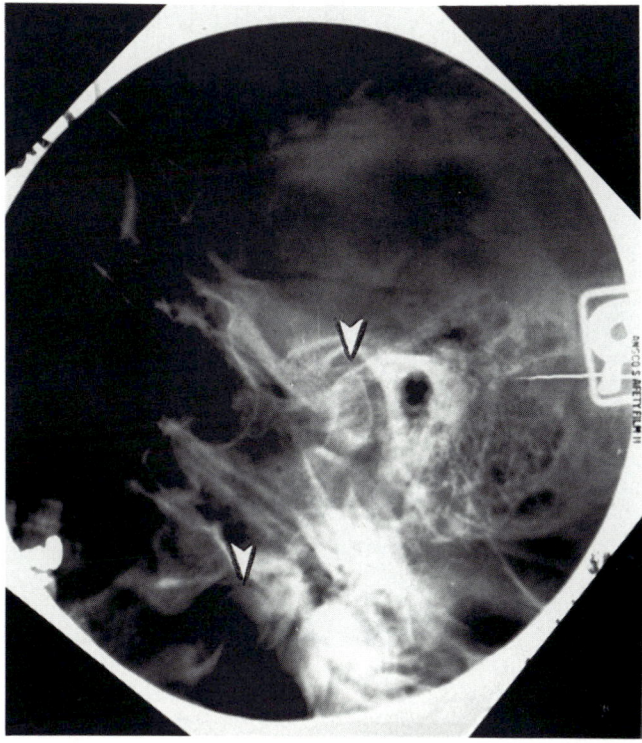

Figure 200. Law's projection with inadequate head rotation (about 10 degrees) places upside TMJ only one inch anterior to downside TMJ (arrows). Proper vertical shift of one and one-half inches indicates correct beam angle.

the understanding that the Arcelin method will magnify the orbit somewhat.

Rotation. With the proper 45 degrees of head rotation, the apex of the petrous pyramid, Figure 202, will be near the lateral rim of the orbit without extending into the orbit. The petrous apex can be located on most radiographs by following the inferior surface of the petrous pyramid as it curves off of the medial mastoid tip until it comes about one-quarter inch from the petrous ridge. If there is be a space between the petrous apex and the orbital rim as in Figure 203, the head was in *too shallow* rotation, too lateral (less than 45 degrees for the mesocephalic skull). If the petrous ridge crosses over the lateral rim and into the orbit as in Figure 204, then the head rotation was *too steep,* greater than 45 degrees.

Flexion/Extension. The petrous ridge should lie horizontally across the film. If the ridge descends toward the face, the head was overflexed as in Figure 204. If the ridge extends upward toward the face, the head was overextended.

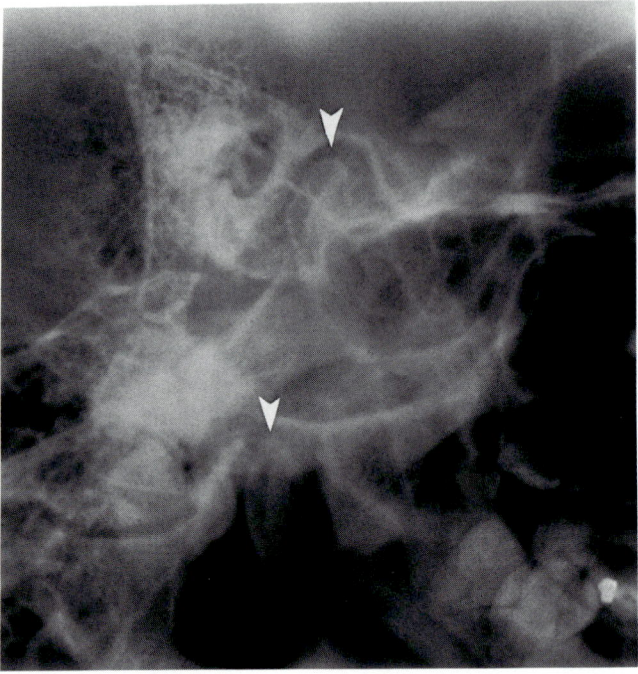

Figure 201. Schuller's method for TMJ's or mastoids shows TMJ's shifted slightly side-to-side, indicating slight head rotation. Two and one-half inch vertical shift indicates proper 25 degree caudal tube angle was used.

TECHNIQUE

Radiographic technique for all skull procedures should provide adequate penetration (kVp) to see details *through* the bones of interest, with relatively high contrast and medium density. For smaller bones such as the zygomatic arches and nasal bones, a technique typical of the PA hand or digits must be used, and of course this will result in the rest of the skull appearing underexposed.

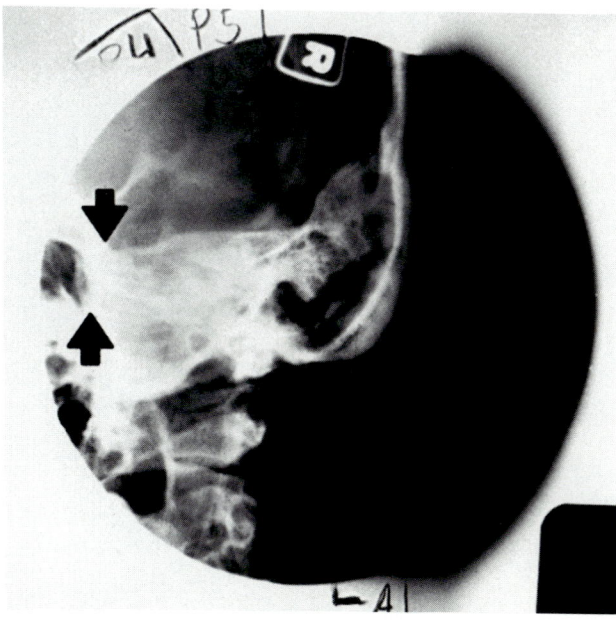

Figure 202. Proper Stenver or Arcelin method for petrous pyramid places apex of petrous pyramid (upper arrow) just to side of lateral orbital rim (lower arrow), with ridge running horizontal.

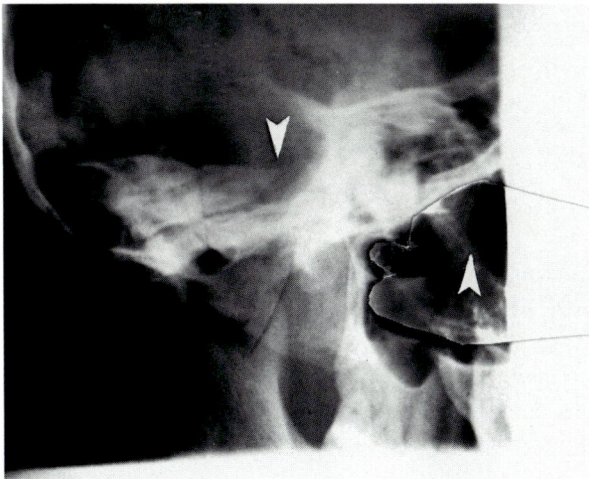

Figure 203. Stenver or Arcelin method positioned with head too lateral (too shallow or less than 45 degrees from tabletop) shows considerable space between apex of petrous pyramid (left arrow) and lateral rim of orbit (right arrow).

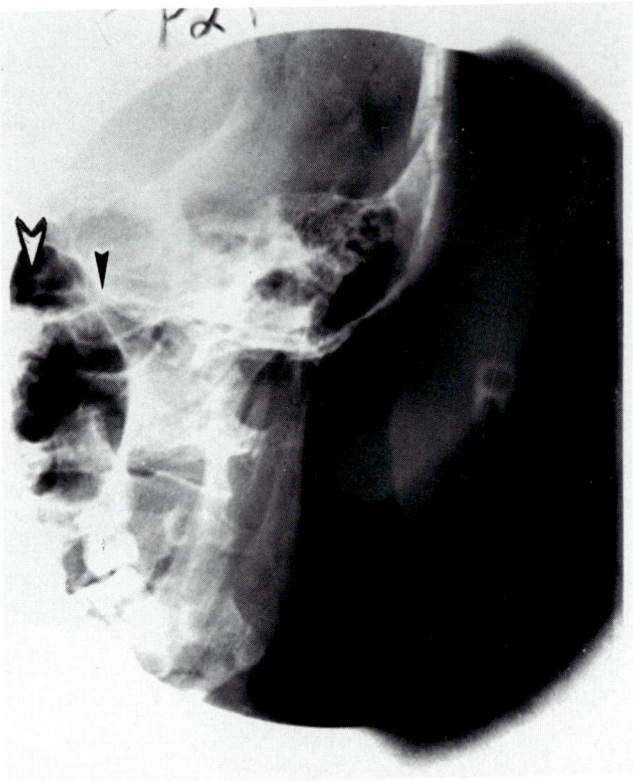

Figure 204. Stenver or Arcelin method positioned with head too steep (greater than 45 degrees from tabletop) shows petrous pyramid (white arrow) running into orbit. Black arrow marks lateral orbital rim. Slight chin flexion causes ridge to not lie horizontal.

REVIEW #2

For each radiograph in Figures 205 through 239, list *all* errors in positioning and alignment. When you are done, check your answers against the key provided in Appendix No. 1. The Appendix also provides additional critiques of the technique employed, if you wish to practice these criteria.

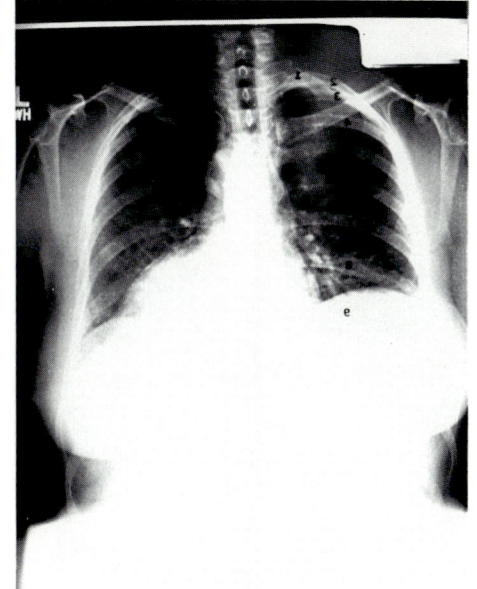

Figure 205.

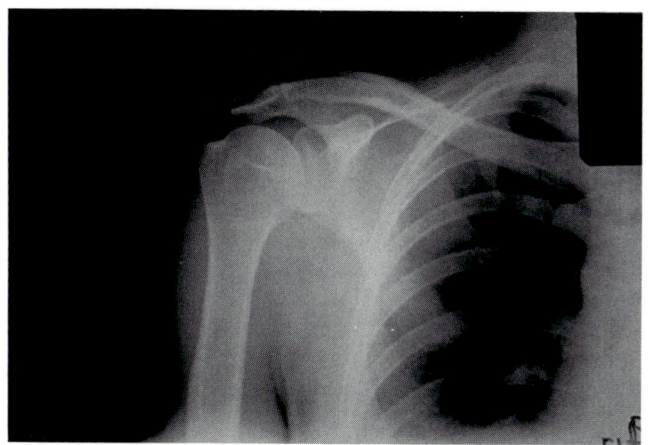

Figure 206.

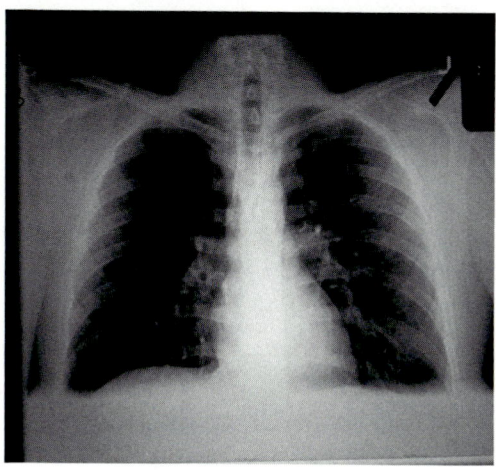

Figure 207.

234

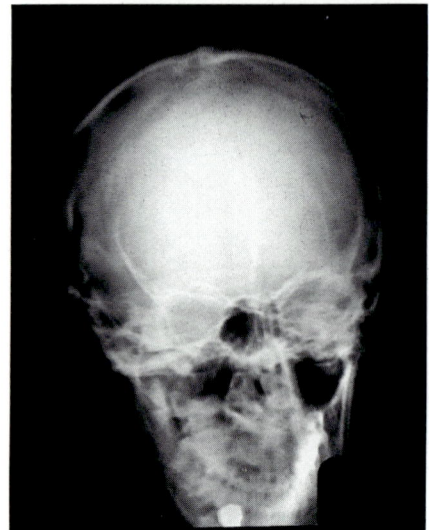

Figure 208.

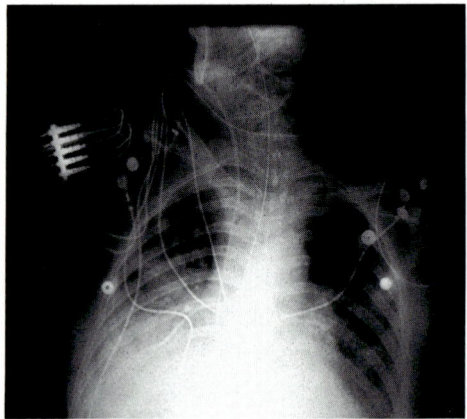

Figure 209.

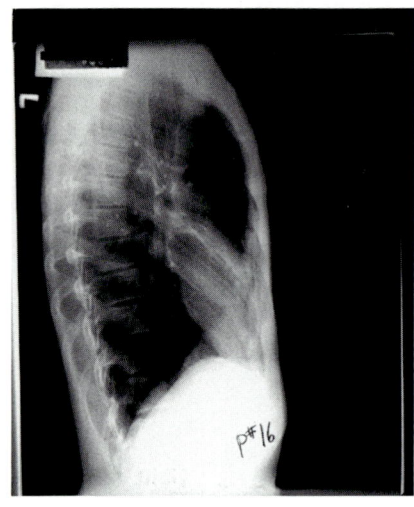

Figure 210.

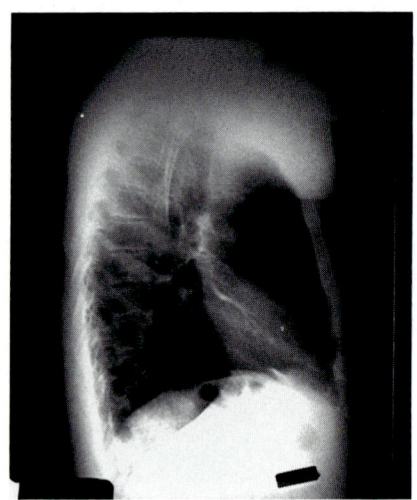

Figure 211.

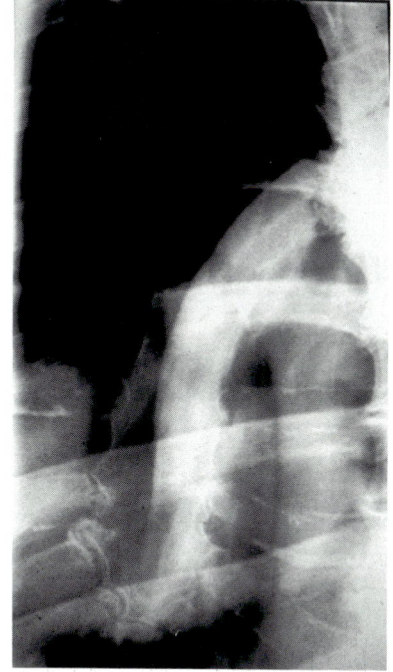

Figure 212.

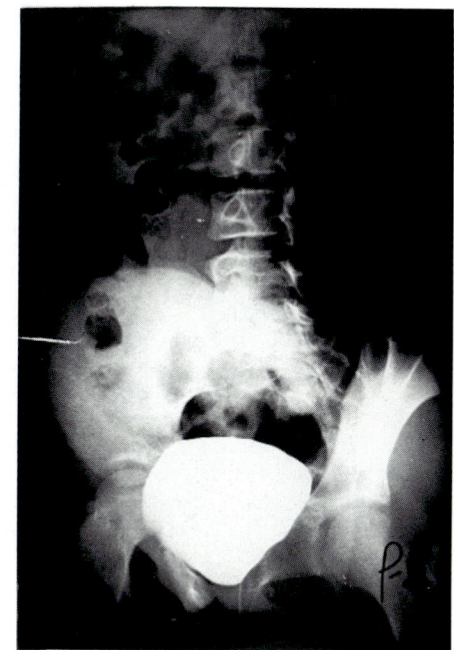

Figure 213.

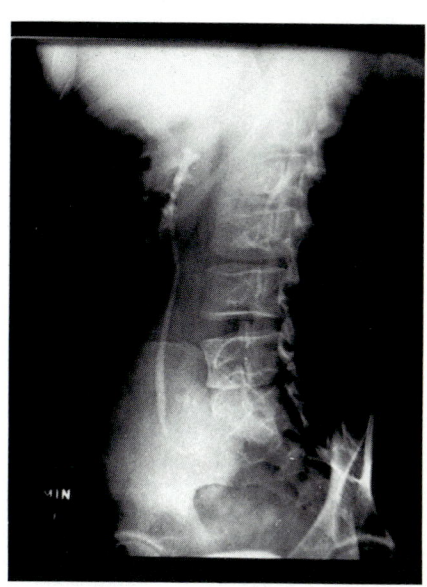

Figure 214.

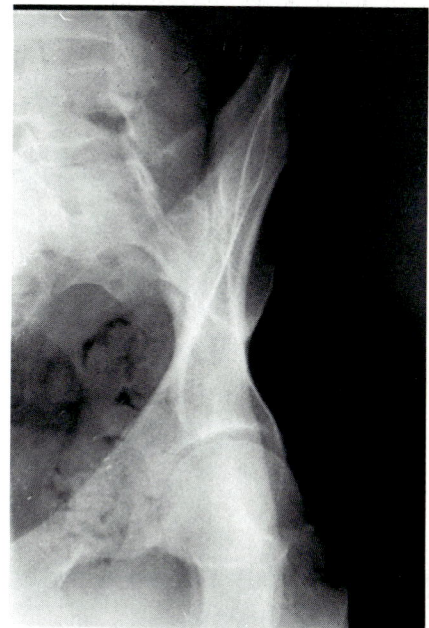

Figure 215.

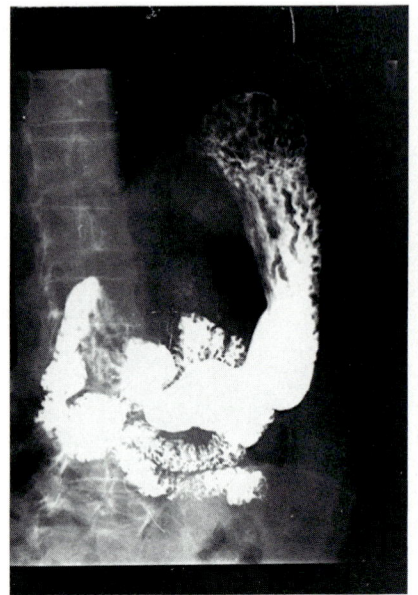

Figure 216.

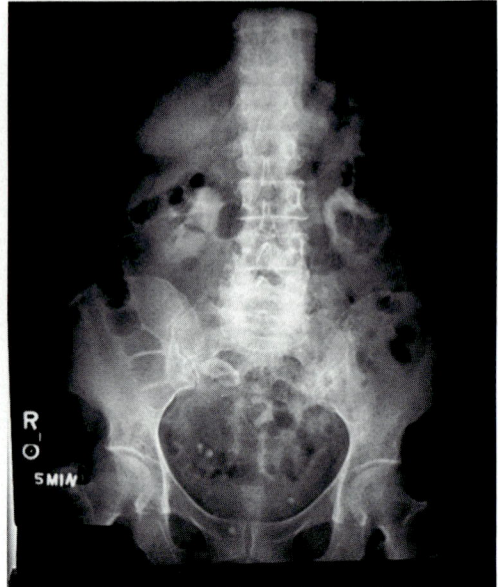

Figure 217.

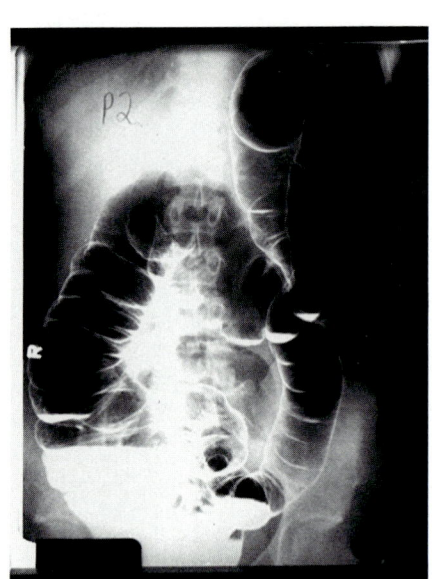

Figure 218.

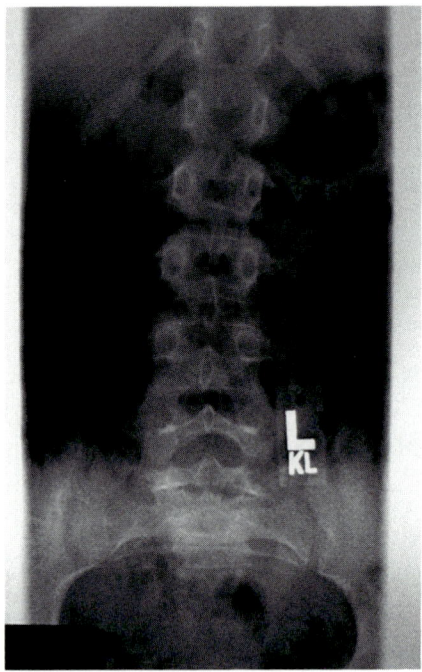

Figure 219.

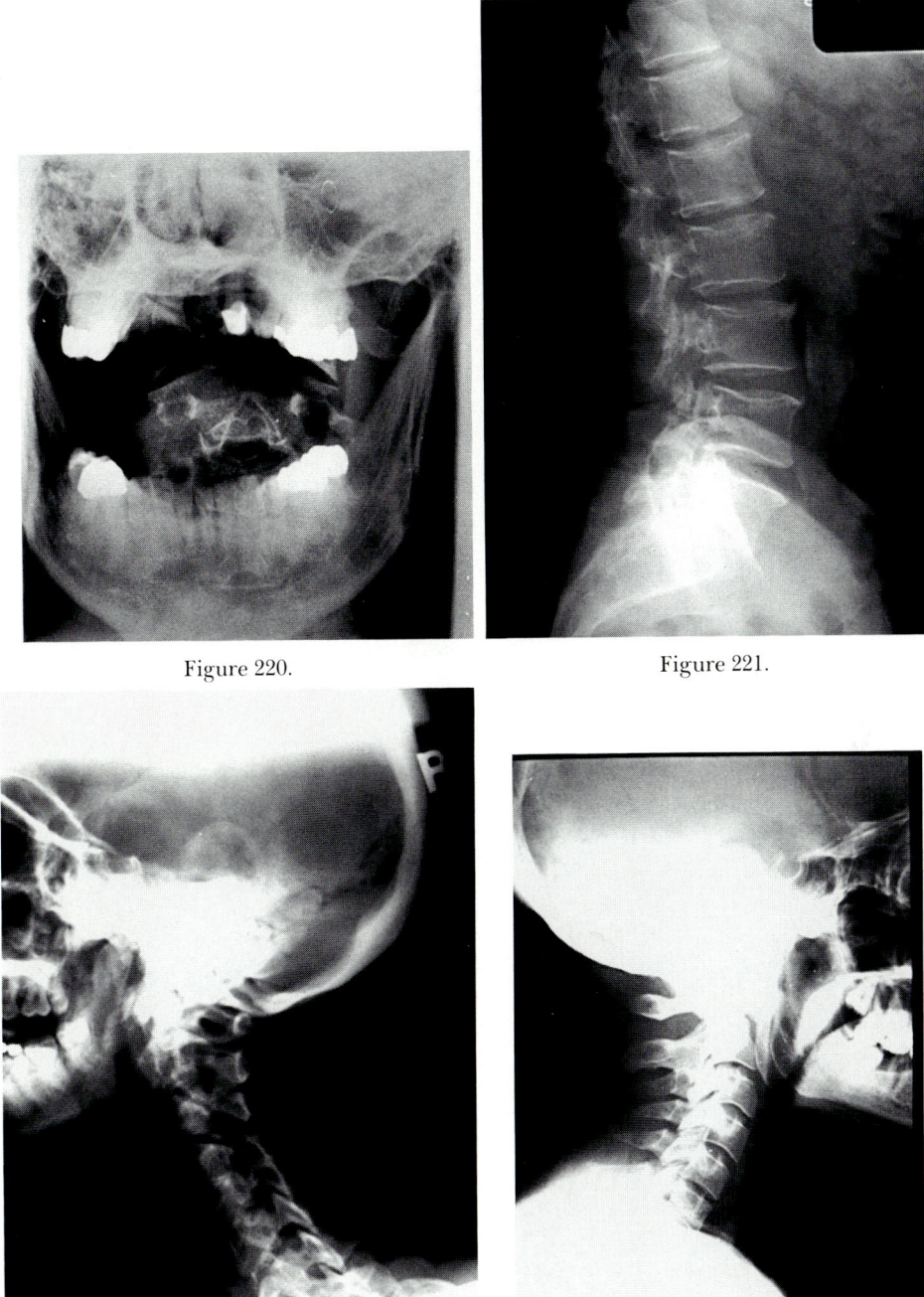

Figure 220.

Figure 221.

Figure 222.

Figure 223.

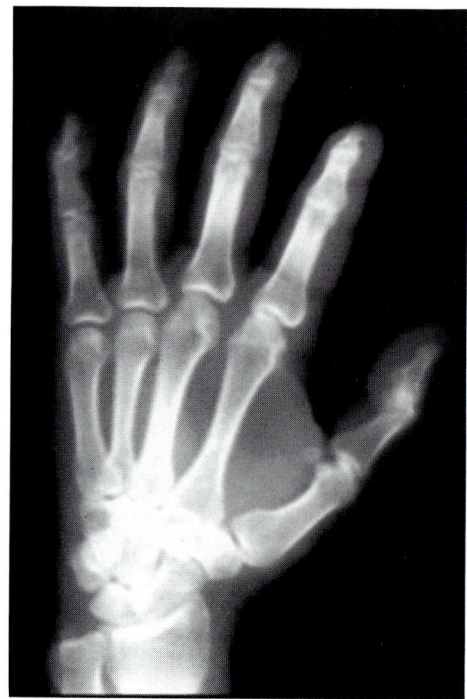

Figure 224.

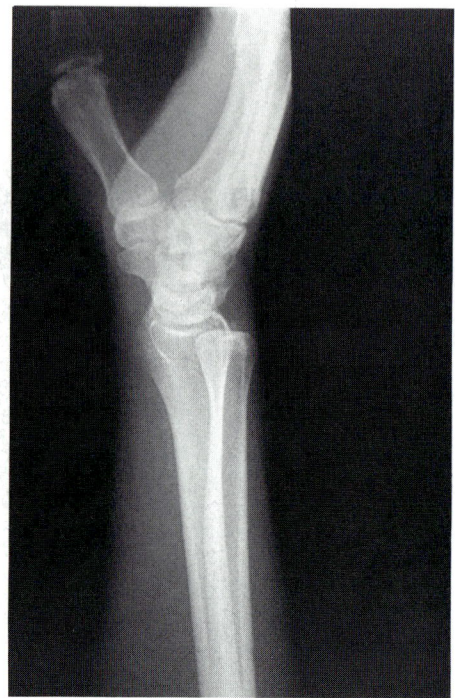

Figure 225.

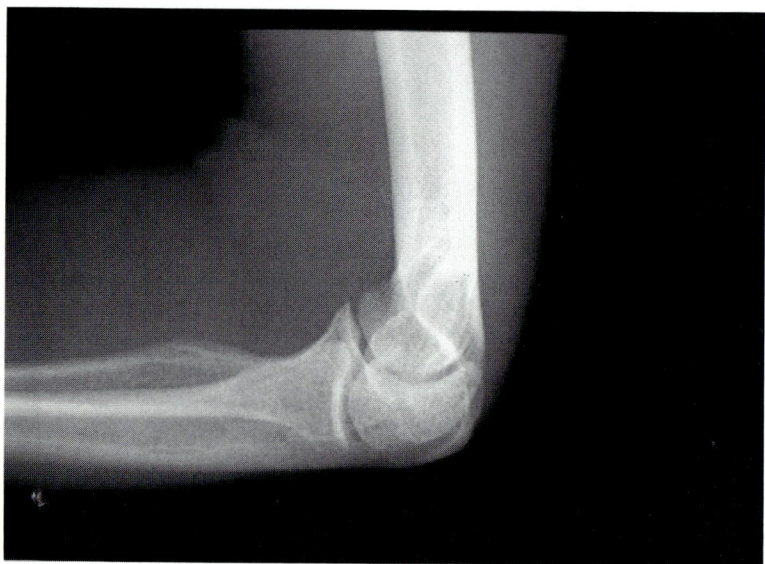

Figure 226.

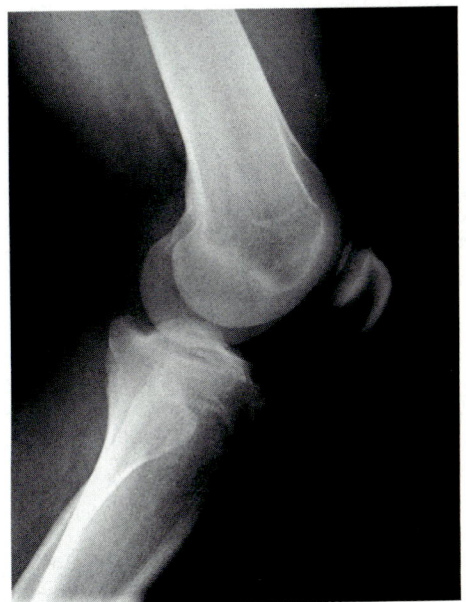

Figure 227.

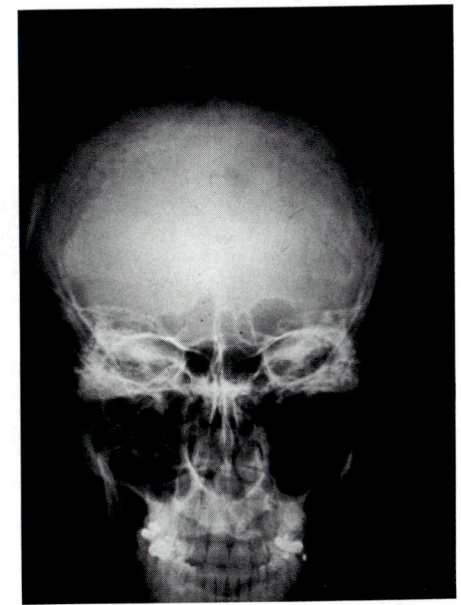

Figure 228.

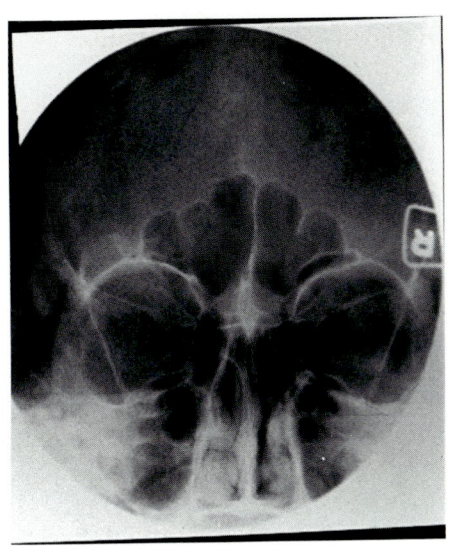

Figure 229.

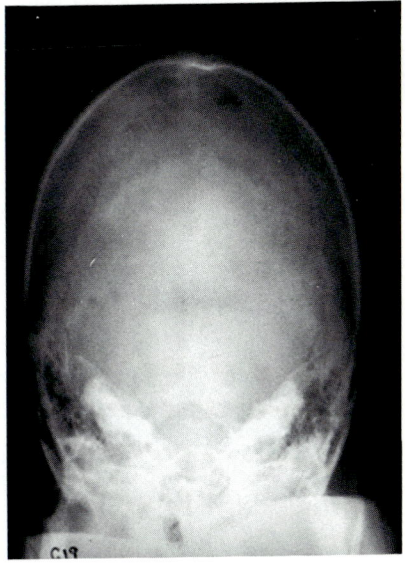

Figure 230.

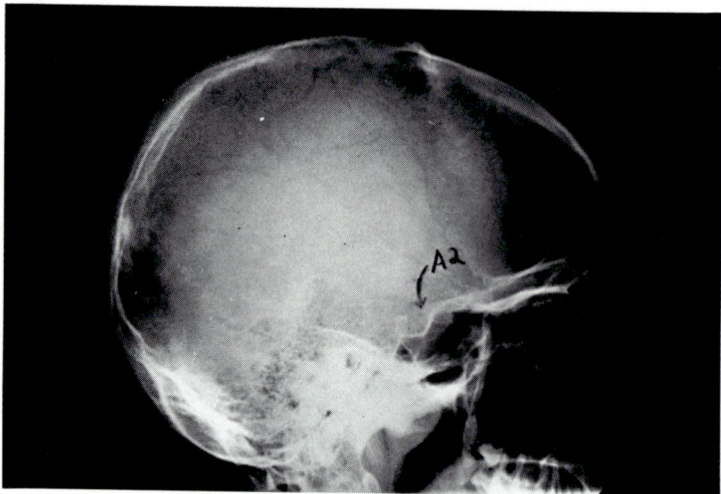

Figure 231.

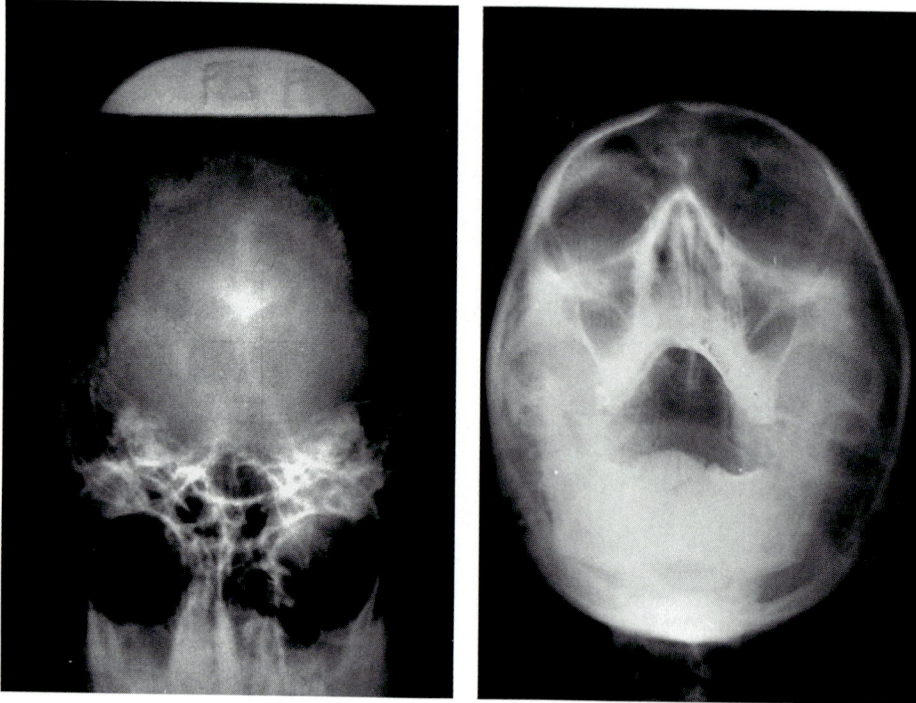

Figure 232.

Figure 233.

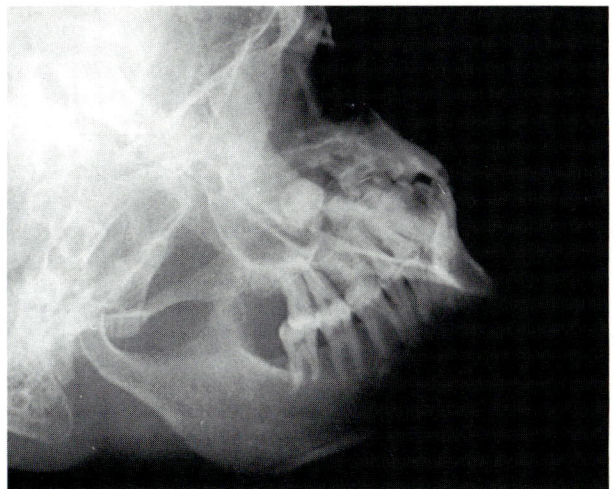

Figure 234.

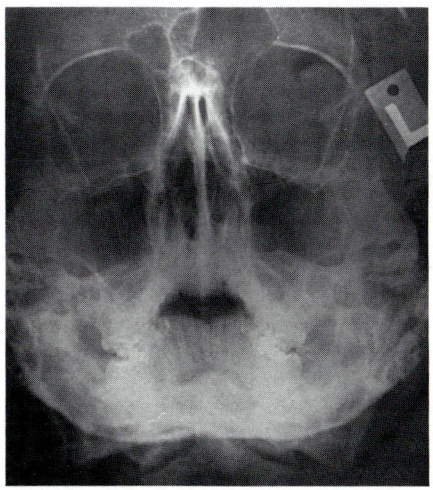

Figure 235.

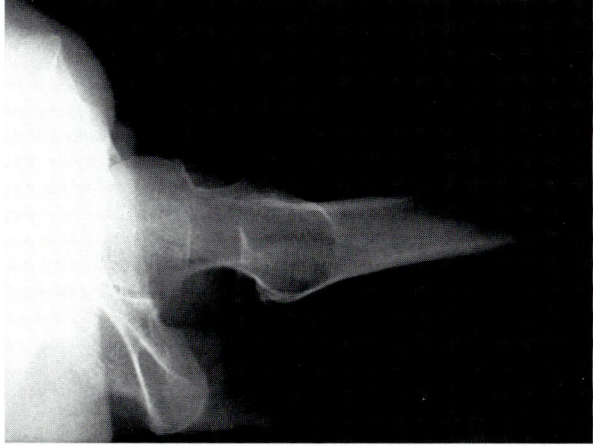

Figure 236.

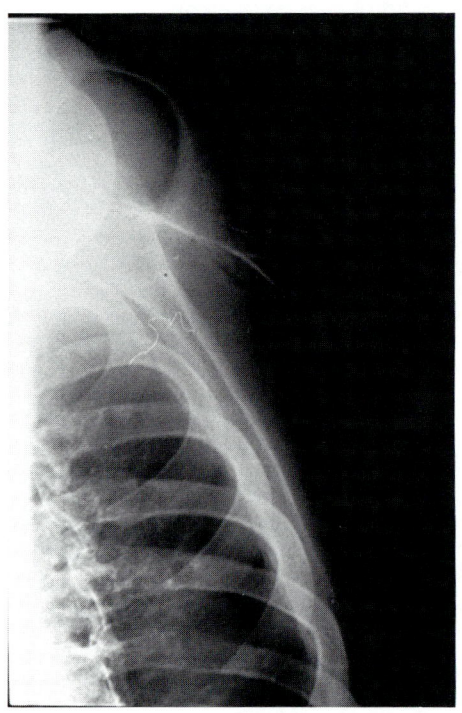

Figure 237.

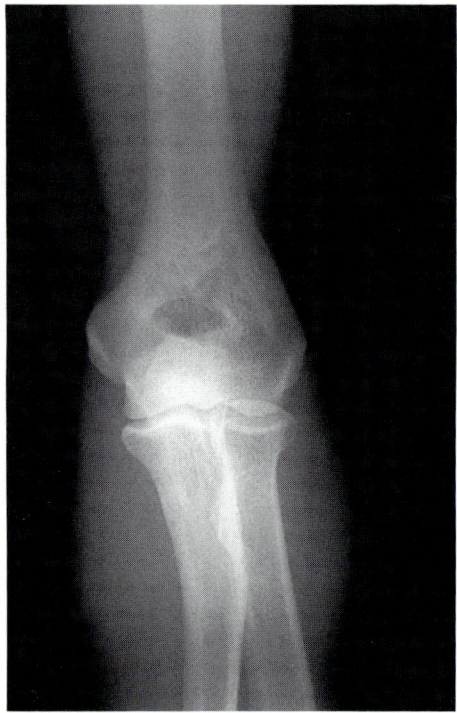

Figure 238.

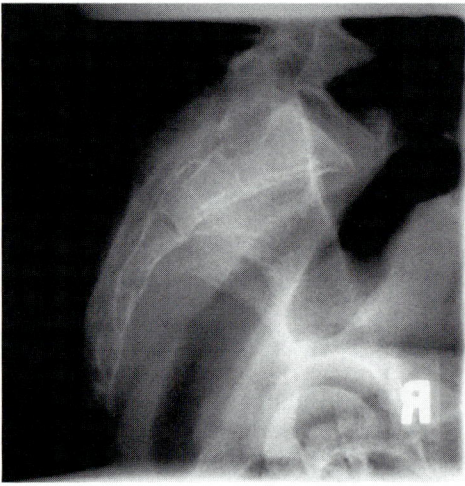

Figure 239.

PART III
TECHNICAL QUALITY

Chapter 10

DENSITY

RADIOGRAPHIC EVALUATION OF DENSITY

The *background* intensity on a radiograph is actually a transparent *white* shade—you see the light shining through its transparent plastic base. The image on it consists of blackened deposits of metallic silver left on the film after processing. The darkest areas represent the greatest exposure (intensity) of radiation striking the film. The amount of blackening present at any given point on the film is referred to as its *density*. Thus, a very dark film is regarded as having high density, and a lighter fflm as having low density. The densities on a film indicate the intensity of the beam of radiation which penetrated the patient and struck the film.

During their passage through a body part, the x-rays are absorbed selectively by various tissue components. This absorption results in the production of a number of *different* silver deposits on the radiograph. Obviously, the greater the number of tones present (correct tone rendition), the greater the number of structural details that can be visualized in the image.

Under standard conditions of illumination, highlights possessing little silver show little detail, and are diagnostically worthless. Also, areas of overexposure may be considered diagnostically useless since the opaqueness of the silver deposit obscures image details when the radiograph is viewed before the light from a standard x-ray illuminator (see Figure 240).

The opposite of density is *tone value.* Tone value refers to the amount of light (from an illuminator, for example) that is able to pass through the film at a given point and strike your eyes. If there is less silver deposited in an area of the film, more light will shine through it, it will appear *whiter* or clearer and has a high tone value. High tone value, then, is the same thing as low density. A device called a densitometer is used to measure the densities on radiographic films. What this device

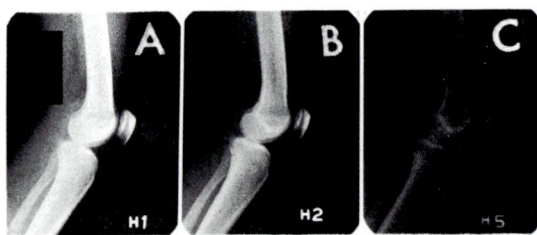

Figure 240. Series of radiographs demonstrating results of underexposure (A), correct exposure (B), and overexposure (C). Note the loss of visible details in the bones at both extremes.

actually does is to detect the amount of light passing through the film at a certain point. So it really measures tone value and then *converts* the measurement into a density reading algebraically. The density values read off of a densitometer range from 0 to 4.0, with a reading of 0 indicating that all of the light striking the film passes through it, and a reading of 4.0 indicating a pitch-black density with virtually no light passing through.

Since neither blank white areas nor pitch black areas on the radiograph contain useful information, those densities that might be considered as "useful" range from a very light gray shade (slightly darker than the film base) to a very dark gray shade just short of black. *This range of useful densities extends from 0.25 to 2.5 as measured on a densitometer.*

In determining appropriate radiographic techniques, we are primarily interested in the apparent *overall darkness* of the radiograph. We are concerned with the image densities *collectively* rather than with each individual shade of gray.

This apparent *overall* darkness of a radiograph is actually dependent upon the *average density.* Theoretically, the average density could be calculated by adding the density values of all shades of gray in the image and then dividing by the number of measurements taken. Figure 241 is a very simplified example comparing two radiographic images which each have only two shades of gray present. The *average density* is for radiograph A is found as $(1 + 2)/2 = 3/2 = 1.5$. The average for radiograph B is $(2 + 4)/2 = 6/2 = 3.0$. Radiograph B is precisely twice as dark as radiograph A.

In Figure 242 note that radiograph B might be described as "grayer" than radiograph A, yet both have the same average density. The average for radiograph A is $(1 + 4)/2 = 5/2 = 2.5$, while the average for radiograph B is $(2 + 3)/2 = 5/2 = 2.5$. "Grayness" is actually a function of

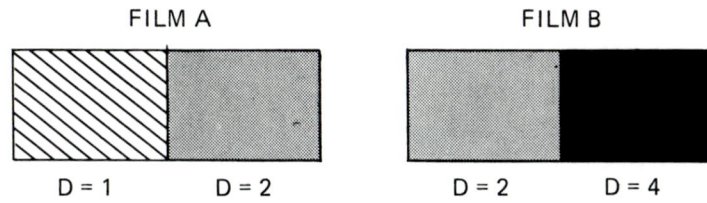

Figure 241. *Average density* for film *A* is $(2 + 1)/2 = 1.5$, while that for film *B* is $(4 + 2)/2 = 3.0$. Overall, film *B* is twice as dark as *A*.

radiographic *contrast,* which will be discussed in the next section, rather than a function of density. In Figure 242, radiograph B appears "grayer" because of a difference in contrast rather than overall density. In other words, a grayer image is not necessarily a darker image, nor is a darker image necessarily gray.

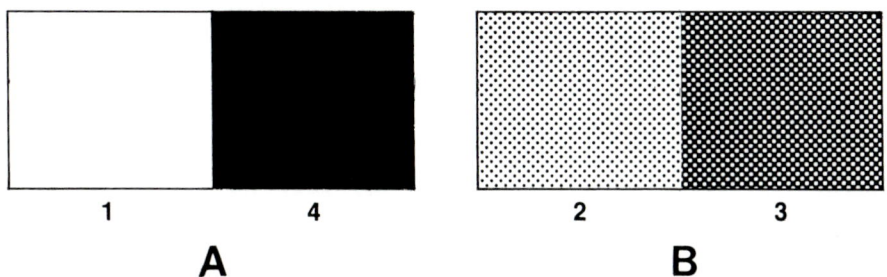

Figure 242. An image such as *B* might be described as "grayer" than *A*, yet have the same overall density. Average density for *A* is $(1 + 4)/2 = 2.5$. Average density for *B* is $(2 + 3)/2 = 2.5$.

Critiquing Radiographic Density

Radiographers must develop, primarily through experience, the ability to accurately assess the density level of the finished radiograph. This ability is *essential* to the control of unnecessary repeated exposures to the patient.

The single greatest technical cause for repeated exposures is improper density levels. Exposed radiographs that are either too light or too dark account for *73 percent* of all repeats in radiology departments without quality control programs, and for *33 percent* of all repeats in departments with quality control.

The exercise in the Review at the end of Part III is designed to help the student develop an ability to visually estimate the needed adjustment in overall technique when repeating an exposure that turned out too light or too dark.

Note that in determining technique adjustments for repeated exposures, it is much more common to *under*estimate the needed change in technique rather than overestimate it. For example, upon repeating a very light radiograph, many radiographers do not increase the technique enough. Although the second image may turn out with "passable" quality, it is frequently still light. Only rarely is the technique overcompensated resulting in a dark radiograph. Generally, then, radiographers need to be *less conservative,* and more daring, about adjusting techniques. Remember that there is no practical purpose in increasing technique by less than 50 percent or in decreasing it by less than 30 percent.

Critiquing Phototimed (Automatic Exposure Control) Density

In evaluating phototimed (automatic exposure controlled) radiographs, many of the rules for manual technique seem to work *backwards.* For example, anything which increases the amount of scatter radiation produced, such as opening the field size too much, results in a *light* radiograph rather than a dark one. One must remember that, in simplistic terms, the phototimer is designed to shut off the exposure when a preset amount of radiation is detected. When the photocells pick up additional scatter radiation, they shut off *sooner.* In effect, the phototimer "thinks" that the film is already dark enough and terminates the exposure early.

Figure 243 is a radiograph produced by improperly attempting to phototime a frontal view of the clavicle. The area of the photocell is drawn in to demonstrate that a small portion of the photocell extended above the patient's shoulder and was exposed to the "raw" x-ray beam. Receiving so much direct radiation, the phototimer "assumed" that the image was dark enough and shut off the exposure early. This resulted in a *light* radiograph. Peripheral anatomy which may not fully cover the photocell should never be phototimed.

The following phototiming errors result in light, *underexposed images:*

1. Phototiming *peripheral* anatomy (Figure 243)
2. Phototiming anatomy which is *too small* to fully cover the photocell(s) used

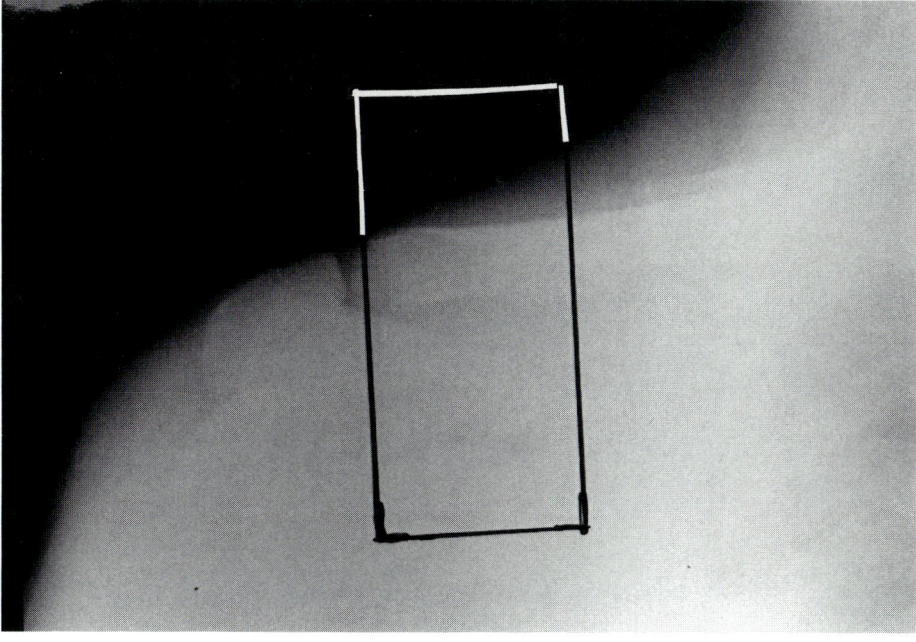

Figure 243. Automated exposure of clavicle with upper portion of photocell exposed to the raw x-ray beam, resulting in underexposure.

3. Phototiming anatomy in which the proper *centering* point results in the photocell not being fully covered with the *tissue of interest*
4. *Inadequate collimation* of the x-ray beam, resulting in large amounts of scatter radiation production
5. Use of *improper photocell configuration* (incorrect selection of the three available photocells)

The following phototiming errors result in dark, *overexposed images:*

1. Phototiming anatomy in which radiopaque *surgical hardware* is implanted (Figure 244)
2. Phototiming anatomy in which the proper *centering* point results in the photocell not being fully covered with the *tissue of interest*
3. Use of improper photocell configuration (incorrect selection of the three available photocells)

A common example of centering complications is the frontal chest view on a patient with pendulous breasts: With typical centering, the two side photocells may be placed over the lower breasts. This thicker anatomy results in the phototimer staying on longer and produces a chest

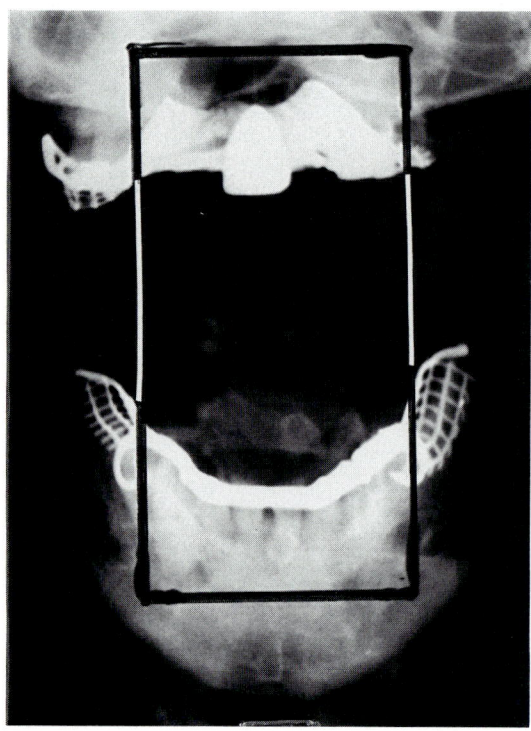

Figure 244. Automated exposure of odontoid projection. The photocell increased exposure time to average density between dental work and anatomy, resulting in overexposure to spine.

view with the lung fields much too dark. A repeated view centered 2 to 3 inches higher will often produce the correct density *with no* adjustment of the "density" knob. *It is not adequate to simply cover the photocells with any anatomy. The photocells must be covered with the tissue of interest* (in this case, the lungs).

Figure 244 illustrates the effect of hardware that cannot be removed. The metal dental devices completely absorbed the radiation in these areas. In effect, the phototimer "averages" the densities within the photocell area. The phototimer in this case stayed on longer in order to obtain some shade of gray under these metal devices. This resulted in an image much too dark for the odontoid process and upper cervical vertebrae.

Automatic exposure controls should only be used when proper positioning and centering will not be compromised. *Phototiming technique charts* are strongly recommended, listing the optimum kVp for each procedure, the correct photocell configuration to use, back-up time or back-up mAs and any notes for the density control knob setting. Automated exposure should *never* continue to be used when repeating a radiograph unless the radiographer fully understands the cause of the improper density and is confident in the adjustment needed. If there is any uncertainty in analyzing the original image, *manual technique* should be used for the repeated exposure.

Use of Wedge Filters

It seems that the use of wedge filters to balance image densities has declined over the years. Figures 147 and 151 demonstrate the impressive results when a wedge filter is used for frontal views of the calcaneus and the foot. The improved image quality and increased amount of diagnostic information are well worth the trouble. Use of a wedge filter is *strongly* recommended for the following views:

1. AP projection of the thoracic spine (thick end toward head)
2. AP projection of the foot (thick end toward toes)
3. PD projection of the calcaneus (thick end posterior)
4. Lateral fetogram (thick end anterior)

Technique must be increased whenever a wedge filter is used, the amount depending on the filter's thickness. As a rule of thumb, *increase 8 to 10 kVp* from normal technique for the wedge filter.

VARIABLES AFFECTING DENSITY

It is outside the scope of this text to analyze the many subtle implications of changing each radiographic variable, and good textbooks on radiographic exposure fully discuss these. A very brief review of those factors directly bearing upon image density is in order. Suppose, for example, that a radiograph were much too light, and on repeating the exposure it were desired to double the image density. Several options might achieve this, including doubling the mA, doubling the exposure time, increasing the kVp by 15 percent, reducing the FFD by 25 to 33 percent, or using a faster intensifying screen speed.

Following is a listing and brief descriptions of the major factors bearing on image density.

Milliamperage

Milliamperage is directly proportional to image density. For example, doubling the mA from 100 to 200 will double the apparent darkness of the radiograph, if all other factors are kept constant and no compensations are made.

Exposure Time

Exposure time is also directly proportional to density. If no compensation is made, increasing the time from 1/20 second to 1/10 second, or from 0.35 to 0.7 second, will double the density.

Milliampere-Seconds (mAs)

The total mAs controls the total density resulting on the film in a directly proportional fashion. Doubling the mAs doubles the density. To see a visible difference in image density, mAs must be altered by at least 1/4 or 25 percent. *The total mAs is the prime factor for controlling image density,* because it does not directly affect other image qualities.

Kilovoltage-Peak

Kilovoltage-peak directly affects image density, according to the *15-percent rule:* A 15 percent increase in kVp causes twice as dark a radiograph (100 percent darker). A 15 percent decrease in kVp results in an image one-half as dark.

Two useful correlaries follow: An 8 percent increase in kVp increases density by one-half or 50 percent, and a 5 percent change in kVp is the minimum required to see a visible difference in image density.

Optimum kVp, however, is essential to allow the production of adequate density: kVp affects density because it controls the *proportion* of the original x-rays which are able to penetrate through the body and reach the film. Adequate density cannot be produced without sufficient penetration.

Machine Phase and Rectification

The type of electrical generators and rectifiers used in x-ray equipment affects the output intensity of the x-ray beam, as well as its average energy, and directly bears upon the resulting density of the image. Operated at the same mAs, three-phase equipment produces twice the density when compared to single-phase machines.

Constant potential generators such as battery-powered mobile units, and high-frequency generators can be equal to or somewhat higher than three-phase units in their efficiency. They often require less kVp to obtain the same density levels.

Compensating Filtration

Compensating filters, such as wedges and troughs, are specifically designed to even out the density on radiographs of anatomy with irregular thickness or absorption characteristics. These filters are as much as five times thicker than protective filtration, and thus result in visible density effects. They can be used to advantage on irregular anatomy to produce more consistent densities across the radiograph.

Field Size Limitation

Collimation of the field size to smaller, confined areas results in a loss of image density. Density may drop by one-third to one-half, depending on how drastic the change is, and should be compensated for by a corresponding increase in mAs.

Patient Condition

Larger body part thicknesses result in a loss of image density, simply because more radiation is absorbed within the patient and less reaches the film. The *four-centimeter rule* should be used to compensate for deviations in patient thickness from the average of 22 cm measured anterior-to-posterior and 30 cm laterally. For every increase of 4 cm, mAs should be doubled. For patients who are thinner than average, cut mAs in half for every 4 cm.

The radiographer must be observant of body habitus, anthropological factors and condition in deriving appropriate techniques to maintain density. Large muscular patients require a much greater increase in technique than hypersthenic patients. Fluid distention requires more technique than obesity. Brachicephalic skulls often require more technique than average. Expiration chest radiographs require more exposure than the normal inspiratory views.

Additive diseases which increase the bone or fluid component of tissue result in a loss of image density, and require increases in technique, typically from one-third to one-half again as much. Destructive diseases which reduce bone or fluid content, or which increase gas or fat content, result in dark images and necessitate a technique reduction. Casts and splints will result in inadequate image density unless technique is increased to compensate for them. Plaster casts require from 2 to 4 times the average technique, while half-casts, wood splints and similar devices require a 50 percent increase.

Extraneous Fog

Scattered radiation, from whatever source, always increases overall image density, and can thus contribute to overexposure. Since fog density is always destructive to the image, field size limitation, optimum kVp, grids, leaded masking sheets, and other methods must be used to control it.

Fogging of the radiograph can also occur from accidental exposure to light, heat or chemical fumes. All fog results in undesirable, darker density.

Grids

The use of grids always lightens the radiographic density unless compensated for. The higher the grid ratio, the more severe the loss of image density. The recommended compensation is an increase in mAs from 2 to 5 times that of a nongrid, tabletop technique, depending on grid ratio.

Misuse of grids can lead to grid cut-off, an unacceptable loss of density over particular regions of the radiograph. Causes of grid cut-off include off-angling, off-centering, FFD outside of the grid radius and grids placed upside down.

Image Receptor Systems

The use of intensifying screens always enhances radiographic density and allows the reduction of patient exposure by compensated techniques. If technique is not compensated, then the higher the speed of the screen, the darker the resulting image density. Special gradient screens can be used to even out the density for radiographs of body parts with irregular thicknesses. Specific speeds and technique adjustments can be obtained from the screen manufacturers and should be followed. Film must also be appropriately matched to the screen system used in accordance with manufacturers' recommendations. The faster the film speed, the darker the density.

Anode Heel Effect

The anode heel effect results in a slight loss of density toward the end of the film nearest the x-ray tube anode. This is used to advantage for wedge-shaped anatomy by placing the thinnest anatomy toward the anode, but is detrimental to radiographs of regular anatomy.

Focus-Film Distance (FFD)

Image density is inversely related to distances in an exponential fashion. This relationship follows the *inverse square law*. Density will be inversely proportional to the square of the change in distance. For example, doubling the distance results in one-fourth the image density.

Object-Film Distance (OFD)

Dramatic changes in object-image receptor distance can cause visible differences in image density. The larger the OID, the less the resulting density.

Processing

If an exposed radiographic film is developed for too long, at too high a temperature, or in chemicals that are too concentrated, it will turn out dark.

Chapter 11

CONTRAST AND GRAY SCALE

RADIOGRAPHIC EVALUATION OF CONTRAST AND GRAY SCALE

In order to see, there must be differing shades of brightness and darkness within your field of view. The greater the difference is between the shade of an object and the shade of the surrounding field of view, the easier it is to see the object. A pure black object against a white background, for example, is a most visible combination. This difference between intensities of reflected light is called *contrast*. For contrast to exist, hence for any image at all to exist, there must be two or more different intensities present. If the differences between the intensities is great, then the image is regarded as having *high contrast*. Some contrast is required for any image to exist.

However, it is possible for an image to have *too much* contrast. This situation is illustrated by the photographs in Figure 245. In photograph *A*, note that you cannot distinguish the edges between the girl's blouse and the background wall, the edges between the stuffed animal and the girl's blouse, or the ruffles in the blouse. These details are visible in photograph *B*. Photograph *A* possesses extremely high contrast—everything in the image tends to be reduced to either black or white, with very few intermediate shades of gray. Objects that should have been depicted as a very light gray, such as the ruffles and shadows of the blouse, are recorded instead as white, and are not discernable against a background of white. Likewise, dark gray objects are depicted as black and will not be distinguishable against a black background. This image has less visible details in it than photograph *B*. Excessive contrast has caused a loss of useful information.

On the other hand, insufficient contrast leads to an image that is not adequately visible. If there is barely any difference between two adjacent shades of gray, it will be difficult for the human eye to detect that there are indeed two shades there. If these gray shades cannot be distinguished

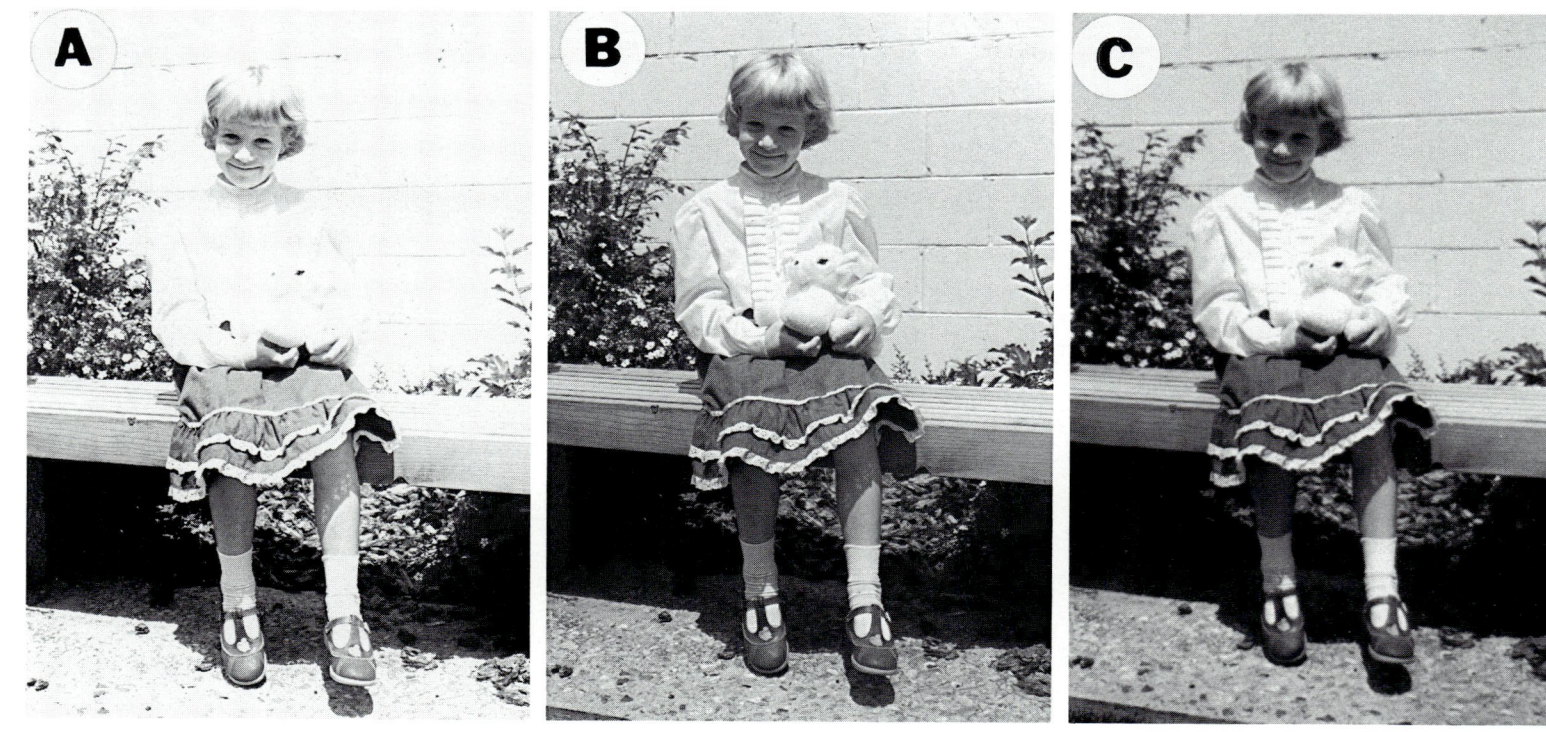

Figure 245. Photographs demonstrating (A) high contrast with short gray scale, (B) medium contrast with longer gray scale, and (C) low contrast with excessive gray scale. Note that details visible in the stuffed animal, blouse and sidewalk disappear with excessive contrast (A). Darker gray details in the leaves, the shadow under the bench and the girl's eyebrows disappear with excessive gray scale (C). Also, note that high contrast can deceptively mimic underexposure: Photograph A appears light at a glance, yet the shadow under the bench is actually *darker* than that in B. The overall density of Photograph A is *not* light, rather it possesses excessive contrast.

from each other, information is again lost. Photograph *C* in Figure 245 demonstrates insufficient contrast, with an overall gray appearance. Note that the subtle dark gray shades of leaves under the bench, visible in photograph *B*, are not as visible in photograph *C*, because there is little difference between them and the dark shadow of the bench.

To summarize, note that the greatest amount of information in Figure 245 is found in photograph *B*, where the contrast level is intermediate. If contrast is too high, gray shades are exaggerated into white or black, and information is lost. If contrast is too low, different gray shades that lie next to each other become difficult to distinguish, and again, information is lost. Excessive contrast can cause as great a loss of information as a lack of contrast. The ideal amount of contrast to maximize the information in an image lies in an intermediate range and is somewhat subject to personal preference.

The word *optimum* is used to describe the ideal level of contrast that an image should have. It refers to an intermediate level which is neither too much nor too little. In radiographic imaging, the goal is not to produce *maximum* contrast, nor *minimum* contrast, but rather to produce *optimum* contrast. The same term should be used to describe the ideal intensity of light for an image: Too little light would be pitch dark, too much would blind us. The ideal amount of light is a medium amount that we would refer to as *optimum intensity.*

Contrast Versus Gray Scale

Radiographic *contrast* is the proportional difference between two adjacent densities, measured as a ratio, not as a subtracted difference. If one density is twice as dark as the adjacent density, the contrast would be measured as 2/1 or 2. A very contrasty radiograph appears to be more *black and white*, whereas a low-contrast radiograph appears to be gray overall. Figure 246 shows how density levels can change without contrast being affected. Note that as long as all densities on the film increase or decrease by the same proportion, the ratios of difference between them remain the same and contrast is equal.

The opposite of radiographic contrast is *gray scale*. There is considerable confusion about the difference between contrast and scale, primarily because of the terminology commonly used. The term *contrast scale* is sometimes used, but combining the word *contrast* with *scale* seems contradictory and is certainly confusing. This book shall

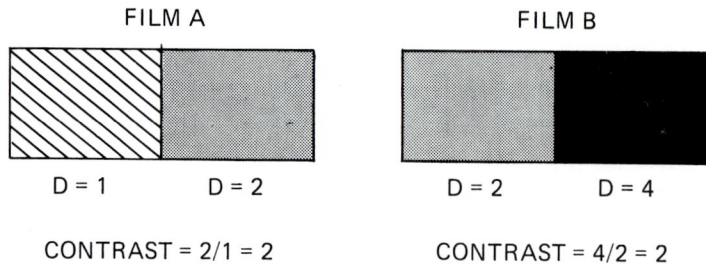

Figure 246. Diagram illustrating a change in density without a change in contrast. The ratio of difference between the two adjacent densities remains the same even though *Film B* is twice as dense overall.

consistently utilize the terms *gray scale* or *scale* to refer to this image quality.

Radiographic gray scale is the *range* of different densities present in an image. When there are many different shades of density (many grays), the radiograph has long scale. Conversely, when few densities are present, the radiograph has short scale. To understand the relationship between contrast and gray scale, consider a 10-foot-high staircase. The staircase may be built to have 10 individual stairs, each one being one foot tall, or it may be built to have only five individual stairs. If there are only five stairs, each one must be two feet tall—there is a greater difference between the stairs. A greater difference from one stair to the next results in fewer total stairs. Conversely, if there are many stairs, there must be a smaller degree of difference from one to the next. With this staircase concept in mind, examine the *aggregate silver deposits* diagrammed in Figures 247 and 248. High contrast implies short scale, because when there are great differences between densities, there can only be a few densities present (Figure 247). With low contrast, there will be long scale (Figure 248).

A good radiograph is one that possesses a correct balance of densities (gradation) over the entire gray scale. The contrast should be such that, with prevailing exposure technics, good differentiation is shown between tissue details portrayed over the whole area of diagnostic interest, without loss of detail in the lighter or darker areas of the radiographic image.

The scale of densities that determines the contrast and the visibility of details is directly influenced by the x-ray wave length which, in turn, is regulated by the factor of kilovoltage. This fact is also demonstrated by Figures 247 and 248. An aluminum stepwedge is shown being irradiated by x-rays; the exposed x-ray film in enlarged cross section is shown

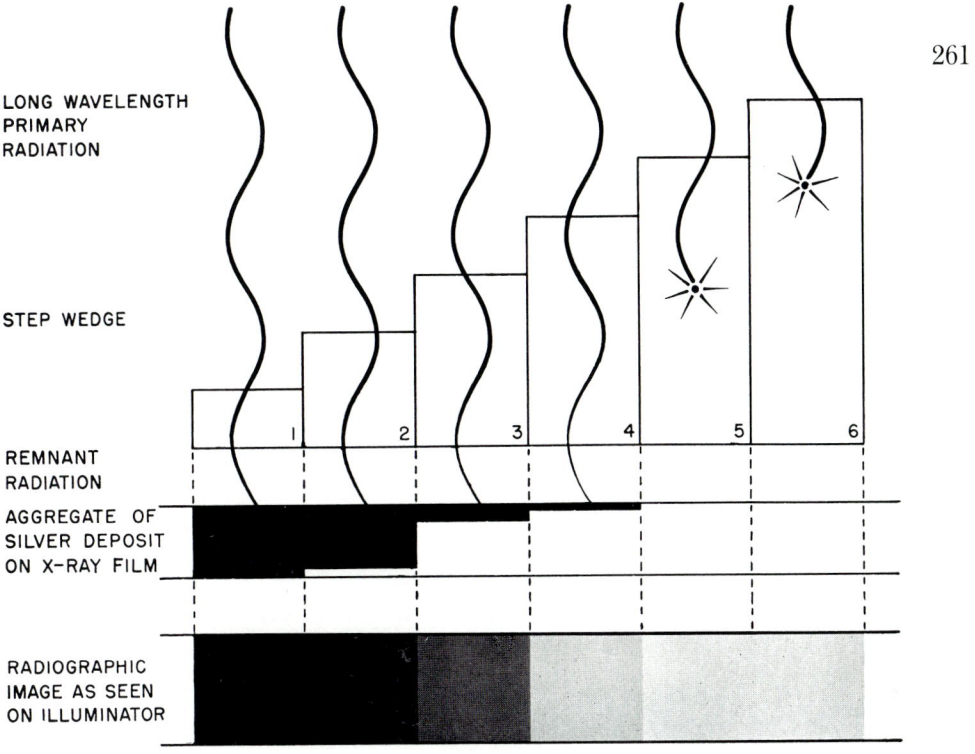

LONG WAVELENGTH
PRIMARY
RADIATION

STEP WEDGE

REMNANT
RADIATION

AGGREGATE OF
SILVER DEPOSIT
ON X-RAY FILM

RADIOGRAPHIC
IMAGE AS SEEN
ON ILLUMINATOR

SHORT SCALE

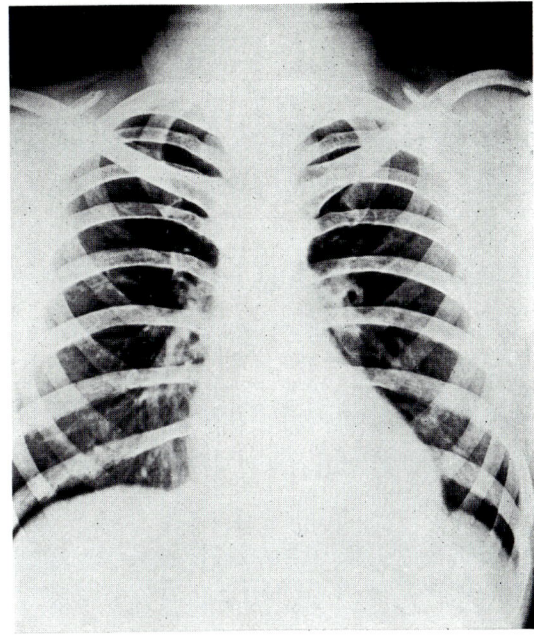

Figure 247. Step-wedge diagram and radiograph illustrating short gray scale.

262

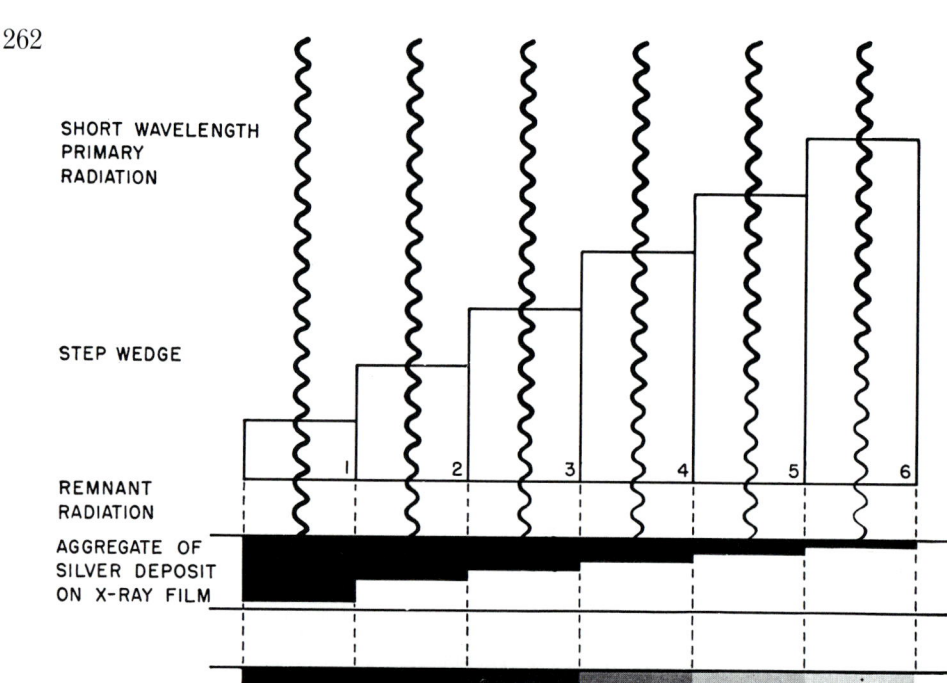

SHORT WAVELENGTH
PRIMARY
RADIATION

STEP WEDGE

REMNANT
RADIATION

AGGREGATE OF
SILVER DEPOSIT
ON X-RAY FILM

RADIOGRAPHIC
IMAGE AS SEEN
ON ILLUMINATOR

LONG SCALE

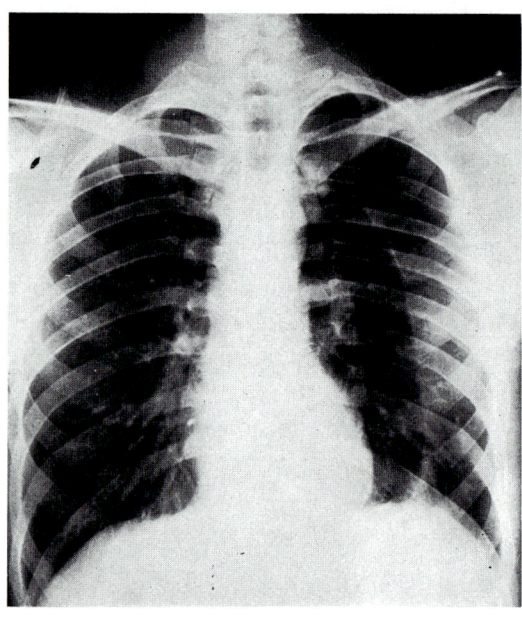

Figure 248. Step-wedge diagram and radiograph illustrating long gray scale.

beneath the step-wedge; and the resulting radiographic image as it appears when viewed on the illuminator is depicted below the film cross section in both illustrations.

Short Scale

The diagram in Figure 247 illustrates the fact that radiographic details of an object cannot be seen in the image unless there are discernible differences in tone value between densities and that there must be a silver deposit on the film if a detail within the object is to be demonstrated. The above situation is typical for *short scale* or high contrast.

When an image of a body part is rendered with densities that are either excessive or virtually nonexistent with a short range of widely different intermediate translucent densities, short scale exists. Such radiographs are pictorially pleasing to look at, for they possess instant eye appeal but they have little diagnostic worth and are economically wasteful.

When low kilovoltage is used for thin tissue parts such as the hand, elbow, etc., greater contrast occurs between the bones and the flesh. In fact, a point may be reached in which the thinner portions such as the skin and subcutaneous tissues and even some muscle detail are obliterated by opaque silver deposits; and, some bone detail may also be lost because the denser bone tissue absorbs so much radiation that little remnant radiation reaches the film. Even when exposures are increased to impractical limits by the mAs factor in order to obtain satisfactory bone detail, opaque silver deposits will still obscure details of the less dense fleshy areas.

On the other hand, when the exposure is decreased to exhibit flesh details satisfactorily, then osseous details are lost. In other words, as kilovoltage is decreased, the number of intermediate tones diminishes and the over-all amount of information diminishes in the same ratio. So only those details in the image produced by exposure factors that happen to be optimum for the area are rendered with maximum visibility and the remainder of the image becomes diagnostically useless.

There are occasions when it seems advisable to shorten the gray scale in a specific area but when this is done, there is always that danger of losing detail visibility in other adjacent areas. On the whole, the entire image exhibiting short scale is invariably incomplete, for details that represent the thinner and thicker portions of the body part are not always shown. Short scale has its place only as a special procedure and in more adequately visualizing details of *small* tissue areas and then only after preliminary survey radiographs have been made. Typical examples of short scale are shown in Figure 249.

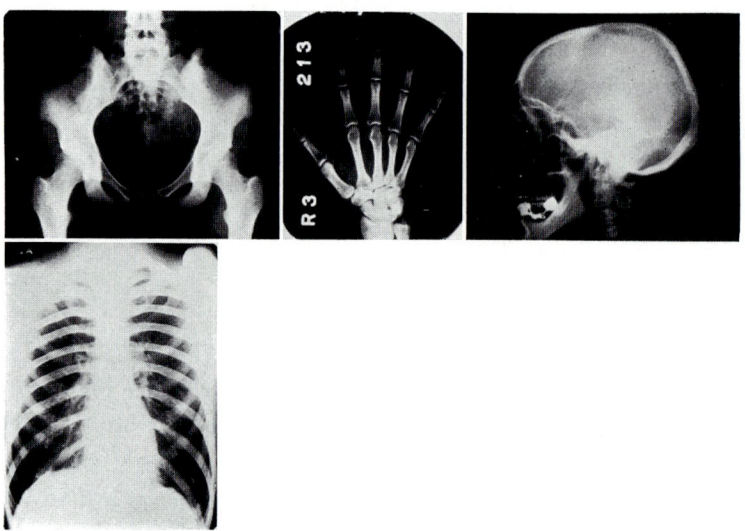

Figure 249. Typical radiographs exhibiting various degrees of short gray scale.

Long Scale

Portraying the same situation as shown in Figure 247, but using *shorter wave length radiation,* the diagram, Figure 248, exhibits a different result. The radiation readily penetrates all portions of the wedge and the selective degree of absorption by each step has permitted remnant radiation to emerge with different intensities that are recorded as separate translucent densities. These densities of varying tone value represent the several steps in the wedge. The transition between tones is gradual and each tone is distinctive. The image is completely informative and is typical of long scale. Desirable long scale is produced when the kilovoltage is adjusted to delineate all normal structures satisfactorily. Absorption of radiation by the silver bromide crystals decreases as the kilovoltage increases and when exposures are correct there is little opportunity to produce excessive densities in the image.

In the case of human radiography, when the scale of densities representing a departure from the normal occurs, the image becomes open to pathologic or physiologic suspicion. In the final analysis, the criterion of good diagnostic contrast is whether one sees all one expects to see.

Compare the radiographs shown in Figures 247 and 248 with the photographs in Figure 245.

Long scale is characterized by a large number of translucent densities of varying tone value, each of which represents some structural element of the part examined. The transition between tones is gradual. Long scale makes possible visualization of small units of image density. The short wave length radiation employed effects greater penetration of the tissues resulting in an abundance of remnant radiation of varying intensity that, in turn, produces a large number of translucent densities (Figure 248). The gray scale, however, should never be so long that differentiation between structures is difficult. If the maximum of diagnostic information is to be obtained in the survey film, a compromise must be made between the radiograph with short scale or that exhibiting the longer scale. Typical examples of long scale are shown in Figure 250.

A medium level of contrast will allow the most information to be visible on a radiograph. Too much contrast can cause the loss of information, just as too much gray scale can do the same.

Figure 251 uses magnetic resonance images of the spine to illustrate these important concepts: Images **A** and **B** both have too short of a gray scale (excessive contrast). **A** was taken with a lighter overall density level, and **B** with a much darker setting, in order to show that *the use of a lighter or darker technique does not correct the image when gray scale is insufficient.* Images **C** and **D** were taken with long gray scale, using similar density settings. Although **C** is light and **D** is dark, *both* of these images demonstrate more details and more information than **A** or **B**. The ideal image would be a relatively long gray scale image with a density level intermediate between **C** and **D**.

VARIABLES AFFECTING CONTRAST AND GRAY SCALE

Kilovoltage-Peak

Kilovoltage-Peak (kVp) should be considered as the prime factor for controlling radiographic image contrast and gray scale. It does so both through its effect upon x-ray beam *penetration* and upon the *proportion of scatter radiation reaching the film.* At higher kVp levels, more different types of tissue are penetrated by the x-ray beam and recorded as shades of gray. With more shades of gray present in the image, there is a smaller degree of difference from one shade to the next, therefore, contrast

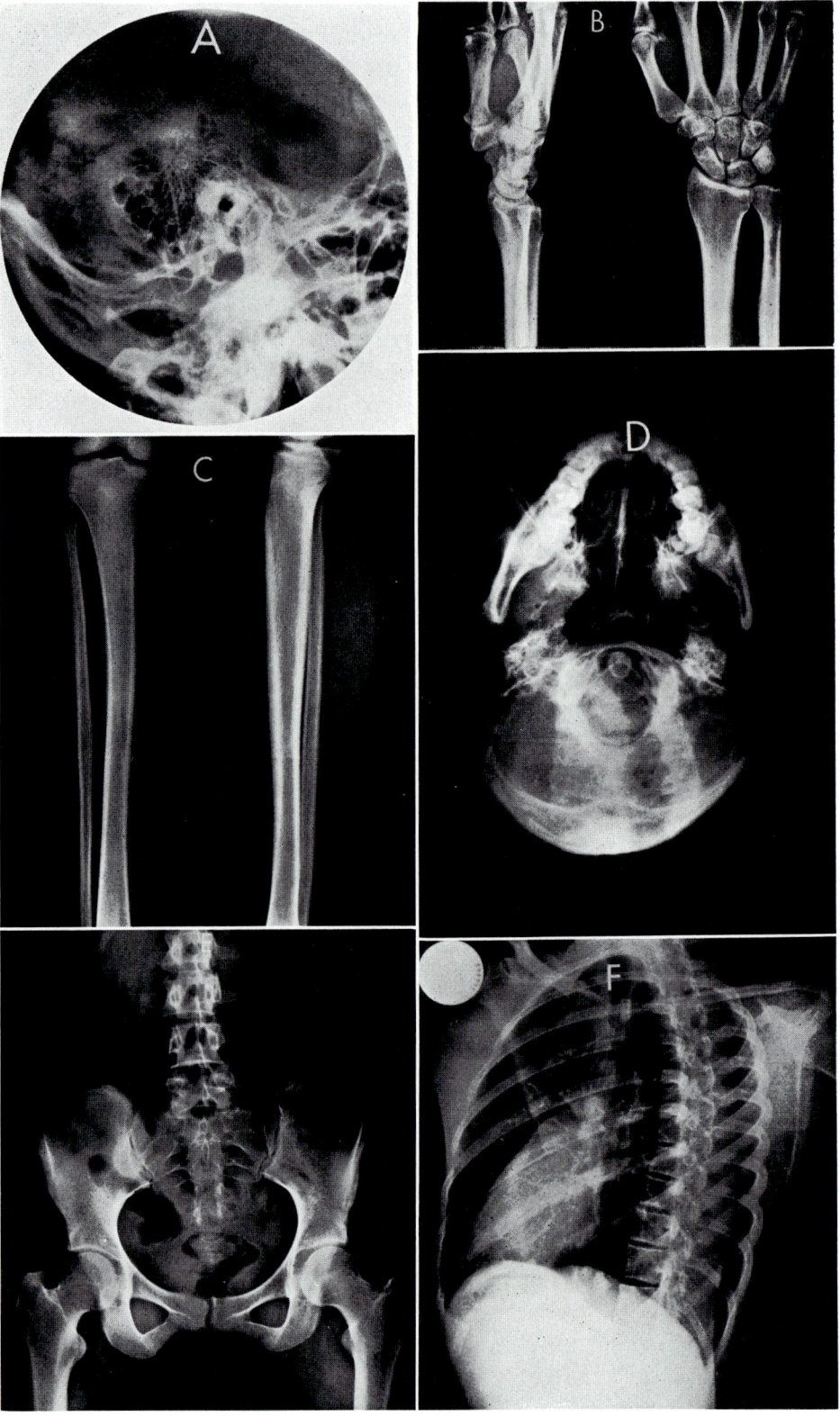

Figure 250. Typical radiographs exhibiting long gray scale. An abundance of details is shown because the kilovoltages used were optimum for the projection.

Patholog

Muscu
tissues, a
scatter, e
effects in

Extraneo

Anythi
the patie
interactic
caused fr
destroys i

An im
When all
will be a
light shad
dark gray

Fog is c
the next c

Grids

Grids
contrast w
exposed t
nate muc
higher the
the highe

Intensifyi

Because
fying scre
technique:
contrast in
the case. S
have on i
mary conc

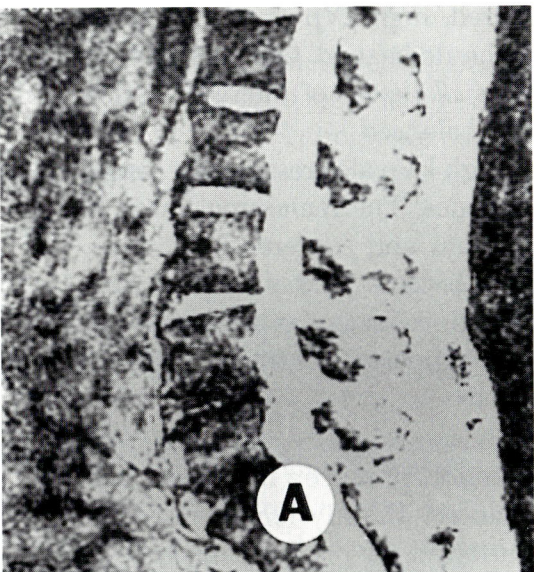
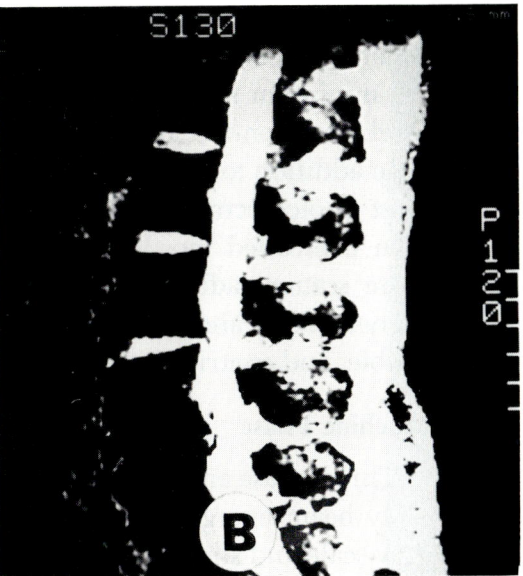
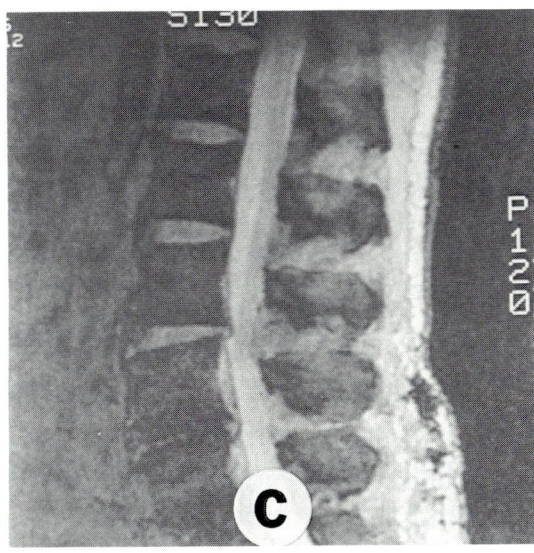
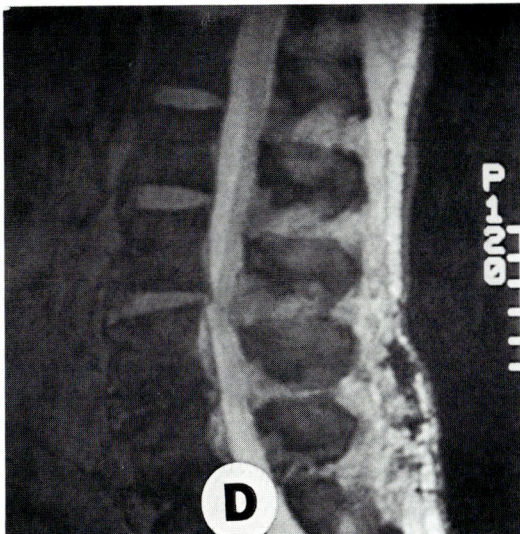

Figure 251. Magnetic Resonance images of the spine showing (A) short gray scale and light density, (B) short gray scale and dark density, (C) long gray scale and light density, and (D) long gray scale and dark density.

ded
Wh
the
lev

I
mo
the
mo
hig
visi

Ma

T
x-ra
gra

Fiel

V
enh
but
the

Pati

V
scatt
mas:
niqu
this
radi

C
ing
agen
opti
throu
are l
mize

Radiographic Film

Generally, higher-speed films also produce higher image contrast. Film can be chemically treated to produce either longer gray scale or higher contrast, according to the needs of the diagnostician. The recommendations of manufacturers should be strictly followed when matching films and screens to obtain a desired image quality.

Object-Film Distance (OFD)

When the OFD is increased, leaving a gap between the body and the film, scattered radiation produced within the tissues and emitted at random angles is allowed to diverge more before reaching the film, in accordance with the inverse square law. The divergence of the primary beam, however, is unaffected by a change in OFD. Hence, the concentration of scattered rays is reduced while the primary beam remains at the same intensity. A smaller proportion of the resulting image will be composed of fog, and contrast will increase. The intentional use of a large OFD for the purpose of enhancing contrast is called the *air gap technique.*

Motion

Motion should not be considered as a *controlling* factor for image contrast. If it is severe enough, however, it can reduce contrast because of the superimposition of different densities across the image. This process is explained in Chapter 16.

Processing

There are optimum times, temperatures and chemical concentrations for processing radiographic film. Although slight increases in any of these may increase contrast, excessive development time, temperature or chemical action will fog the film and destroy contrast as a rule.

Chapter 12

FOG AND NOISE

RADIOGRAPHIC EVALUATION OF FOG AND NOISE

One more factor affects the visibility of an object in your field of view: If it is raining heavily between yourself and the object, you may not be able to see it well. The rain represents unwanted information which obstructs the visibility of the wanted information. Undesirable information that interferes with the subject of interest is referred to as *noise.* Interference and static on your TV screen are examples of noise in an image. In radiography, fogging of the film by heat or light, static discharges and artifacts from foreign objects are forms of noise. The most common form of image noise in radiography is fogging of the film by random radiation known as *scatter.*

When a primary beam of x-rays traverses an object, some of the x-rays are absorbed while others pass directly through it; a considerable percentage, however, is scattered in all directions by the atoms of the material struck—very much as light is dispersed by a mist (Figure 252). These secondary rays comprise what is known as *scatter radiation* and are radiographically effective. Scatter radiation strikes the film from random directions and produces a fairly uniform deposit of silver over an *entire* image. This veil of silver overlays the image density produced by the remnant radiation and is, in reality, a form of noise known as scatter *fog.* When fog is present, the effect is as if image details were being viewed through a mist. In other words, the quality of the image is degraded. A radiographic example of scattered radiation fog is shown in Figure 253-B. Observe (1) the characteristic dull gray appearance of the images and (2) the absence of important details.

Virtually the whole question of radiographic quality is related to the effect of scatter radiation fog on the visualization of detail. Its effect is greatest on those elements of an object that are farthest from the film. Visibility of these details may be greatly lessened and on occasion they may not even appear in the image. By controlling the amount of scatter

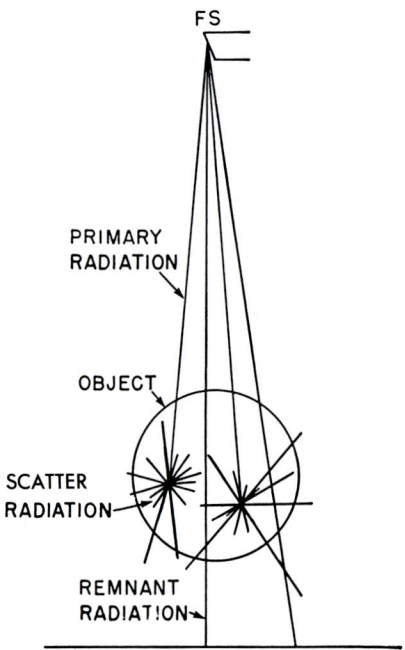

Figure 252. Diagram illustrating manner in which scatter radiation is generated when x-rays strike any form of matter.

radiation reaching the film during an exposure, details become more pronounced with resultant improvement in image quality. Rendition of all anatomic details, then, becomes more in accord with the actual absorption properties of the tissues irradiated. Also, reduction in fog makes possible easier visualization of details representing small differences in tissue absorption.

The scatter radiation reaching the film has more of the quality of the longer wave lengths (lesser penetration) than the remnant radiation. Its intensity is modified either (1) by the *absorbing action* of the tissues through which it must pass, or (2) by the *distance* from the film to its origin in the tissues. Scatter radiation originates from a multiplicity of sources and is, therefore, unfocused and random. Even with present-day accessories, it is not always possible to control it completely. The supplemental density superimposed by this radiation on the image is like a veil; it actually increases the over-all density of the image and limits the ability to see radiographic details clearly. In fact *a desirable range of densities (gray scale) is usually destroyed and important detail is obscured by this common form of image noise.*

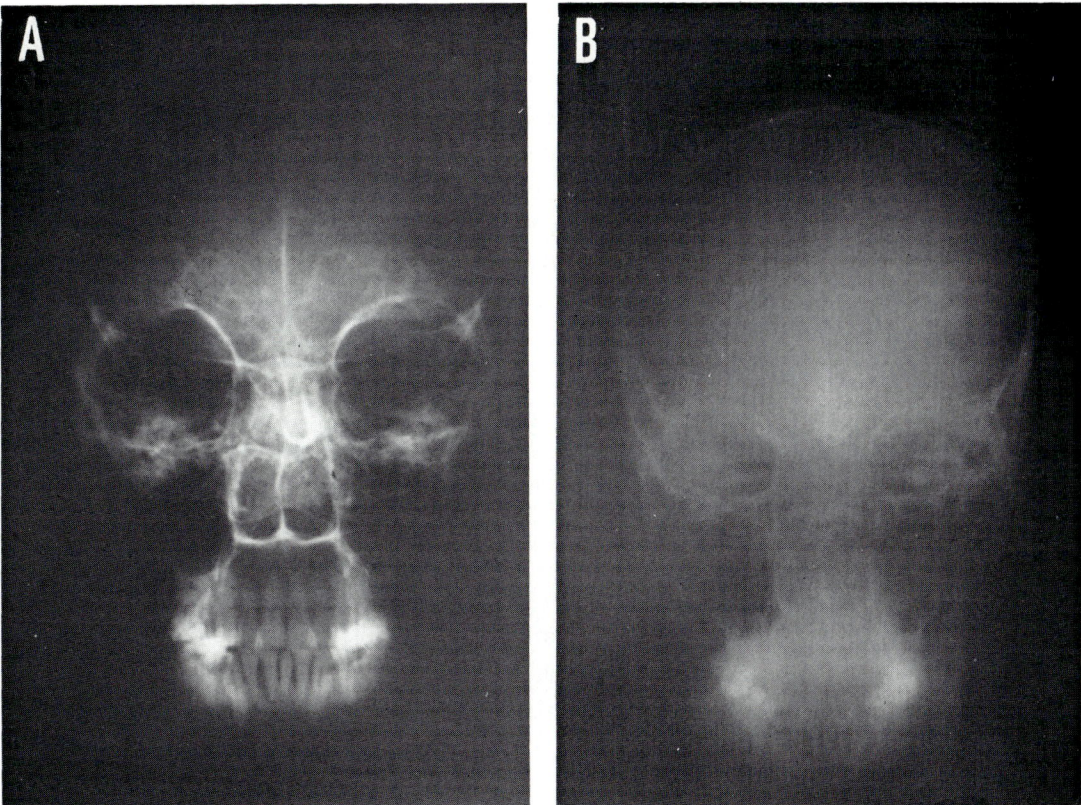

Figure 253. Radiographs demonstrating the difference in appearance between an overexposed image (A) and a fogged image (B). Note that a fogged image can be lighter in overall density (as at the top portion of this skull).

Gray Scale, Fog and Density

It is essential to understand that every "gray" radiograph is not necessarily fogged. Long gray scale is often desirable in an image. Fog is never desirable. Yet, both make the image appear more "gray." Long gray scale can improve the image, or in excessive amounts it can degrade the image, but fog is *always* destructive.

When gray scale is increased, contrast is reduced. But, when fogging occurs, *both gray scale and contrast are reduced.* This is possible because fog is a *blanket* of density which covers *every* useful density on the radiograph. Therefore, those densities which should have been a very light gray shade are completely lost to the image as the fog darkens them, and there are less densities altogether present.

It is quite easy to confuse an overexposed *burned-out* radiograph with a fogged radiograph, so it is important to understand that a darker film is not necessarily a *fogged* one. Fogging is caused by scattered radiation. It is possible to simply overexpose a film with too much radiation without scatter levels changing. Figure 253 shows the difference between an overexposed radiograph and a fogged radiograph. Note that a fogged radiograph is not necessarily very dark but can be quite light and still present a *washed-out* gray, low-contrast appearance. An excessively dark film may be simply overexposed, or it may be both overexposed and fogged.

Desirable Gray Scale Versus Fog

Gray scale is a desirable, *indeed an essential,* component of the radiographic image. Any portion of the image which is blank white presents *no* information at all (except at its edges), and is diagnostically useless. (Figure 254 illustrates such a radiograph, with unpenetrated barium in the stomach.) The same may be said for portions of an image that are pitch black—they are diagnostically useless. The ideal radiograph possesses a range of gray shades from a very dark gray to a very light gray, with no blank areas. This means that every type of tissue depicted must be at least partially penetrated by the x-ray beam.

Optimum kVp results in at least some penetration of the beam through *all* tissues, resulting in a fairly long gray scale. An image with long gray scale has many different shades of gray and depicts many different types of tissue. *Quantitatively, an image with long gray scale has more information in it than a short-scale image.* Of course, gray scale can be *too* long, but unless all tissues are penetrated to some degree, the gray scale is too short.

Fairly long gray scale is, therefore, desirable. Such images contain much information, but are not immediately appealing to the eye. They have an overall gray appearance. It is important to understand that the apparent "grayness" of such an image is *not due to fog.* Figure 255 compares an unfogged image with long gray scale to a fogged image. Not every "gray" radiograph is a fogged radiograph. Optimally long gray scale is desirable, fog is not.

Gray scale is, by definition, the opposite of contrast. *Image contrast is reduced at a higher kVp. This would be true whether scattered radiation were present or not.* Fog can, however, *contribute* to lower image contrast in a very destructive way. There are several ways in which an image

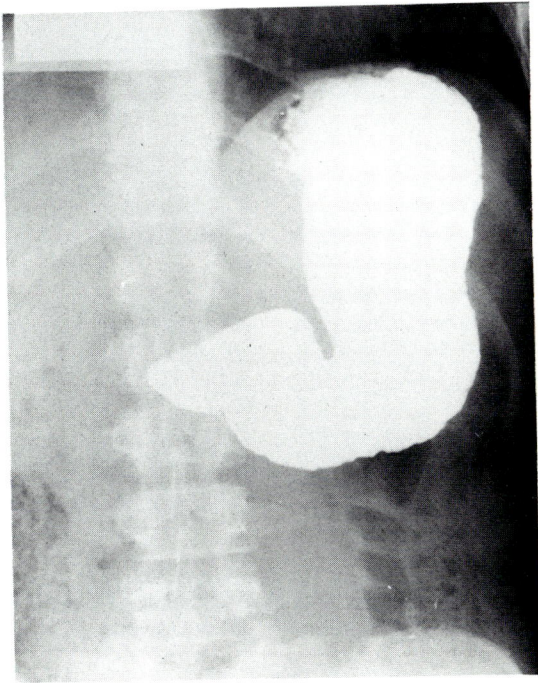

Figure 254. Radiograph of barium-filled stomach taken with 80 kVp. Note that with inadequate penetration through the barium, the only details visible in the stomach are those at the very edge of the barium bolus. Such a silhouette image is of little diagnostic value.

can be fogged, but the most important one to the radiographer is scatter radiation.

Causes of Scatter Fog

Let us briefly consider each of the three factors that increase the amount of scatter radiation reaching the film. They are:

1. High kVp levels
2. Large field sizes
3. Large tissue thicknesses

1. High kVp Levels. At high kilovoltages, slightly *less* scattering interactions occur in the patient. However, that scattered radiation which is produced has higher energy, and it is emitted in a more forward direction. With an increased proportion of the scattered rays penetrating through to the film, and with an increased proportion of them directed toward the film, *the net result is an increase in scatter radiation reaching the film, increasing image fog.*

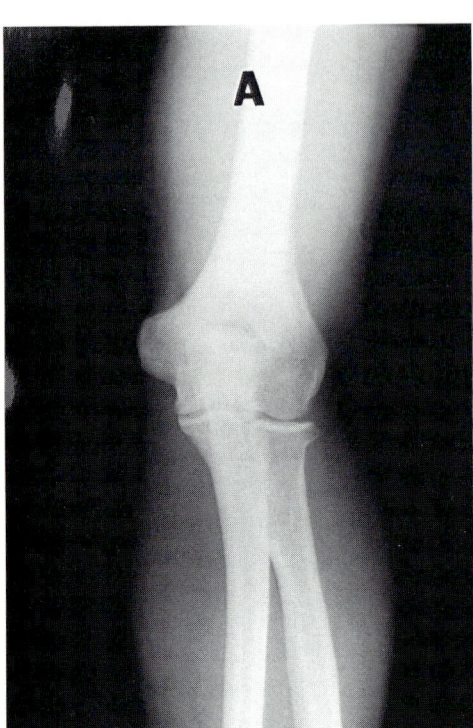
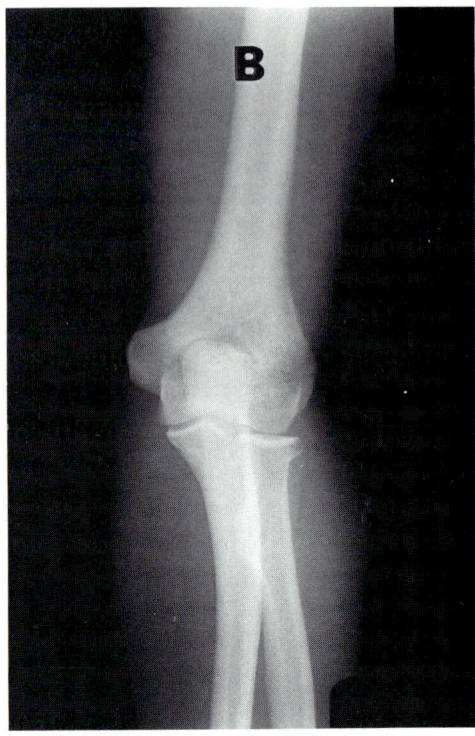
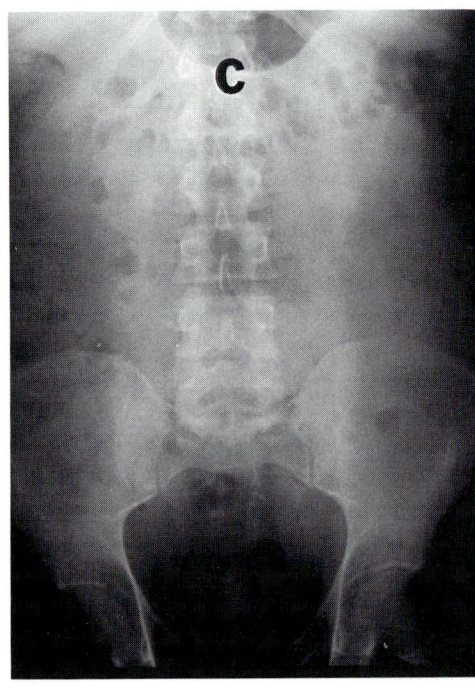
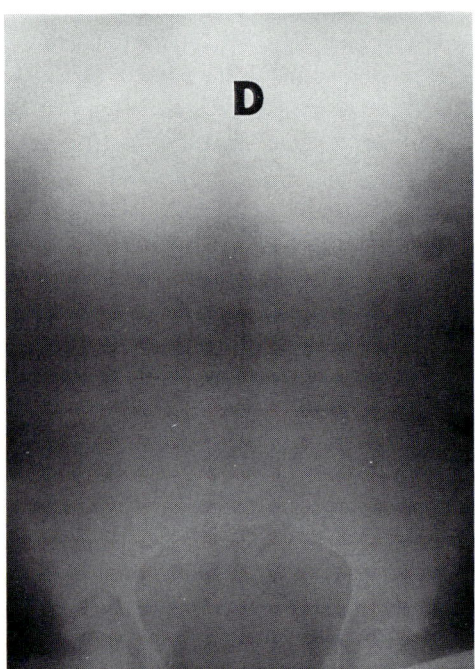

Figure 255. Radiographs demonstrating gray scale versus fog. From (A) to (B), increased "grayness" is due to a desirable increase in penetration and gray scale, with no fog. From (C) to (D), increased "grayness" due to undesirable fog.

But, high kVp settings are required to obtain adequate *penetration* for the radiographic studies using contrast agents and for those body parts with high proportions of bone tissue. Furthermore, high kVp is frequently desirable in order to produce longer *gray scale* in the image. In most cases, these two benefits outweigh the gradual increase in fog at higher kilovoltages. Therefore, the selection of kVp should be based primarily upon the penetration and gray scale desired, with scatter radiation only as a secondary consideration.

2. **Large Field Sizes.** Larger field sizes allow greater amounts of exposed tissue to generate more scatter radiation, while the concentration of the primary radiation is unaffected. Excessive proportions of scatter radiation are also produced in the x-ray table any time the light field is allowed to extend well beyond the anatomy. As long as the field size is adequate to include all anatomy of interest, there is *no benefit* to further increasing the field size, and no reason for accepting an image fogged in this manner.

3. **Large Tissue Thicknesses.** Larger patients or larger body parts present more exposed tissue to generate scatter radiation, even while the primary beam is further attenuated. The loss of useful rays combined with the increased scatter results in a dramatic increase in visible image fog.

For some procedures (particularly fluoroscopic procedures), the radiographer or radiologist may be able to reduce tissue thickness by using a *compression paddle* or similar compression device. But for the most part, tissue thickness is outside the control of the radiographer.

Of these three causes of scatter radiation then, high kVp levels have advantages which outweigh the fog produced, and tissue thicknesses are not usually under the radiographer's control, leaving *field size limitation (collimation) as the primary method of preventing scatter radiation.*

Two methods are available to help eliminate scatter radiation *after it has been produced,* but before it reaches the film and fogs it. These are the use of grids, discussed in the next chapter, and the use of the "air gap technique".

Effects on Density and Contrast

Scattering is a *random* event, and therefore, when it occurs in sufficient quantity, it results in a relatively *even density deposit* across an area of the film, if not across the entire film. (Of course, by inverse square law, this deposit will gradually decrease at greater distances from the scattering source; nonetheless, a silver deposit will result both directly under the scattering object and under adjacent structures.)

Figure 256 is a density trace diagram showing the "blanket" effect of scatter fogging. The diagram is a cross-section of the thickness of the silver deposit on the x-ray film. A thicker silver deposit would be seen as a darker density. The white box represents a high-contrast object, such as a bone, being projected onto the film and showing a lighter density. Contrast is measured as the *ratio* of the background density to the density under the object of interest. In this diagram, the background density would normally be 3, and the image density 1. The normal contrast would be $3/1 = 3$.

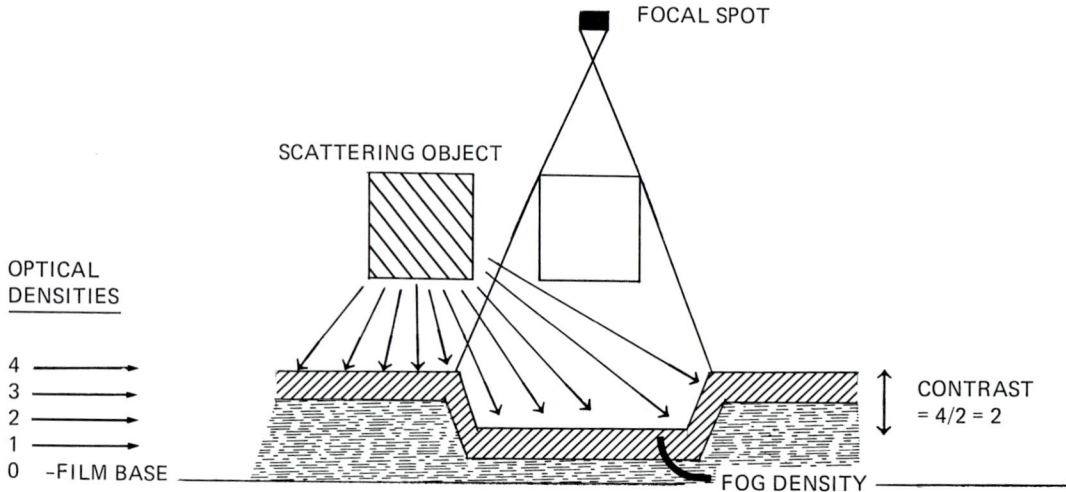

Figure 256. Effect of scatter radiation upon image contrast. Prior to fogging, background density is 3.0, density under the object of interest is 1.0, and contrast is $3/1 = 3$. After scatter radiation lays down an additional "blanket" density of 1.0, background density is 4.0 and image density 2.0. Contrast for the fogged image is $4/2 = 2$, reduced from the original contrast of 3.

However, if a scattering object is placed within the x-ray beam near to the object of interest, the scatter radiation produced lays down a blanket of density across the film, covering *both* the area directly under itself and adjacent areas under other structures. In the diagram this added density has a value of 1. The background density is increased to 4, and the image density is increased to 2. The image contrast after fogging is $4/2 = 2$. Contrast has been reduced by scatter fog.

Fog increases density anywhere it occurs on the film. The addition of fog density to those areas depicted as dark grays may be sufficient to turn them pitch black, resulting in a loss of radiographic information. Fog increases density, but in a destructive way, reducing image quality.

It is possible for a radiograph to be both *light* and *fogged* (Figure 257). This frequently occurs with very large patients. The large volume of tissue results in excessive scattered radiation, which would normally fog and darken the film, but, at the same time, such thicknesses of tissue reduce the amount of primary radiation reaching the film. The total exposure to the film is reduced, yet a greater *proportion* of that exposure is attributable to fog densities. The result is a "washed out" appearance, underexposed and gray at the same time. Such radiographs are of little diagnostic value.

Fog Versus Blur

There is also a common misconception that scattered radiation "undercuts the edge" of an image, causing it to become "blurred." It has even been asserted that grids reduce blur by eliminating scatter. These are false and misleading statements. The *resolution* of details (the ability to distinguish them as separate from each other) is reduced by a loss of contrast, but this is due to less *visibility,* not to a lack of geometrical integrity. The sharpness of the edges of an image depends on the width of the *penumbra.* Anything which does not change the spread of the penumbra cannot be said to affect sharpness.

Scatter is a completely random phenomenon. It does not "select" the edges of an image to affect, but lays down a blanket of density over the *entire* image. Blurring, on the other hand, is geometrically predictable through penumbra and absorption diagrams and relates specifically to the edges of the image. Scatter, emanating from the patient, cannot and does not affect the alignment of the primary rays projected from the x-ray tube.

To develop this concept, let us separate a fogging event and the projection of the original image in time. A film may certainly be fogged before or after it is used for an exposure. For example, it may be fogged in the dark room during storage. Would such a fogging affect the way that image edges are projected onto the film during an exposure taken at a later time? Clearly the answer is no. The visibility of the image would be compromised because of the fogging, but the projection of the penum-

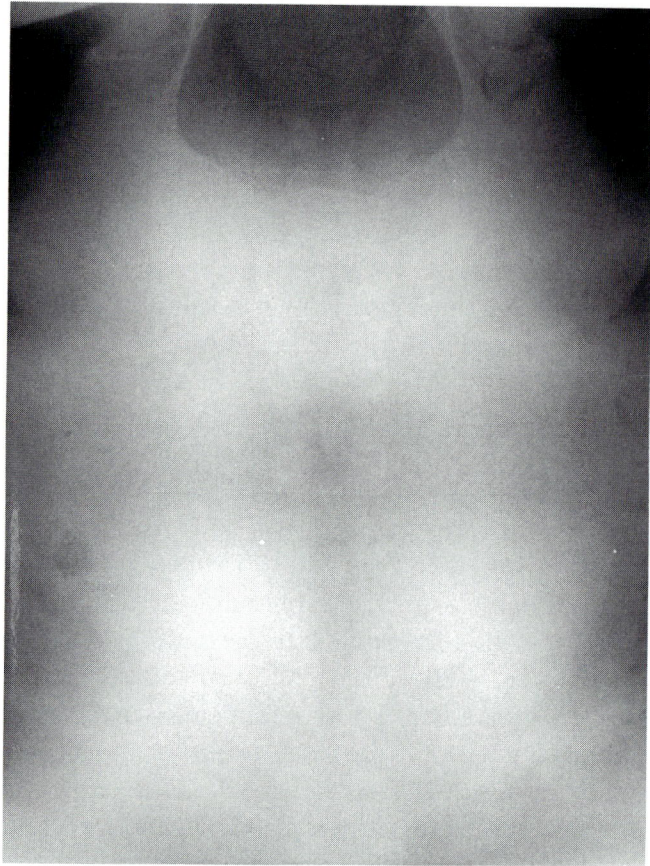

Figure 257. Radiograph of large patient demonstrating both fog and underexposure. An image can be light and yet fogged.

bra and umbra of the image during regular exposure is affected only by primary beam geometry.

Figure 258 illustrates that scatter radiation is a phenomenon separate from the geometry of penumbra formation, and does not change image sharpness or blur. Figure 259 demonstrates that images can be fogged without blur, or blurred without fog. Because scatter is random in nature, it cannot affect *any* of the geometrical factors in the image—sharpness, magnification or distortion.

Artifacts

Any impertinent, useless, grossly distorted, or false information which obscures the useful details in an image may be referred to as

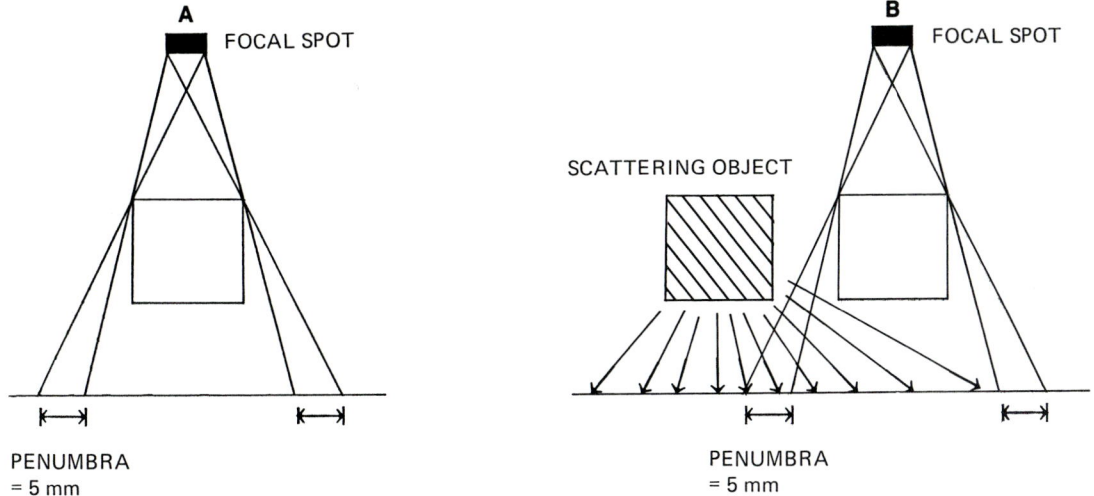

Figure 258. Diagram illustrating that scatter radiation does not affect sharpness of recorded detail. The spread of the penumbral shadow is 5 mm prior to fogging (A), and is still 5 mm after fogging (B). Although *visibility* is reduced by the scatter, blur is unchanged, and sharpness is equal.

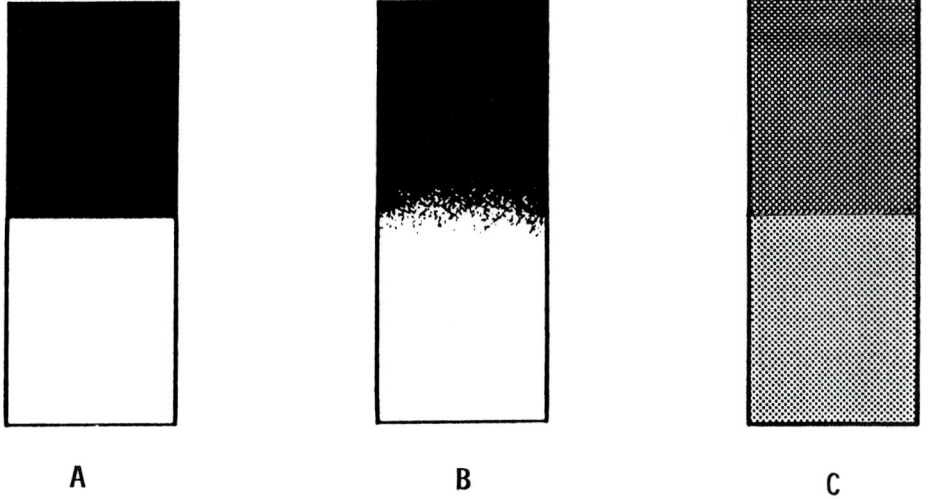

Figure 259. Blur versus fog. Image A shows no blur and no fog, image B shows blurring, but no fog, while image C shows poor contrast due to fog, but no blur.

noise. Scatter fog has already been described as the most common form of radiographic noise. In addition, a radiograph may be fogged from exposure to white light or excessive exposure to darkroom safelights, or it may be *chemically* fogged from excessive temperatures, excessive development times, or improper solution concentrations during processing.

Many other artifacts too numerous to list here constitute forms of image noise. A few examples are torn paper or dirt inside screen cassettes, iodine or barium spilled onto sponges or patient gowns, removable objects in or on the patient such as hairpins, dentures and jewelry, scratches and splashed chemicals on the film.

Static electricity discharges on the film can be caused from rough handling, pressure from stacking boxes of film on their sides rather than on end, automatic film conveyor systems and low humidity. These discharges cause branching or radiating black exposure marks on the finished radiograph, one of the most common and destructive types of artifacts. Another type of artifact which is often misunderstood is the *false* image. False images are images created by patient motion, tomographic movements or other geometrical anomalies that blur and superimpose true images into each other. Although these images are often referred to as distorted images, it should be clarified that they are newly *created* images which do not represent any real anatomical object at all and, therefore, are completely *false*.

Regardless of origins or causes, all of these artifacts obscure the visibility of the useful portions of the radiographic image and, therefore, constitute image noise.

Examples of the many types of artifacts caused by the patient, by exposure or by processing are illustrated and discussed in Chapters 3 and 4.

VARIABLES AFFECTING FOG AND NOISE

Milliampere-Seconds (mAs)

Insufficient mAs leaves such a light exposure reaching the film that the uneven distribution of x-rays within the beam becomes visible on the finished image. The resulting blotchy or freckled appearance in the image is called *quantum mottle,* and is a form of image noise because it interferes with the visibility of details.

Kilovoltage-Peak

Because of the loss of photoelectric interactions at high kVp levels, the remaining image is composed only of penetrating rays and scattered rays. Further, a higher proportion of those scattered rays that are produced will reach the film, because they have more energy and are emitted in a more forward direction. Fog in the image becomes more apparent. A high proportion of fog interferes with the visibility of image details. Therefore, high kVp may be considered as a contributor to image noise.

Field Size

Larger field sizes increase the amount of exposed tissue producing scatter radiation. The scatter creates noise in the image in the form of fog. This noise is reduced by limiting field size to the anatomy of interest.

Patient Status and Pathology

Large patients also increase the amount of exposed tissue creating scatter radiation, causing more noise in the form of image fog.

Artifacts and Casts

Artifacts include any object or substance inadvertently left within the passage of the x-ray beam which impedes visibility of image details. A few examples are objects or clothing left on the patient, removable devices on the patient's person such as dentures, objects left on the x-ray table or film, particles of dirt or paper inside intensifying screens, and contrast agents soaked into positioning sponges from previous spills. Casts and splints also interfere with the image quality, and constitute noise, even though they may not be removable.

Extraneous Fog

Fog on the radiograph, whatever the source, constitutes noise since it reduces visibility of details.

Intensifying Screens and Film

The use of extremely high speed intensifying screens can lead to very low mAs values. As previously explained, this will lead to quantum mottle, a form of noise. Clumping of crystals in the manufacture of emulsions for screens or for radiographic film can cause a mottled appearance in the finished radiograph that is unrelated to the x-ray beam itself. This type of image noise is referred to as screen mottle or as film mottle, respectively.

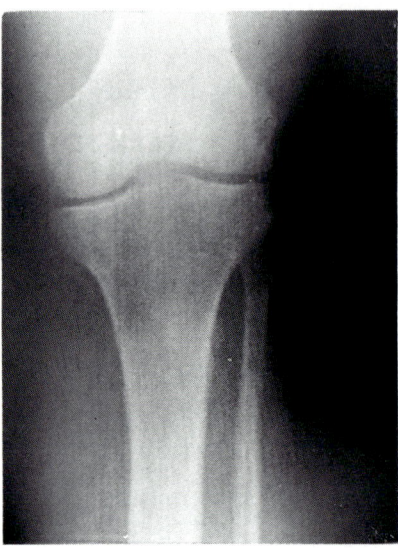

Figure 260. Radiograph of a knee with the central ray off-centered two inches to a 12:1 stationary grid showing grid lines (thin, vertical white streaks).

Motion

In addition to its blurring effects, motion of the patient, the x-ray tube or the film during exposure can cause the production of false images such as streaks. False images can obscure the anatomy of interest, and are a form of image noise.

Grid Lines and Cut-Off

Grid Lines

Grid cut-off may be considered an extreme case of artifacts occluding the image. But stationary grids such as those taped to cassettes during mobile procedures will result in grid lines even when they are used properly. On close inspection, one can see the clear white lines where grid strips absorbed radiation, reducing the amount of information reaching the film, Figure 260. Grid lines interfere with details and are a form of noise.

They can never be completely eliminated when stationary grids are used. The employment of a Potter-Bucky diaphragm blurs out the grid lines, but there is still a loss of density called *grid cutoff,* caused by their absorption of the remnant radiation. Special care must be taken when using stationary *wafer* grids and *grid cassettes* to keep the interference of grid lines to a minimum. When improper distances are used or when the beam is not properly aligned to stationary grids, the grid lines recorded become much wider than necessary, obscuring larger amounts of information in the image (Figure 261).

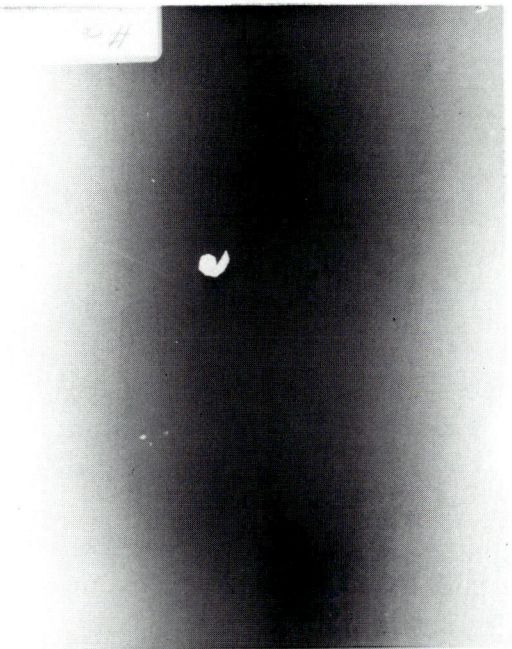

Figure 261. Radiograph demonstrating grid cutoff from placing the x-ray tube at 20 inches FFD with a 12:1 40-inch radius focused grid.

Any time the focus-film distance used is not within the grid radius, the density pattern resulting on the radiograph will be a darker strip of density down the middle of the lengthwise axis of the film, with a loss of density toward both lateral sides equally, as long as other factors and centering were correct (Figure 262).

The proper placement of the stationary grid is also critical in minimizing grid cut-off and information loss. With wafer grids, a common error is to place the grid upside down over the film cassette. With a focused grid, the effect is to obliterate the densities toward both lateral sides of the film equally. This effect is similar to placing the x-ray tube outside of the grid radius, but much more severe (Figure 262)

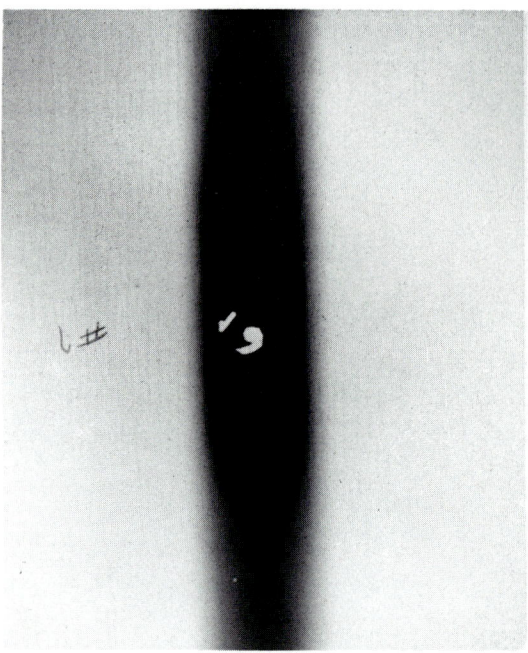

Figure 262. Diagram and radiograph showing the grid cutoff caused by placing a focused stationary grid upside down.

Alignment of the Beam and Grid

When performing portable radiographs with stationary grids, two other common problems are placing the grid and film tilted so that they are not perpendicular to the central ray (equivalent to angling the central ray across the lead strips) and off-centering the central ray or grid in relation to each other. Off-centering or angling across the lead strips have the same effect. While there may be some loss of density toward both lateral sides of the film, the loss will be much greater toward one side than the other, as demonstrated in Figure 263. Again, these problems become more severe when working with selective, higher grid ratios than with lower grid ratios.

Only when off-centering or angling the central ray *across* the lead strips (in a direction perpendicular to the strips) do visible grid cutoff problems occur. Lengthwise tube angles and off-centering can be used when using the Potter-Bucky diaphragm but the beam must not be angled or off-centered across the table.

Figure 263. Radiograph demonstrating the grid cutoff caused by off-centering the central ray by two inches across the strips of a 15:1 stationary grid. The effect of angling the beam or tilting the grid would be similar.

Chapter 13

SHARPNESS OF RECORDED DETAIL

RADIOGRAPHIC EVALUATION OF SHARPNESS

Sharpness of recorded detail may be described as the *abruptness* with which the edges of a particular image *stop.* To better visualize this principle, imagine yourself moving across a black-and-white photograph, perhaps in a microscopic sports car: You are passing from a white image onto a black background. If you suddenly find yourself over the black part, the edge of the white image was sharp and *stopped* abruptly. If you gradually pass from white to gray to black, then the edge of the white image is blurred and is not sharp.

Theoretically, if shadows could be cast from a *point* source of light, there would never be any blur. There would be a single, pure shadow with sharp edges. But when the source of light is an *area* such as the sun or a flashlight bulb (or an x-ray tube focal spot), there will always be partial shadows cast around the edges of the *pure* shadow. This occurs because the shadow of any given edge of the object is projected at several different angles from several different points within the area of the light source.

Figure 264 illustrates this effect. Note that when the light comes from a single point, a pure shadow with sharp edges is projected behind the object. However, single point sources of light are not found in nature. The sun, for example, has a surface *area,* and light can be emitted from many different regions across that area. This means that the shadow of a particular edge of the object will be projected by different beams of light coming from different angles. The edge of the shadow will then be projected onto the background in more than one place, resulting in an unsharp appearance called *blur.*

The *pure* shadow of an object is named its *umbra.* The partial shadow of the edge of an object is called its *penumbra.* Penumbra is synonymous with blur—the more penumbra that is present, the more blurry the edge appears. To demonstrate umbra and penumbra, hold your hand over an

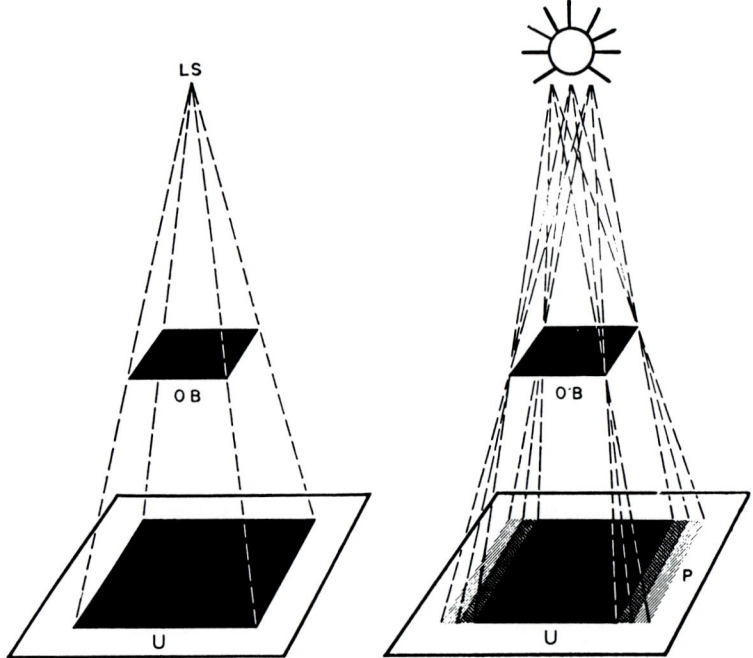

Figure 264. Diagram illustrating a pure umbra image from a theoretical point source of light (*left*) compared to the production of penumbra (p) at the edges of a shadow image by an area light source such as the sun (*right*).

overhead projector or in front of a flashlight, move it away from the light and then toward the light and observe the shadow cast. As you move your hand back and forth from the light source, you will see the blurry penumbra at the edges grow and shrink. Note that the penumbra does not only grow outward but also inward, causing the umbra portion to shrink. With enough penumbra present, you would not be able to recognize the image as the shadow of your hand.

Now consider the problems caused with recognizability when observing a very blurry image of two closely adjacent objects. As penumbra grows, the edges of the two images recorded will blur into each other and overlap. The penumbra also replaces a portion of the umbra, so that the umbra diminishes in size. When two shadows overlap in this way, they may appear as one shadow of one object, even though there are really two objects.

Since increasing penumbra invades the umbra, it is even possible for an image to deteriorate until it is all penumbra and virtually no umbra, effectively disappearing, with only a nebulous area of blurry density left in the area of the image.

Sharpness may be destroyed not only by the geometrical growth of penumbra but also by blurring due to motion. An example of motion blurring of the hand is found in Figure 265. Sharpness of recorded detail has a strong impact upon our ability to recognize images.

In radiography, a very common misconception occurs when the *visibility* of edges is confused with the *sharpness* of edges in an image. Compare the two chest radiographs in Figures 247 and 248 and see if you can determine which radiograph has sharper edges between the ribs and the background lung density. The answer is that they are both equally sharp. High-contrast radiographs are not only deceptively appealing to the human eye but they also create the *false* impression that they are sharper. The longer-scale radiograph is not blurred, and the edges of the ribs have no more penumbra present than those in the short-scale radiograph. They *stop* just as abruptly. However, the rib edges in the long-scale radiograph are less *visible* than those in the short-scale version, because they possess less contrast, which is a visibility function. Edges of image details, just like all of the other parts of the image, have both visibility and recognizability components. Edges that are more visible must not be construed as necessarily being sharper. Conversely, penumbra or blur must not be confused with fog.

Figure 259 in the previous chapter illustrates the difference between unsharpness (blur) and poor contrast such as might be caused by fog. In this illustration, **A** shows a high contrast image with a sharp edge between the two densities. In **B,** the high contrast is still present, but the edge is blurry, gradually changing from one density to the other. In **C,** very poor contrast causes the edge between the two densities to become less *visible,* but it is still sharp, because it "stops" abruptly. Blur is not present in **C.**

Geometrical penumbra and motion are the two most important causes of blur or unsharpness. Blur may also be caused by poorly constructed film and intensifying screens, referred to as "materials unsharpness," or by absorption defects at the edges of an object. To summarize the types of unsharpness, they are (1) geometrical penumbra, (2) absorption penumbra (see chapter 16), (3) motion unsharpness and (4) materials unsharpness.

292

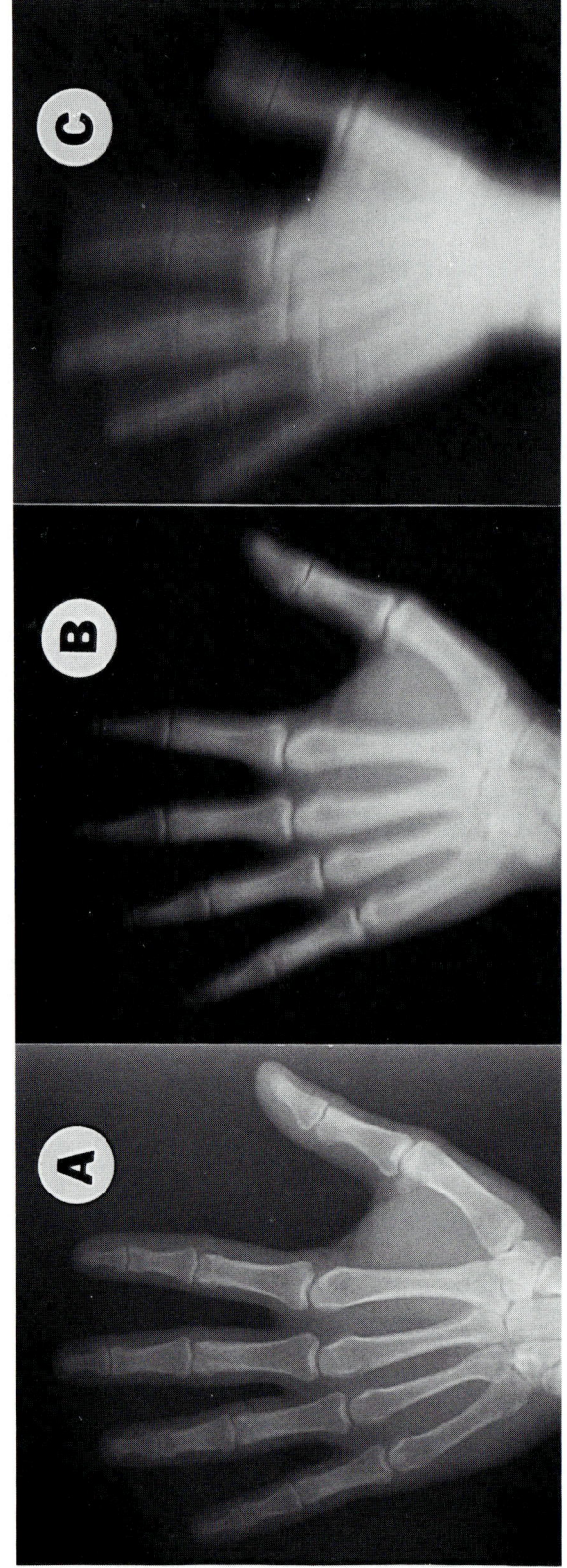

Figure 265. Radiographs of the hand showing (A) a sharp and high contrast image, (B) a blurred image due to motion, and (C) a severely blurred image showing a loss of contrast.

VARIABLES AFFECTING SHARPNESS
OF RECORDED DETAIL

Focal Spot Size

The size of the focal spot should be considered as the primary control for sharpness of recorded detail in the image, for two reasons: (1) It is the only variable that *exclusively* affects sharpness, without affecting any other image characteristic, (2) It is readily manipulated by the radiographer. The smaller the focal spot, the sharper the recorded detail. The relationship is inversely proportional: If the focal spot size is reduced to one-half the original, sharpness of detail doubles.

Radiographers should be conscientious enough to utilize the small focal spot whenever high detail resolution is of essence, (for example, whenever "extremity" cassettes are used). The large focal spot must be employed whenever high techniques might overheat the x-ray tube.

Anode Bevel

Through the line-focus principle described in Chapter Seventeen, steeper anode bevels (at a smaller angle from vertical) result in smaller projected focal spot sizes, and therefore contribute to sharpness of recorded detail.

Focus-Film Distance (FFD)

Focus-film distance is directly proportional to the sharpness of recorded detail produced in the image. If the distance is doubled, the sharpness is doubled, provided all other factors are equal. FFD should not, however, be considered as a primary control for sharpness, because it affects other image qualities as well, and because it cannot always be easily modified.

Object-Film Distance (OFD)

When the distance from the object to the image receptor is increased, sharpness of recorded detail is reduced. If all other factors are kept equal, the sharpness is inversely proportional to the OFD. When OFD is doubled, sharpness is cut to one-half due to a doubling of the penumbra. The OFD should always be kept at a minimum.

FFD/FOD Ratio

The ratio of FFD to FOD is directly proportional to sharpness of recorded detail. If both the FFD and the OFD are doubled, the FOD will also be doubled. The FFD/FOD ratio will therefore be unchanged, and image sharpness will remain equal.

Positioning

If the body is positioned so that the anatomy of interest is further from the film than necessary, sharpness of recorded detail is diminished. This effect is due to a change in the OFD where the "object" is restricted to the specific anatomy of interest. Radiographers must utilize those positions which place the anatomy as close as possible to the image receptor.

Motion and Exposure Time

Motion blurs the image and is therefore the prime enemy of sharpness of recorded detail. Radiographers must use communication skills, immobilization and short exposure times to reduce the probability of motion occuring.

Long exposure times are not the *direct cause* of motion. But in chest radiography, for example, heart motion is unavoidable, and can only be eliminated radiographically by the use of very short exposure times. In addition, the longer the time, the greater the chance for peristaltic motion, breathing motion or movement of the patient to occur. Therefore, exposure time should be considered as a *contributing cause* of motion during radiographic procedures. Generally, the shorter the exposure time, the sharper the recorded detail.

Intensifying Screens

The use of an intensifying screen always results in less sharpness of detail than the use of direct exposure holders, because light from a screen diffuses prior to reaching the film. When changing from one screen speed to a higher speed, image sharpness *may* be compromised depending on the manufacturing method by which the higher speed was achieved. If a thicker emulsion or larger crystals were used, sharpness will be reduced. If chemical differences were used, sharpness may be unaffected, or even enhanced if the resulting emulsion layer is thinner. As a general rule, the higher the speed, the less the sharpness.

Image Receptor Systems

Usually, the higher the speed of a radiographic film, the lower the sharpness of recorded detail. As with screens, chemical changes will not affect sharpness. But most speed differences in films are due to crystal size or emulsion thickness. Any increase in these will reduce sharpness.

Duplitized film is less sharp than single-emulsion film, because of the parallax effect of viewing two images in two separate emulsions.

Single-screen cassettes result in better sharpness of detail than double-screen cassettes, due to the elimination of the cross-over effect.

Chapter 14

MAGNIFICATION

RADIOGRAPHIC EVALUATION OF MAGNIFICATION

Magnification

Excessive magnification of the size of an image may make it difficult to recognize what real object the image represents. It is hard to tell what kind of a building you are looking at when you are standing one inch from the wall. In photography and in radiography, *magnification* may be defined as the difference between the size of a real object and the size of its image on the *picture*. Magnification is often referred to as *size distortion* and classified under the general heading of *distortion*. However, for the sake of clarity, the word *distortion* shall be used in this book only with regard to changes in the apparent shape of an image. *Magnification* shall be consistently used to describe changes in the *size* of the image.

Magnification of a radiographic image can be quantitatively measured by detecting a difference between its size and the actual object's size in *both dimensions or axes,* lengthwise *and* crosswise, Figure 266. If the length or width of the image is equal to the same measurement on the real object, no magnification is present. In a magnified image, both the length and the width of the image will measure larger than the object by equal proportions. For magnification to be present, the *umbral* portion of the image must increase in size. When the penumbra expands *without* the umbra increasing, the image is not magnified but only blurred.

VARIABLES AFFECTING MAGNIFICATION

Focus-Film Distance (FFD)

The FFD is inversely related to magnification, but not proportional to it. A longer FFD projects the image of the object with more parallel beams, and results in less magnification. The reduction in magnification, however, is relatively small compared to the change made in the FFD.

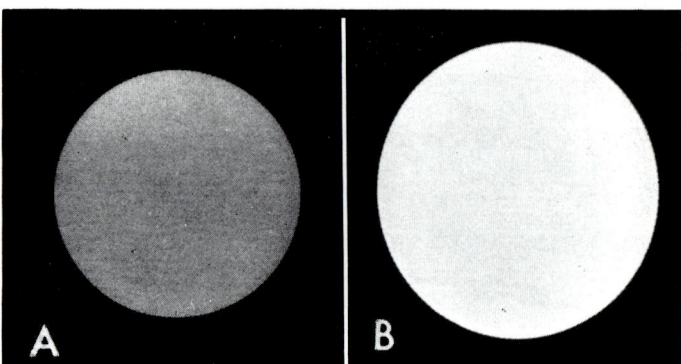

Figure 266. Radiographs of discs demonstrating effects of magnification (A) disc on film; (B) disc and emitter 5 inches above film, causing enlargement of image.

The longest feasible FFD should always be used to minimize image magnification.

Object-Film Distance (OFD)

The OFD is directly related to magnification, but again, is not proportional to it. The greater the OFD, the greater the magnification. If the OFD is doubled, the image size will not double, but it will increase (by about 30 per cent). The OFD should always be minimized to control magnification.

FFD/FOD Ratio

The FFD/FOD ratio should be considered as the primary controlling factor for magnification of the image size. The FFD/FOD ratio is directly proportional to the magnification factor.

For example, a 20-inch FFD and a 15-inch FOD yields a magnification factor of 20/15 = 1.25 or 25 per cent magnification. Doubling the FFD to 40 inches without changing the object-film distance results in an FOD of 35 inches, and the magnification factor becomes 40/35 = 1.14 or 14 per cent magnification.

To minimize magnification of the image, the FFD/FOD ratio should always be kept as low as possible. This is accomplished by long FFDs and short OFDs.

Positioning

Since positioning of the patient may place the anatomy of interest nearer to or further from the film, effectively changing the OFD, it can result in unnecessary magnification of the anatomy of interest. To minimize magnification, radiographic positioning should always be done with an eye to placing the anatomy of interest as close to the film as possible.

Chapter 15

SHAPE DISTORTION

RADIOGRAPHIC EVALUATION OF SHAPE DISTORTION

Shape Distortion

S*hape distortion* is defined as the difference between the shape of a real object and the shape of its image on a radiograph or photograph. In a given axis of direction, shape distortion will consist of either a foreshortening of the image or an elongation of the image. When a square object, for example, is projected onto a two-dimensional film as a rectangular shadow due to angling or off-centering of the camera or x-ray tube, the true nature of the object is not recognizable and information recorded on the film may be misleading and misinterpreted (Figure 267).

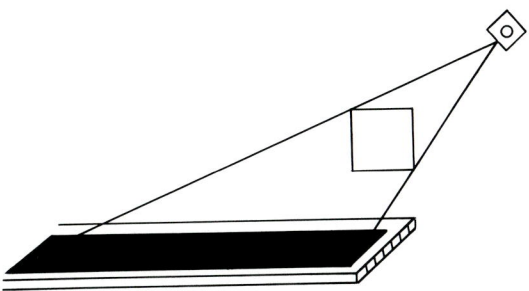

Figure 267. Diagram demonstrating shape distortion. Misalignment or angling of a beam of light will project the shadow of a square object as a distorted rectangular image.

Good recognizability or geometrical integrity in an image is determined, then, by maximum sharpness of detail and minimum magnification and shape distortion.

If the length of an image should measure differently than the length of the real object it represents while its width is unchanged, the image is *shape distorted*, it is not magnified. The shape of an object might be grossly represented as the ratio between its length and its width. For example, if the length and width are equal, their ratio would be 1:1 and

301

you might have a square or a circle shape. If the length is twice as long as the width, however, their ratio would be 2:1 and you might have a rectangle or an elipse shape. The shape only changes when this ratio changes.

For example, the radiographic "shadow" of a spherical object will be a circle with equal width and "length," having a *shape ratio* of 1:1, Figure 268-A. Suppose that the circular image measures *both* 20 per cent longer and 20 per cent wider than the real object. The *shape ratio* of the image is now 1.2:1.2 = 1:1 = 1. The ratio of length to width is unchanged from that of the real object, and there is *no shape distortion* present. There is, however, *magnification.* The image is larger, but still has the same circular shape, Figure 268-B.

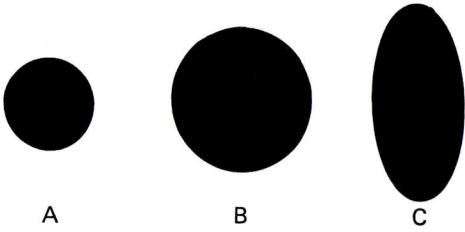

A   B   C

Figure 268. Diagram showing difference between magnification and shape distortion. If image measurement changes in both axes (length and width) equally, a magnified but still circular image results. Only when one axis changes *more* than the other does shape distortion occur, producing an oval shadow.

For *shape distortion* to be present, one dimension (axis) of the image must be changed by a different proportion than the other dimension. Length must change *more* than width, or vice versa. In Figure 268-C, the *width* of the image measures the same as the original width in *A,* but the *length* of the image is increased. If the length is doubled, the new *shape ratio* (length/width) is 2:1 = 2. This is different from the original shape ratio of 1, and indicates that distortion has occurred. If the length were cut in half while the width remained at 1, the new shape ratio would be 1/2:1 = 1/2, again indicating shape distortion. Any time one dimension or axis of the image changes differently than another, the result will be a different shape.

Suppose that *both* the length and width increase, but the *length* grows three times longer while the width only doubles. The new shape ratio is 3:2 = 1.5, and shape distortion has occurred. In this case, however, magnification has *also* occurred because *both* dimensions were increased. This image was both magnified and distorted.

Specifically, if the image measures longer in *one* axis than the real object, it is said to have *elongation* distortion. If it measures shorter in *one* axis, it is said to have *foreshortening* distortion. If it changes equally in *both* axes, it is *magnified.*

Blur, magnification and distortion reduce the recognizability of information, can cause misleading information or create false information, and can lead to the complete loss of some information on a radiograph.

VARIABLES AFFECTING SHAPE DISTORTION

Beam-Part-Film Alignment and Positioning

The *only* variable which affects shape distortion in radiography is beam-part-film alignment. Nonetheless, this variable has several aspects including positioning of the patient, the actual shape of the anatomy of interest, centering of the central ray, angulation of the x-ray beam, and proper placement of the film holder or image receptor. Beam-part-film alignment is the controlling factor for distortion. The effects of various angling and centering problems are illustrated in Figure 269.

If the anatomy of interest is thick and spherical or cubical in general shape, any distortion of it will be exacerbated. If it is thin and flat, linear, tubular, or wedge-shaped, with a distinct long axis, then distortion effects will not be as severe. When the long axis of an object is angled in relation to the film, while the beam is perpendicular to the film, foreshortening distortion will occur.

When the object and the film are parallel to each other, any angling of the x-ray beam so that it is not perpendicular to them will cause elongation distortion. However, if the object is angled in relation to the film, distortion is minimized by using Ceiszynski's law of isometry: Angle the central ray one-half of the angle formed between the object and the film.

Off-centering of the central ray from the anatomy of interest causes distortion effects similar to angulation. Positioning must be performed with an eye to maintaining a perpendicular beam-film relationship and a parallel part-film relationship whenever possible.

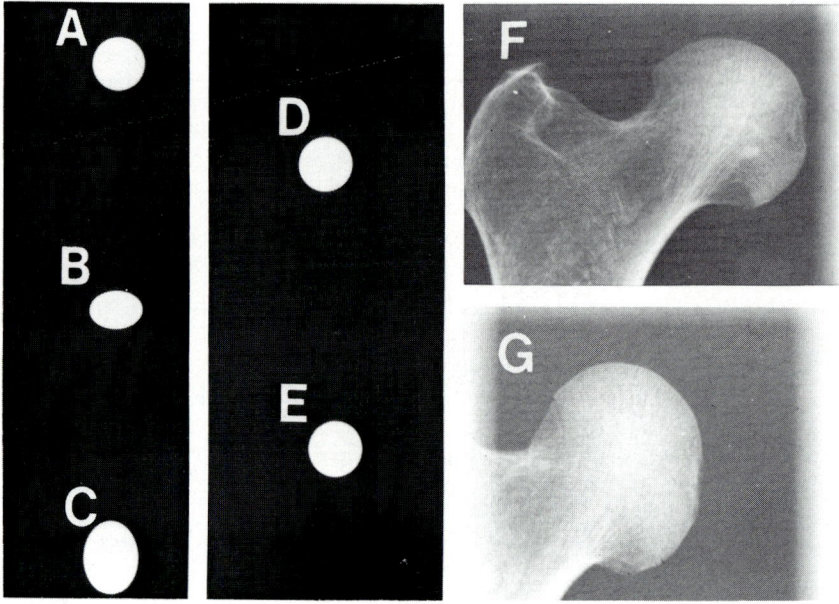

Figure 269. Radiographs demonstrating various cases of shape distortion from beam-part-film alignment changes: (A) flat coin parallel to film with beam perpendicular; (B) coin tilted and beam perpendicular to film showing foreshortening; (C) coin tilted and beam perpendicular to coin showing elongation; (D) coin tilted 45 degrees with beam angled isometrically at 22.5 degrees showing no distortion; (E) coin parallel to film with beam angled 30 degrees showing no distortion; (F) sphere (head of femur) with beam perpendicular to film; (G) sphere with beam angled 30 degrees showing elongation distortion.

Chapter 16

RESOLUTION: OVERALL IMAGE QUALITY

RESOLUTION

The ability to distinguish two adjacent details as being separate and distinct from each other is called *resolution*. A well-resolved image detail will have *both* high visibility and optimum recognizability. The two most important aspects of the resolution of a particular image detail are its *contrast* compared to other details nearby, and its *sharpness* or acutance against background details.

Contrast and sharpness are closely related to each other, because they both affect the resolution of the image. In other words, both sharpness and contrast are essential to the *resolution* of image details.

Nonetheless, contrast and sharpness are different image qualities, and they must not be confused, even though they are related. High contrast images can still have poor resolution if edges are blurred. Sharp images can still have poor resolution if contrast is low, as illustrated in Figure 259 in Chapter 12.

Thus, the resolution of information in the image depends upon both visibility and *geometrical integrity* (recognizability).

We depend upon the geometrical integrity of the image to recognize what real object it represents. If the image is blurry, or if it's size or shape is grossly distorted, we may not be able to tell what it is, even though it is visible. Recognizability or geometrical integrity is made up of three components: sharpness of recorded detail, magnification and shape distortion. Visibility is also composed of three parts: density, contrast and noise.

The actual measurement of the resolution in a radiographic image can be made by exposing resolution pattern templates (Figure 270). Made of lead foil, such templates provide an image of black-and-white line pairs which gradually diminish in width, Figure 271. The smaller the line pairs which can be visibly distinguished on the radiograph, the greater is the resolution. In a *blurred* image, the penumbral shadows at the line

305

edges will grow into each other so that the smaller lines cannot be distinguished. In a *fogged* image, the smaller lines will be less visible.

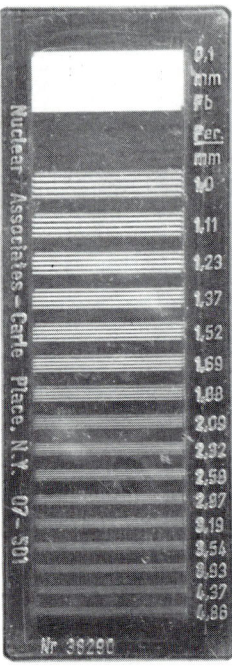

Figure 270. Photograph of test template used to measure the resolution of detail recorded on a radiograph. The smaller the line pairs which are seen clearly as separate lines, the higher the image resolution.

The smaller the lines that can be clearly recorded on the film, the more pairs of these lines would fit into a certain area on the film. A functional unit of measurement for image resolution can thus be derived. This unit is *line-pairs per millimeter,* abbreviated *LP/mm.* The more line-pairs per millimeter that can be resolved clearly, the greater the resolution of detail.

The overall image quality may be defined as the total amount of diagnostic information resolved in the image. Overall image quality is dependent upon the entire imaging system—the combination of a particular type of film and cassette with the x-ray machine used and all related variables.

In evaluating the overall quality of any image, the concept of resolution is of essence. A dictionary may define optical resolution as the "ability to distinguish the individual parts of an object or closely adja-

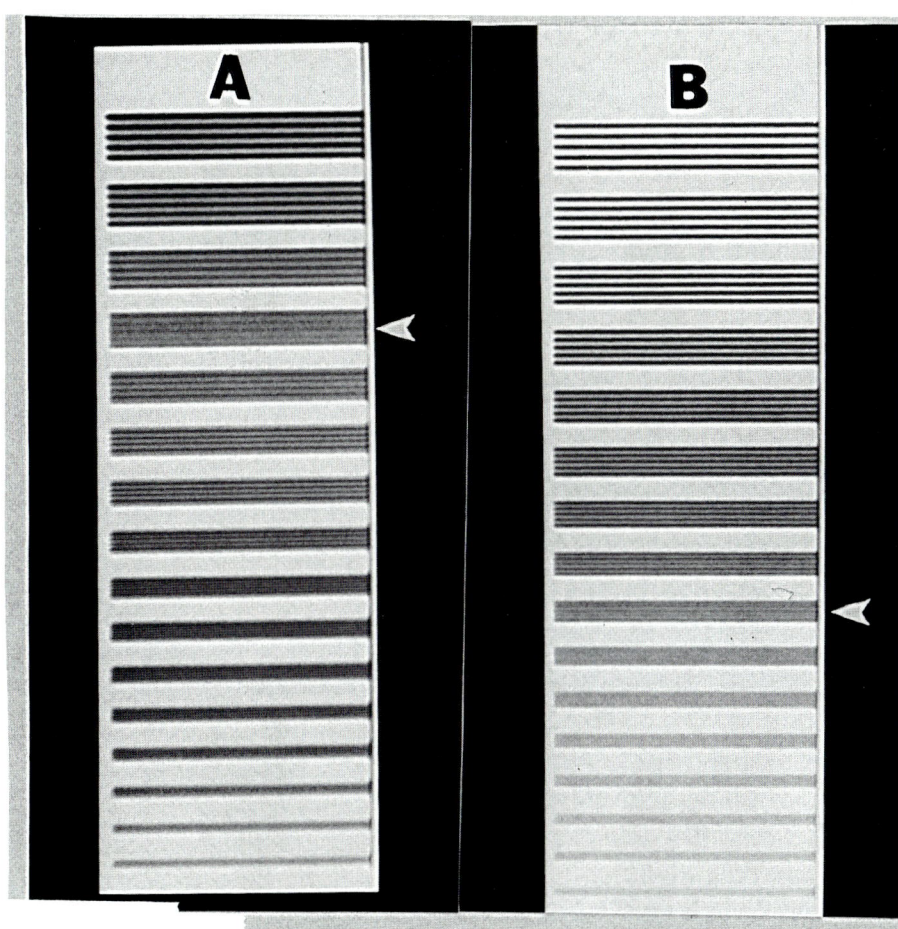

Figure 271. Radiographs of resolution test template taken with a fixed OFD of 8 inches. Arrows demarcate blur points. Exposure (A) was taken at 22 inches FFD and resolved 1.23 line pairs per millimeter. Exposure (B) was taken at 44 inches and resolved 2.46 line pairs per millimeter, double that for (A) and showing a directly proportional relationship between FFD and resolution. Changes in focal spot size have similar effects on resolution.

cent images," as being separate from each other. On a radiograph, in order for two small, closely adjacent details to be recognized as distinct and separate from each other, density and contrast must be optimal, sharpness of recorded detail must be high, and magnification, distortion, and noise must be minimal. *All of the image qualities affect resolution.*

To fully understand resolution, these six qualities must be considered collectively, in relation to each other, rather than individually. A helpful aid in studying these interrelationships is the density trace diagram.

Density Trace Diagrams

Density trace diagrams are simple diagrams of a physical "cross-section" of the radiographic film emulsion after development. They demonstrate the thickness of metallic silver deposit remaining on different areas of the film. Where the thickness of the silver is great, the film would appear dark, thinner regions would appear gray, and areas with little or no silver thickness would appear nearly clear or "white".

Contrast can be defined as the ratio of difference between two adjacent densities. This difference is shown on a density trace as the *vertical* distance through which the image edge drops (Figure 272). This contrast measurement must be taken at the center of the image, as compared to the density outside the image.

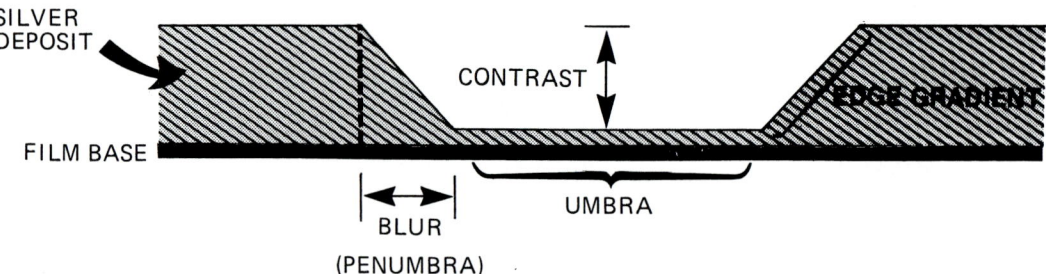

Figure 272. Density trace diagram. Image contrast is indicated by differences in vertical depth of the silver deposit on the film, comparing the middle of the image to the background deposit. Edge gradient is the slope in the silver deposit at the edges of the image. Penumbra or blur is indicated by the *horizontal* spread of the edge gradient.

One can see that the density at the edge of a radiographic image does not drop straight down. Rather, it drops more or less gradually, forming a slope of decreasing silver deposit on the film. This slope is called the *edge gradient,* Figure 272. The edge gradient can be measured by dividing the height of the slope by its width. For example, if the silver deposit drops 10 microns over a horizontal distance of 2 microns, the edge gradient is $10/2 = 5$ (*A* in Figure 273). If it takes 4 microns of horizontal distance for the silver deposit to drop 10 microns, the edge gradient is $10/4 = 2.5$ (*B* in Figure 273). A high edge gradient indicates a steep slope, a low edge gradient indicates a gradual slope.

The abruptness of the edge of a radiographic image is called its *acutance,* how *acutely* it drops off. Acutance is closely related to the

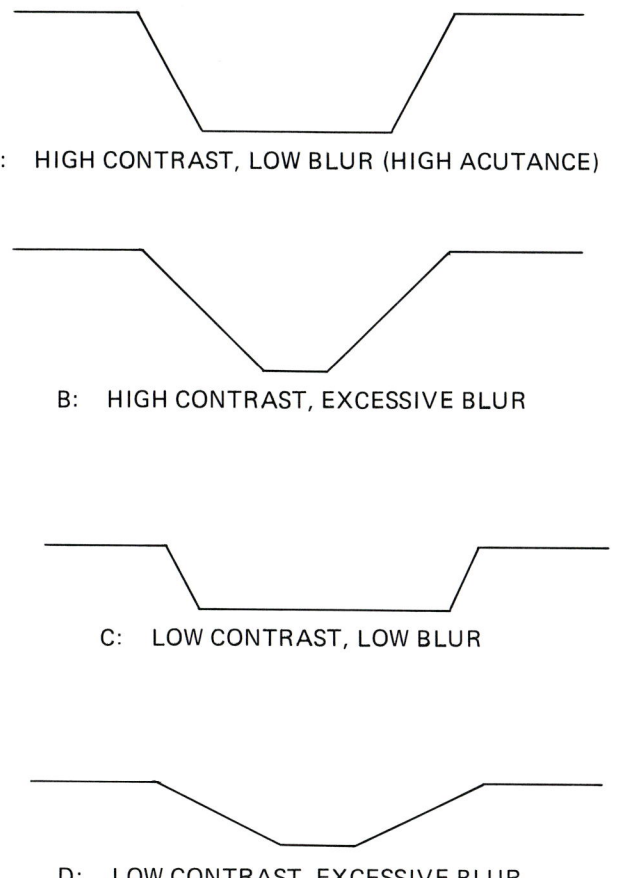

A: HIGH CONTRAST, LOW BLUR (HIGH ACUTANCE)

B: HIGH CONTRAST, EXCESSIVE BLUR

C: LOW CONTRAST, LOW BLUR

D: LOW CONTRAST, EXCESSIVE BLUR

Figure 273. Density trace diagrams for various contrast and sharpness levels. (A) would be the best resolved image, with high contrast (vertical density drop) and high sharpness (steep edge gradients). (B) shows blur, but still has high contrast. (C) shows a loss of visibility through low contrast, but has sharp edges. (D) is the poorest image, with both low contrast and excessive blur.

sharpness of recorded detail. A steep edge gradient indicates high acutance, and results in a high level of image sharpness.

Sharpness is defined in terms of the *horizontal* distance through which the edge gradient passes. More precisely, the horizontal measurement of the edge gradient represents penumbra or blur from *un*sharpness, Figure 272.

Motion blur and parallax blur (from double-coated film) are actually both superimposition processes which result in *horizontal* spreading of the edge (Figure 274). Motion should not be considered to affect image

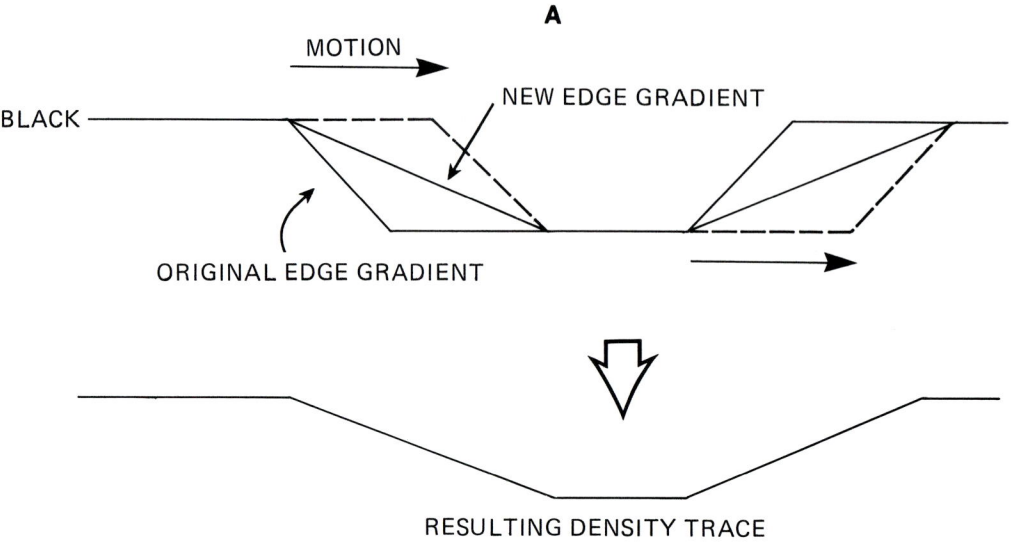

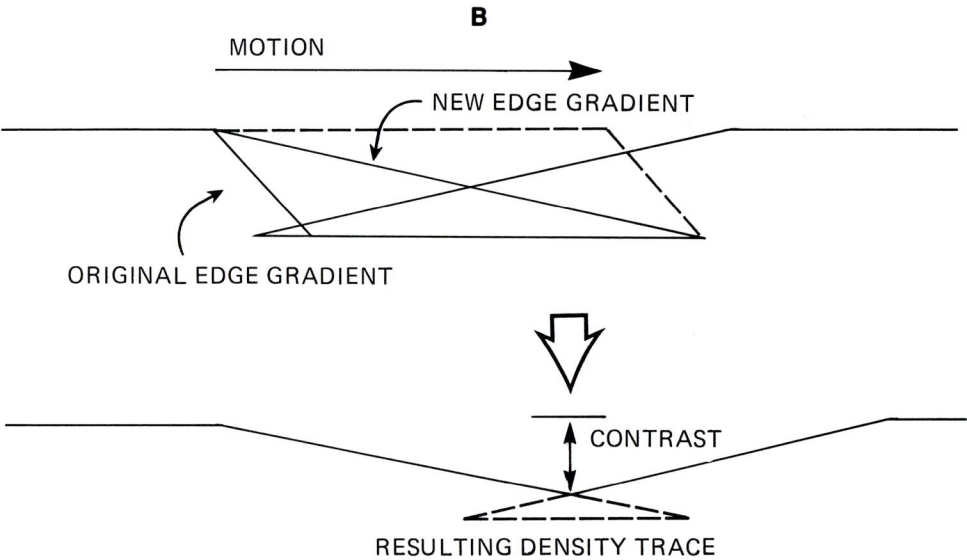

Figure 274. Density trace graphs illustrating the effects of motion on image sharpness and contrast. Slight motion (A) increases the horizontal spread of the edge gradient, reducing sharpness, but contrast at the middle of the image is unchanged. With *severe* motion (B) the edge gradients may begin to overlap, causing a loss of contrast.

contrast unless it is so severe that this horizontal spreading crosses the middle of the image, effectively reducing the vertical component of the density trace at mid-image (Figure 274-B).

At this point, one can readily see that contrast and sharpness are closely related to each other, because they both affect the slope of the edge gradient. In other words, contrast and sharpness are both essential to the *resolution* of image detail. Resolution of detail depends upon both sharpness and contrast.

Nonetheless, contrast and sharpness are different image qualities, and they must not be confused, even though they are related. Figure 273 illustrates the traces for various images with different contrast and blur levels. High contrast images can still have poor resolution if edges are blurred (Figure 273-B). Low contrast images can be sharp in spite of poor visibility (Figure 273-C).

In defining the slope of the edge gradient, density trace diagrams provide a simplified way to measure the resolution of a single image detail, calculated as the ratio of contrast to unsharpness, C/U. But remember that overall image resolution depends on more than just contrast and sharpness. Adequate density and control of noise, magnification and distortion also affect the ability to distinguish details.

Modulation Transfer Function

Physicists use a complex measurement of the total resolution capacity of an imaging system called *modulation transfer function* or *MTF*. A full discussion of MTF is not necessary for radiographers, but it is worth noting that MTF is very similar to density trace diagrams. If one were to expose a resolution test template, the density trace diagram for the resulting silver deposits on the film would be essentially identical to an MTF graph. A high MTF indicates that the imaging system produces high resolution, and therefore provides images with maximum diagnostic information. A low MTF indicates poor overall image quality.

Geometrical Penumbra

X-rays can be emitted at various angles and from different points within the area of the focal spot, and yet record the same edge of an object on the film. This means that the same edge of the object will actually be recorded several times in various different locations on

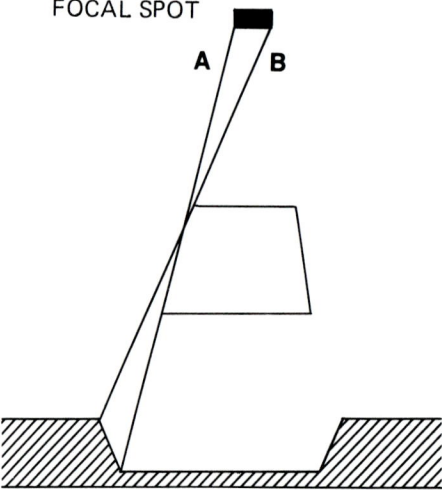

Figure 275. Density trace diagram illustrating geometrical penumbra. The extent of penumbra is represented by the horizontal spread of the edge gradient slopes.

the film, Figure 275. This "spreading" of the edge constitutes blur or *penumbra.*

In Figure 275, between "A" and "B" absorption of the x-ray beam is *partial,* increasing toward the object. Hence, "penumbra" may be thought of as a *partial absorption* process (bearing in mind that "partial" refers to a portion of the total amount of x-rays which the object in question is capable of absorbing, not to a portion of the total x-ray beam).

Absorption Penumbra

"Absorption unsharpness" or "absorption penumbra" is a blurring of the edge of an image due to the relationship between the shape of the object being radiographed and the diverging x-ray beam. Suppose that several objects having different shapes, but made out of the same, homogeneous material, are to be radiographed:

The "ideal" shape for an object to be radiographed would be a trapezoid whose slanted sides coincide exactly with the angles of the diverging x-rays (Figure 276-A). All portions of the x-ray beam striking such an object will be attenuated by the same thickness of material. The density trace diagram in Figure 276 shows that there will be no blur due to absorption unsharpness at the edge of the image produced. Note that the black silver deposit on the film drops off straight down at the edge of this image. The image of the trapezoid is as "white" just inside the edge as it is in the middle. This "sudden" change in density at the edge of the image represents a sharp edge with no blur.

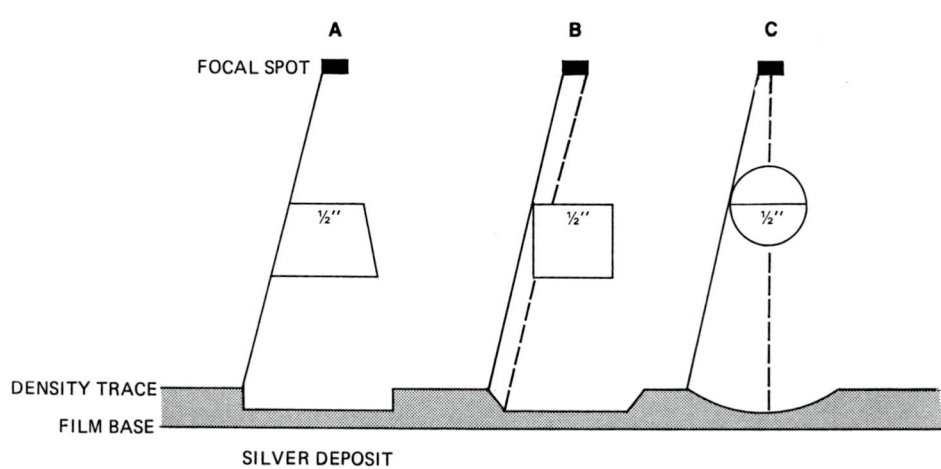

Figure 276. Density trace diagrams for absorption penumbra, using objects of equal width but different shapes. The trapezoid object (A) will produce geometrical penumbra as shown in Figure 275, but will have no *absorption* penumbra as shown here. The square object (B) absorbs most radiation at the thickest portion of its projected edge, causing a penumbral edge gradient. For a spherical object (C) the edge gradient (penumbra) extends to the middle of the image.

Imaging a *cube* of the same material (Figure 276-B) yields different results: Note that the lateral diverging x-rays pass through only a small thickness of material at the upper corners of the cube. Little absorption occurs, and the density trace shows a reduced but still dark deposit of silver. As inner beams pass through thicker portions, the density trace drops until the full thickness of the cube is reached at the lower corners (dashed line). On observing this image, the density would gradually change from dark to light as one scans across its edge. This effect is identical to geometrical blurring, even though it is caused by a different process.

Worse yet is the spherical object (Figure 276-C), whose full thickness is found only at the center. The density trace shows that the drop in density is very gradual and the edges of the image very indistinct.

Referring to Figure 276, note that all three objects are of the same thickness in the center, and should have identical absorption and identical contrast at this point. Indeed, the density traces have dropped the same vertical distance in the center of each image.

Total Penumbra

A representation of total blur or penumbra may be obtained by combining the diagram for geometrical blur with that for absorption blur (Figure 277), using a cube or a spherical object. In this case, all beams are not absorbed at the inside penumbral line, but rather at the (dashed) absorption line. Within the penumbral (solid) lines, absorption varies primarily because the beams originate at different points within the focal spot. Within the dashed lines, absorption continues to vary, but strictly because of changing object thickness. *Total penumbra is comprised of geometrical penumbra plus absorption penumbra.*

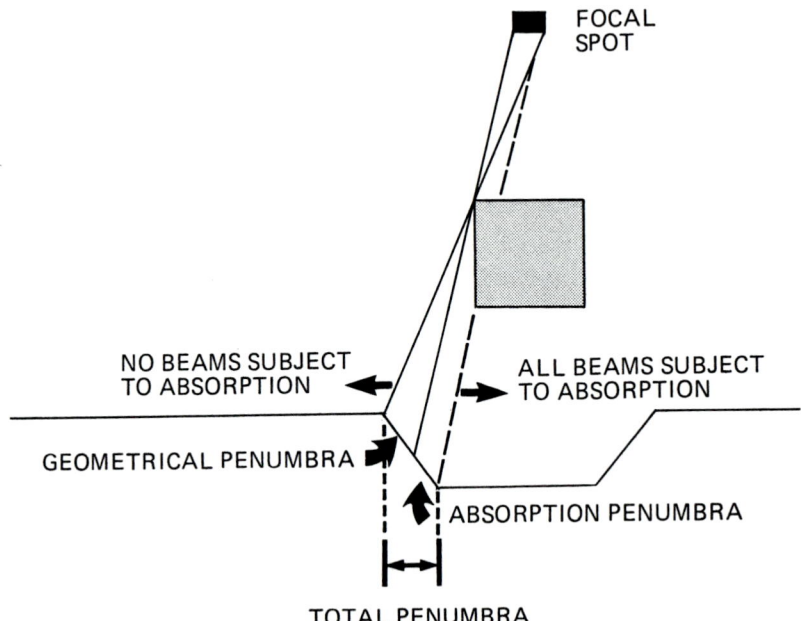

Figure 277. Density trace diagram combining the effects of geometrical penumbra and absorption penumbra in producing the total penumbra or total amount of blurring at the image edge.

Magnification, Distortion and Noise

Magnification or distortion of an image does not cause any change in edge gradient. The slope of the edge will drop at the same rate.

(Many of the same variables that create magnification also cause unsharpness, and it is easy to mistake the two as being directly related to each other, but they are not. If the magnification of an image is accompanied by increased blur, that is, if the expansion of the umbra is accompanied by an expansion of the penumbra, then adjacent details may overlap and image resolution will be lost. But, this loss of resolution is due to the *blurring*, which does affect the slope of the edge gradient, *not* to the magnification. Desirable magnification techniques, such as those used in angiography, can be employed without a loss of sharpness.)

Clearly, the enlargement of any image makes it more visible overall, but results in an inaccurate representation of its true size. The value of magnification depends on whether the diagnostic emphasis is on measurement or simple detection.

Noise, such as an artifact or fog, superimposes and obscures the visibility of the anatomy of interest. This does not change the slope of the edge gradient, but since details are obscured, overall image resolution is lost.

SUMMARY

To summarize, any image must be both visible and recognizable in order to possess high resolution. The visibility of the image is best when its intensity (density) is adequate, its contrast and gray scale are balanced, and its noise is minimal. The image is most recognizable when its geometrical integrity is maintained with the real object it represents. This occurs when sharpness of recorded detail is maximized and when magnification and shape distortion are minimized.

Hierarchy of Image Qualities

An overview of the relationship between all of the radiographic image qualities is presented in graphic form in Figure 278, and a concise table of definitions of imaging terms follows.

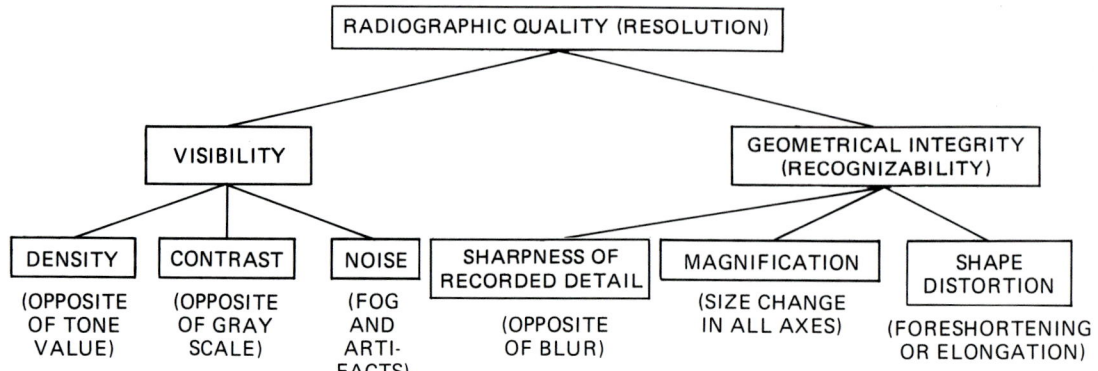

Figure 278. Hierarchy of radiographic image qualities.

Definitions of Image Qualities

1. **Density:** The degree of *blackness* in an area of the image, determined by the amount of silver deposited on the film in that area.

2. **Tone Value:** The amount of light that is able to pass through an area on the film, or its *translucency.* The opposite of density.

3. **Contrast:** The *ratio* of difference between two adjacent densities on the film.

4. **Gray Scale:** The *range* or number of different densities present on the film. The opposite of contrast.

5. **Noise:** Any unwanted, *useless information* recorded on the film which obscures the visibility of the desired image. Includes fog, static and artifacts.

6. **Fog:** A form of noise, fog is a veil of *useless density* covering portions of the desired image. It is caused by randomly scattered radiation which carries no useful signal or image.

7. **Sharpness of Recorded Detail:** The *abruptness* with which the edges of an image stop. Also, the lack of penumbra in an image.

8. **Blur:** See **Penumbra.** The lack of sharpness, or the presence of penumbra, in an image.

9. **Penumbra:** A *partial shadow* at the edges of an image, whereby its transition into the adjacent density is gradual rather than abrupt.

10. **Magnification:** The *difference* between the *size* of a real object (measured in all axes) and the size of its umbral image on the radiograph.

11. **Distortion of Shape:** The *difference* between the *shape* of a real

object and the shape of its image on the radiograph, consisting of either *elongation or foreshortening* of the image in one axis.

12. **Visibility Factors:** Those factors which directly affect the ability to *see* an image, including density or tone value, contrast or gray scale, and noise including fog.

13. **Geometrical Integrity (Recognizability) Factors:** All those *geometric* factors in an image which directly affect the ability to *discern* the nature of the real object it represents. These include sharpness of detail, magnification, and shape distortion.

14. **Resolution:** The ability to distinguish adjacent details as being *separate* from each other, controlled by both visibility factors and geometrical factors.

15. **Radiographic Image Quality:** The total amount of useful diagnostic information resolved in an image, controlled by all of the visibility and geometrical factors.

REVIEW #3

A: CRITIQUING DENSITY AND REPEATING RADIOGRAPHS

Radiographers must develop, primarily through experience, the ability to accurately assess the technical qualities of the finished radiograph — its density level, contrast, gray scale, noise level, sharpness of recorded detail, and any magnification or distortion present. This ability is *essential* to the control of unnecessary repeated exposures to the patient.

The following exercise is designed to help the student develop an ability to visually estimate the needed adjustment in overall technique when repeating an exposure that turned out too light or too dark. In each of two series of radiographs, (Figures 279 and 280), a radiograph with optimum density level is first shown for comparison. The following numbered radiographs were taken at precisely selected techniques at rounded out values, such as double the original mAs or one-third the original mAs. For each of the numbered radiographs, estimate the *overall technique change* required to restore density to the optimum level. All answers are in factors of 2, 3 or 4. Check your answers using the Appendix.

1. For the series of chest radiographs in Figure 279, compare each of the *numbered* radiographs to the *optimum* radiograph first shown.

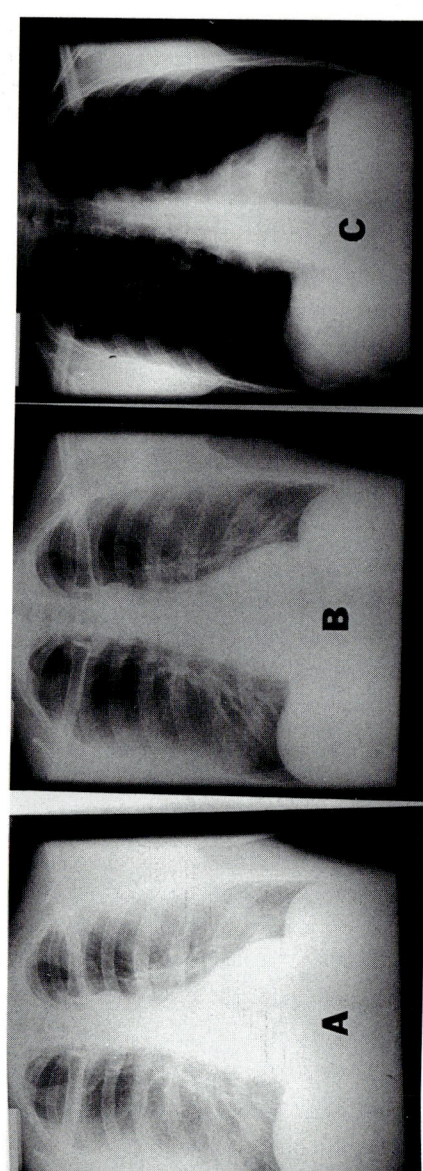

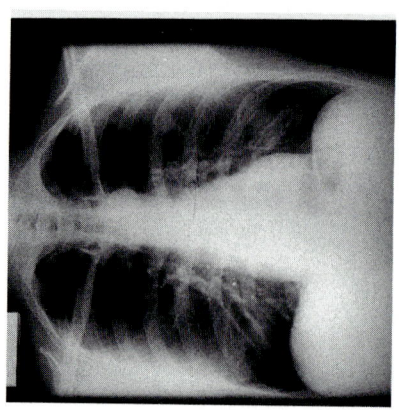

Figure 279. Chest radiographs for density change estimation.

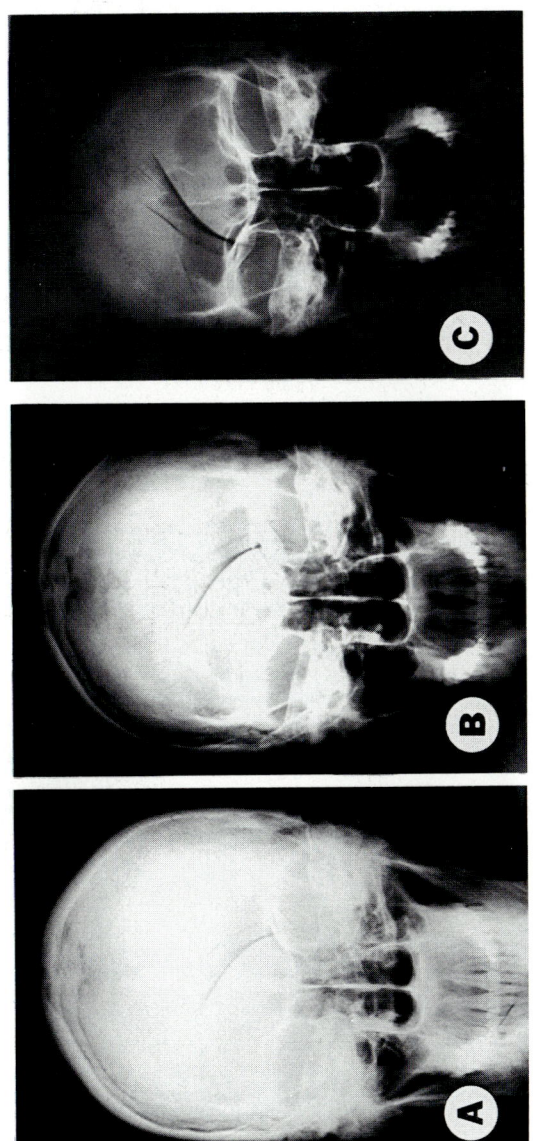

Figure 280. Skull radiographs for density change estimation.

List the *factor* to which the density for each numbered radiograph should be changed to restore it to optimum density. The correct answer will be *4X, 3X, 2X, 1/2, 1/3 or 1/4.*

2. For the series of skull radiographs in Figure 280, compare each of the *numbered* radiographs to the *optimum* radiograph first shown. List the *factor* to which the density for each numbered radiograph should be changed to restore it to optimum density. The correct answer will be *4X, 3X, 2X, 1/2, 1/3 or 1/4.*

B: CRITIQUING IMAGE QUALITIES

Referring to the four radiographs in Figure 281:

1. Which of the four has the longest gray scale?
2. Which of the four has the highest contrast?
3. Which of the four is fogged most?
4. Which of the two elbows shows better penetration?
5. Which of the two elbows shows resolution of more detail?
6. Which of the two abdomens is lighter overall?

Referring to the four magnetic resonance images in Figure 282:

7. Which of the four magnetic resonance images in Figure 282 demonstrates the greatest amount of resolution of details overall?

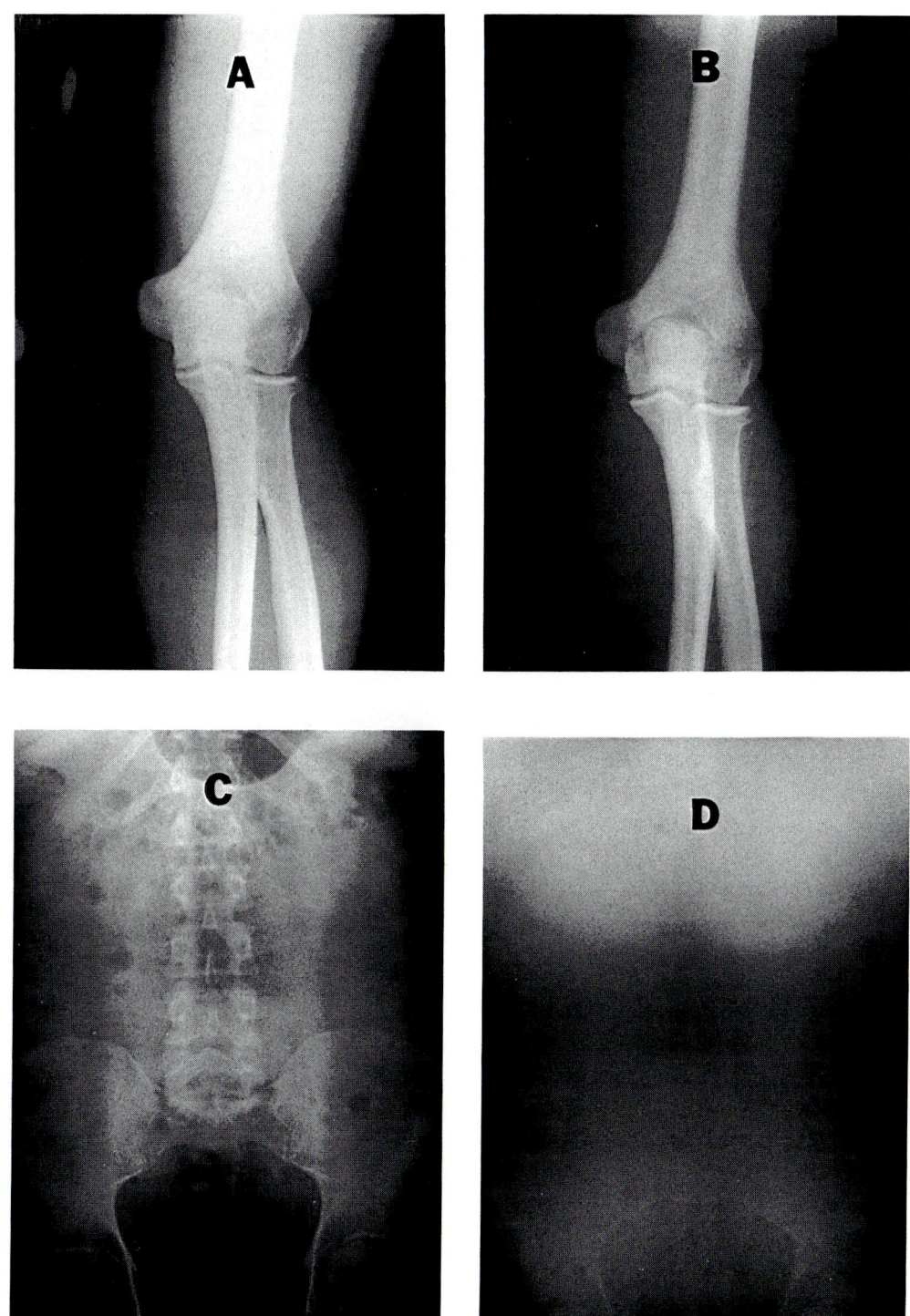

Figure 281.

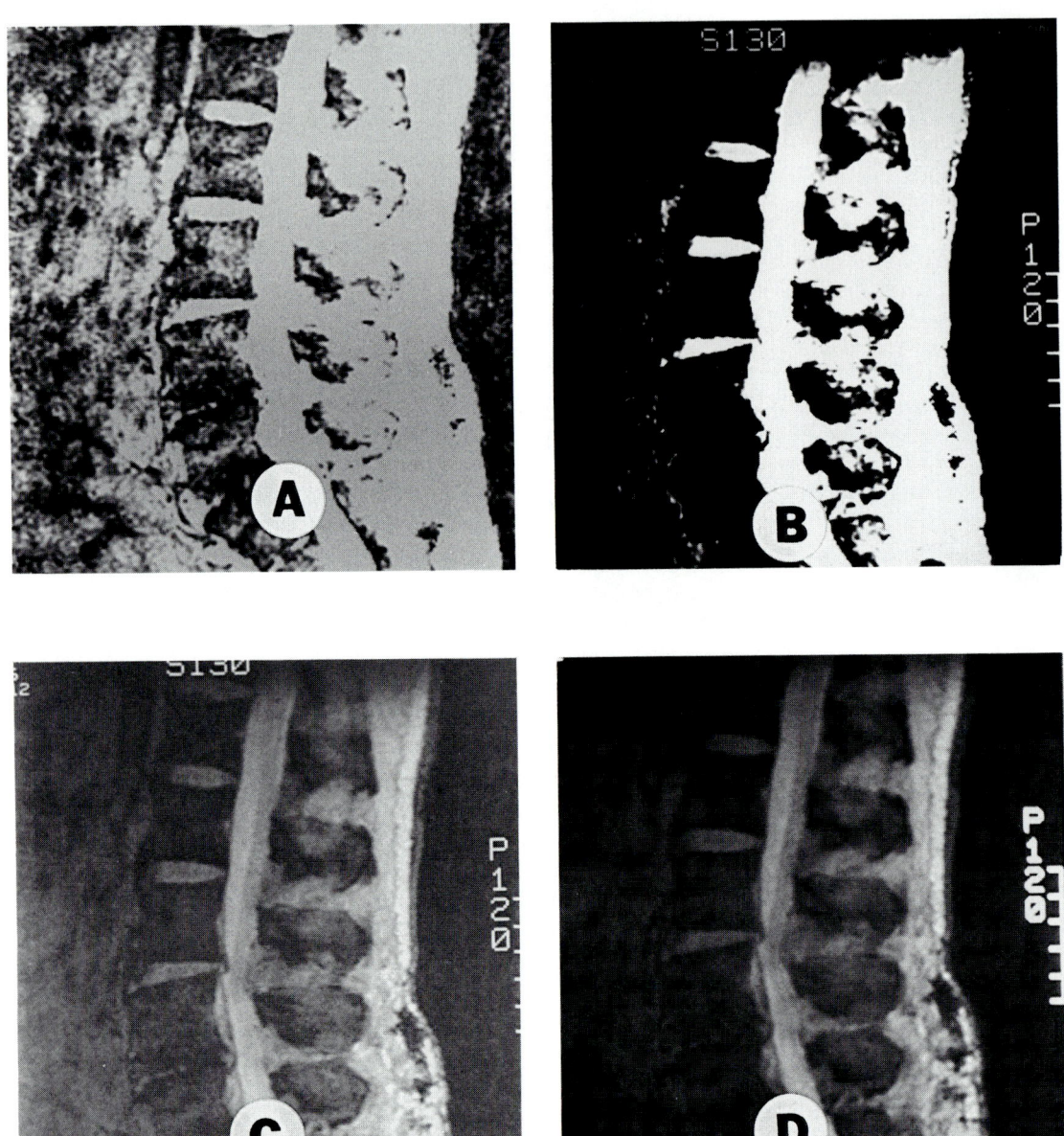

Figure 282.

APPENDIX 1

REVIEW 1

Figure Number **Critique**

40. Centered high, clipping both the hip prosthesis and the ischial tuberosities.
(Slight pelvic rotation due to scoliosis.)

41. Excessive film and field size.
No gonadal shielding.
Coils of wire leads unnecessarily over anatomy.
(Rotation in chest.)

42. Artifact (patient's nose) superimposing breast tissue.

43. Respirator hose and connection over patient's mediastinum.
Electrical leads crossing lung fields unnecessarily.
(Rotated position, and centered high clipping bottom of lung.)

44. Breathing motion (Note blurriness of diaphragms and kidneys).
Centered slightly low with circular field, clipping right diaphragm.

45. Voluntary motion of entire torso (Note that spine and ribs are are blurred as well as lung details).
(Anterior costophrenic angle is clipped due to patient learning back.)

46. Intravenous line caught between patient and film (Note relative sharpness of IV line, indicating closeness to film).
Fog from exposure to light across lower left lung field.

47. Guide shoe scratches (Note that they run parallel to the direction of film travel).

48. Roller marks with linear fogging patterns due to stopping movement of film through developer tank (Note that they run perpendicular to the direction of film travel).
Artifact (hair pin or pen) over upper right lung.

49. Double image caused by double exposure (internal and external rotation views) of shoulder. Motion can cause similar double images, but in this case, the darkness of the image and the shape of the head of the humerus can be used to determine double exposure.

50. Overcollimation resulting in clipped anatomy of interest. (This view is centered properly, close to the PIP joint.)

51.   "Tree" static electricity marks (top) and "smudge" static marks (bottom) due to friction from rough handling.

REVIEW 2

Figure Number   Critique

205.   Inadequate inspiration, showing only eight ribs above diaphragm. Film hung up reversed right-to-left.

206.   Blocker over sternal extremity of clavicle due to placing it medially and centering film too laterally.

207.   Clipping of costophrenic angles due to centering of *field* too high and possibly also from vertical overcollimation.

208.   Rotation of head to patient's left. Slight head tilt.

209.   Rotation of entire torso to patient's right. Film centered much too high, clipping left costophrenic angle. Unnecessary amount of lead wires over lung fields.

210.   Rotation of entire torso about one-half inch, resulting in one inch of shift of posterior ribs and costophrenic angles. Film centered slightly low, placing blocker in lung field.

211.   Inadequate abduction of arms, placing soft tissue of arm over upper lung field. Blocker improperly placed down, just running into left posterior costophrenic angle.

212.   Over-rotation, placing sternum four inches from spine and resulting in unnecessary obliquity of sternum.

213.   Proper 35 degrees of rotation for female cystogram.

214.   Too steep rotation for an IVP, placing upside kidney and ureter directly over spine. Centered high, clipping floor of bladder and upper rim of pubic bones.

215.   Too steep rotation, closing off SI joint and placing iliac crest on end.

216.   Good centering and collimation. (Position is RAO.) Shallow obliquity for purpose of opening C-loop.

217.   Improper patient preparation, leaving stool and excessive gas in colon.

218.   Upright view during air contrast barium enema. *Right* marker placed in poor location, superimposing it over ascending colon.

219.   *Left* marker placed too far medially on film, superimposing transverse process of fifth lumbar vertebra.

220.   Head rotation to patient's right, placing left upper teeth over C1 and atlantoaxial joint.

Slight flexion of head, placing upper teeth lower than occipital bone and obscuring odontoid process.

221. Slight rotation of torso, but not enough to repeat.
Fog pattern obliterating posterior spinous processes, which could have been corrected by using lead sheet behind patient on table.

222. Rotated too steep (too lateral) for oblique C-spine, causing narrowing of intervertebral foramina.
Centered film two inches too high, but not clipping C7.

223. Failure to depress shoulders to demonstrate C7.

224. Blurred due to motion.
Interphalangeal joints closed off due to improper flexion of fingers to rest fingertips on film.

225. Rotated toward pronation for lateral wrist, placing ulna posterior to radius. Hand, which is in true lateral position, should be supinated 5 degrees in order to place wrist in true lateral.

226. Tilted elbow due to improper abduction of humerus (failure to get shoulder down at level of film with 90 degrees of shoulder abduction).

227. Tilted condyles obscuring knee joint due to failure to use 5 degree cephalic beam angle.
Medial rotation of knee, due to failure to roll leg out and down toward table enough.

228. Hyperflexion of head for PA skull view, placing petrous ridges above superior rims of orbits.

229. For Caldwell view, 5 degrees of head *extension* OR 5 degrees *too much caudal angle* places petrous ridges at lower rims of orbits.
Coned field centered too high, clipping floor of maxillary sinus.
Coned field off-centered side-to-side, also contributing to clipping off of one maxillary sinus.
(There is no rotation in this view, only off-centering.)

230. Collar obscures lower petrous pyramid.
Slight head rotation, but proper beam angle and flexion/extension of head.

231. Tilted (but not rotated) lateral view, displacing orbital plates of frontal bone vertically.

232. For Townes view, insufficient caudal tube angle OR presence of head extension causing less than one-half of foramen magnum to rise over junction of petrous pyramids and leaving petrous ridges at an obtuse angle.
Rotation to patient's right.
Low centering of *field* clipping off top of cranium.
Technique too dark.

233. Insufficient head extension for open-mouth Waters view, leaving upper teeth over sphenoid sinus.
Slight rotation.

234.   Good position for oblique mandible.
            Technique a bit dark.
235.   Insufficient extension of head for Waters view, placing petrous
            ridges over lower maxillary sinuses.
            Centered a bit too low clipping top of frontal sinuses.
236.   Failure to *abduct* unaffected thigh left soft tissue density obscuring
            acetabulum and head of affected femur for groin lateral
            projection.
237.   Too steep body rotation for lateral scapula view placing lateral
            border of scapula over lateral ribs.
238.   Improper flexion of elbow during frontal view resulting in head of
            radius overlapping capitellum of humerus.
239.   Combination of improper beam angle and centering too high
            resulted in closing off of lumbosacral joint.

REVIEW 3

Part A: 1.   A.   3X
               B.   2X
               C.   1/2
          2.   A.   4X
               B.   2X
               C.   1/3
Part B: 1.   C
          2.   A
          3.   D
          4.   B
          5.   B
          6.   D
          7.   C

APPENDIX 2

REVIEW QUESTIONS

Chapter 1

1. Legally, which of the following is the most credible form of radiographic labelling:
   a. written ink
   b. sticker
   c. lead marker
   d. written china marker
2. Who has the primary responsibility for determining any modifications in routine, positioning or technique that should be made for a particular patient:
   a. nurse
   b. referring physician
   c. radiologist
   d. radiographer
3. A radiograph will turn out light if technique is not increased for:
   a. excessive aeration
   b. additive diseases
   c. asthenic body habitus
   d. wood slivers
4. A radiograph will turn out dark if technique is not decreased for:
   a. postmortem radiography
   b. presence of barium
   c. muscular build
   d. a patient who is 4 cm thinner than average
5. "Right" and "left" lead markers may be used to label:
   a. the position the patient is in
   b. which side is down for decubitus views
   c. anatomy
   d. all of the above

Chapter 2

6. Mismatching of films and screen cassettes results in repeated exposures because the image turns out:
   a. light

    b. dark

    c. unsharp

    d. mottled

7. The difference in the radiation dose received by an organ when it lies *within* the x-ray beam compared to lying just outside the edge of the beam is:

    a. two times greater

    b. 10 times greater

    c. 100 times greater

    d. 1000 times greater

8. Generally field size should be about:

    a. 5 percent larger than the anatomy of interest

    b. 20 percent larger than the anatomy of interest

    c. 33 percent larger than the anatomy of interest

    d. 2 inches beyond the anatomy of interest on all sides

9. Lead shielding should NOT be used if:

    a. no critical organs lie within the x-ray field

    b. the patient is not of child-bearing age

    c. it would obscure the gonads

    d. it would obscure the anatomy of interest

10. Which of the following practices does NOT help reduce repeat rates:

    a. using automatic exposure controls on all procedures

    b. using manual technique charts

    c. continuing education

    d. processor quality control monitoring

Chapter 3

11. A radiograph shows a white exposure artifact which is slightly blurred and slightly magnified. The location of the object causing the artifact was most likely:

    a. within the film cassette

    b. behind the patient

    c. on top of the patient

    d. near the x-ray tube

12. Which of the following situations would result in a dark radiograph:

    a. double technique for a mixed fiberglass/plaster cast

    b. triple technique for a wet plaster cast on a knee

    c. 50 percent increase in technique for a thick wood splint

    d. no change in technique for a sheet of plexiglass

13. An upper GI radiograph demonstrates blurriness around the duodenal bulb, but sharply defined ribs, diaphragm, and spine. This is a case of:

    a. heart motion

    b. breathing motion

    c. peristaltic motion

    d. voluntary motion

14. An upper GI radiograph demonstrates blurriness of all anatomy including the bones. If the patient did not move, this could be a case of:
    a. failure to engage the Potter-Bucky mechanism
    b. failure to lock the x-ray tube
    c. heart motion
    d. breathing motion

Chapter 4

15. X-ray film will be fogged most quickly:
    a. in storage before the box is opened
    b. after exposure but before processing
    c. after opening the box but before exposure
    d. after processing
16. Pressure can cause which of the following artifacts on a radiograph:
    1. dark marks
    2. light marks
    3. crescent-shaped marks
    4. static marks
    a. 1 and 3 only
    b. 1 and 4 only
    c. 1, 3 and 4
    d. 1, 2, 3 and 4
17. Tree or crown static can be caused by:
    1. low humidity
    2. rough handling
    3. invisible electrical discharges
    4. visible electrical discharges
    a. 1 and 2 only
    b. 4 only
    c. 1, 2 and 3
    d. 1, 2, 3 and 4
18. Guide shoe scratch marks will show up on the radiograph as:
    a. white lines perpendicular to the direction of film travel, at even intervals
    b. white lines parallel to the direction of film travel, at even intervals
    c. white lines parallel to the direction of film travel, at uneven intervals
    d. dark lines perpendicular to the direction of film travel, at even intervals
19. A small black spot occuring at regular intervals in a line parallel to the direction of film travel is caused by:
    a. a grain of dirt embedded in a roller
    b. dirty wash water
    c. quantum mottle
    d. reticulation
20. Uneven sheen on a radiograph is caused by improperly seated:
    a. dryer tubes
    b. rollers

    c. guide shoes

    d. feed rollers

21. When the developer solution thermostat is not functioning, radiographs will emerge from the processor:

    a. dark

    b. light

    c. mottled

    d. stained

Chapter 5

22. Crosswise placement of the cassette for a PA chest projection is indicated for:

    a. all male patients

    b. obese patients

    c. broad-shouldered patients

    d. no patients

23. Which of the following is an acceptable placement of the "right" or "left" marker for the oblique view of the cervical spine:

    a. upper anterior

    b. lower posterior

    c. lower anterior

    d. none of these

24. A frontal view of a child's chest shows all four edges of the field within the film area. One inch of the *right* costophrenic angle of the lung is cut off laterally, yet one-half inch of the *left* costophrenic is also clipped off. Which of the following are causes of the cut off:

    1. too small film size

    2. collimated too tight

    3. field off-centered to the patient

    4. patient off-centered to the film

    a. 1 only

    b. 1 and 4 only

    c. 2 and 3 only

    d. 2, 3 and 4

25. A Townes (Grashey) view of the skull shows the blocker placed at the bottom, obscuring part of the occipital bone, while there are two inches of exposed film above the skull. Which of the following contributed to the obscured anatomy:

    1. film placement (CW or LW)

    2. blocker placement (up or down)

    3. film centering

    4. x-ray beam centering

    a. 1, 2 and 3

    b. 2 and 3 only

    c. 2 and 4 only

    d. 1, 2, 3 and 4

Chapter 6

26. For frontal or lateral radiographs, a side-to-side shift of a pair of identical anatomical parts indicates what type of body movement:
    a. rotation
    b. flexion/extension
    c. tilt
    d. abduction/adduction

27. During positioning for a Townes (Grashey) view of the skull with the patient supine, angling the x-ray beam caudal is equivalent to:
    a. extending the chin
    b. flexing the chin
    c. tilting the top of the head toward the film
    d. rotating the face away from the film

28. During positioning for lateral view of the skull, angling the x-ray beam cephalic would be equivalent to:
    a. extending the chin
    b. flexing the chin
    c. tilting the top of the head toward the film
    d. tilting the top of the head away from the film

29. For a lateral radiographic view, vertical (up or down) shift of a pair of identical anatomical parts indicates which type of body movement:
    a. rotation
    b. flexion
    c. extension
    d. tilt, abduction or adduction

30. Anatomical criteria selected to evaluate positioning on a radiograph should be a pair of identical parts which lie:
    a. close to the central ray location
    b. close to each other
    c. close to the midline of the body
    d. close to the film

31. Anatomical criteria selected to evaluate positioning on a radiograph should be a pair of identical parts which lie:
    a. perpendicular to the film
    b. perpendicular to each other
    c. perpendicular to the expected direction of shift
    d. parallel to the central ray

32. In critiquing a rotated frontal view of the chest, the *amount* of apparent shift of the sternoclavicular joints depends on:
    a. the thickness of the patient's body
    b. the amount of rotation
    c. the focus-film distance used
    d. all of these
    e. none of these

Chapter 7

33. For a lateral projection of the chest, the patient's shoulders are placed in line, but the patient has one foot placed in front of the other. On the resulting view, this will result in:
    a. assymetrical sternoclavicular joints
    b. desuperimposed upper posterior ribs
    c. desuperimposed posterior costophrenic angles of lungs
    d. desuperimposed scapulae

34. For the lateral view of the chest, five degrees of rotation will shift the right and left posterior ribs how far off of each other:
    a. ¼ inch
    b. ½ inch
    c. 1 inch
    d. 2 inches

35. A posterior oblique view of the ribs shows the heads of the downside ribs overlapping the spine. The position was:
    a. too steep
    b. too shallow
    c. just right
    d. tilted

36. An RAO sternum view shows the sternum shifted 3 inches away from the spine. The position was:
    a. too steep
    b. too shallow
    c. just right
    d. tilted

37. A "portable" AP projection of the chest shows the clavicles over the first ribs and a straightened, linear appearance to the posterior ribs. This view was most likely taken with the:
    a. patient sitting up too erect
    b. tube angled too caudal
    c. tube not angled caudal enough
    d. tube and patient correctly positioned

38. For a premature infant in a newborn intensive care unit, how many posterior pairs of ribs should be visible above the diaphragms:
    a. 6
    b. 8
    c. 10
    d. 12

39. An RAO projection of the sternum shows blurring of the lung markings. This indicates:
    a. proper technique
    b. voluntary motion
    c. improper distance

    d. excessive exposure time

40. At 30–35 degrees of rotation of the pelvis, the upside iliac crest usually appears:
    a. flat and broad
    b. flat but somewhat foreshortened
    c. "looped"
    d. fully on end

41. On a KUB radiograph, the right obturator foramen appears foreshortened compared to the left foramen. This indicates:
    a. rotation toward the patient's right
    b. rotation toward the patient's left
    c. cephalic tube angulation
    d. caudal tube angulation
    e. diagonal alignment of the body on the table

42. An oblique view during an IVP shows the upside ureter overlapping the spine. The position was rotated:
    a. too steep
    b. too shallow
    c. the correct amount

43. An upright projection is taken during an acute abdomen series with the patient and table tilted back 15 degrees from vertical, so the patient can lean back against the table. Which of the following beam angles and centering should be used:
    a. beam angled 15 degrees downward, perpendicular to the table, centered to the level of the iliac crests
    b. beam angled 15 degrees downward, perpendicular to the table, centered 1–2 inches above the iliac crests
    c. beam horizontal, centered 3–4 inches above the iliac crests
    d. beam horizontal, centered at the level of the iliac crests

44. During a barium enema, which position should be centered 3–4 inches above the iliac crests:
    a. AP
    b. decubitus
    c. LPO
    d. RPO

45. A radiographic view from an air contrast barium enema shows barium pooling in the rectum and along the entire length of the ascending colon. The position used was:
    a. erect
    b. left posterior oblique
    c. left lateral decubitus
    d. right lateral decubitus

46. Which of the following oblique views during an upper GI series best demonstrates the C-loop of the duodenum, laying it out parallel to the film:
    a. steep LPO

    b. shallow LPO

    c. steep RPO

    d. shallow RPO

47. A frontal view during a cystogram shows the floor of the bladder superimposed over the pubic bones. Which of the following is true:
    a. the position was performed correctly
    b. the CR should have been angled caudally
    c. the CR should have been angled cephalic
    d. the pelvis was tilted so as to arch the patient's back

48. Which of the following is NOT an indicator of rotation on frontal spine views:
    a. symmetry of the pedicles over the vertebral body
    b. centering of the spinous process over the vertebral body
    c. double edges seen at the posterior vertebral bodies
    d. superimposition of the head of one rib over the vertebral body

49. Closure of the joints of the spinal column can be caused by:
    1. improper flexion/extension of the spine
    2. improper spinal tilt
    3. off-centering of the x-ray beam
    4. improper angulation of the x-ray beam
    a. 1 only
    b. 1 and 4 only
    c. 1, 3 and 4
    d. 1, 2, 3 and 4

50. An oblique view of the lumbar spine shows one pedicle placed over the posterior half of the vertebral body. The position was:
    a. rotated too steep
    b. rotated too shallow
    c. tilted
    d. positioned correctly

51. A frontal view of the cervical spine shows the chin superimposed over the third cervical vertebra and the lower intervertebral joints closed. Which of the following caused this:
    a. head flexed too much
    b. head extended too much
    c. failure to angle the x-ray beam
    d. correct positioning

52. An open-mouth odontoid view shows the occipital bone and the bottom edge of the upper incisor teeth superimposed, yet an upper right molar tooth superimposes the joint space between the atlas and the axis. The patient's head was:
    a. improperly flexed
    b. improperly tilted
    c. rotated to the patient's right
    d. rotated to the patient's left

53. An oblique view of the cervical spine shows *all* of the intervertebral foramina

fully opened, but the gonion of the mandible superimposes the second cervical vertebra. The most likely cause was:

    a. improper rotation of the body

    b. improper rotation of the head

    c. chin flexed

    d. chin extended

    e. head tilted

54. The recommended method for assuring that an infant's chin does not superimpose the apices of the lungs during a supine AP chest projection is to:

    a. angle the beam cephalic

    b. angle the beam caudal

    c. drop the head off the top of the film

    d. place a 15-degree angle sponge under the shoulders

55. Which of the following is strongly recommended for use on the frontal projection of the thoracic spine:

    a. breathing technique

    b. wedge filter

    c. cephalic beam angle

    d. angle sponge

Chapter 8

56. An oblique view of the hand shows the heads of metacarpal bones overlapping, but spaces are seen between the *shafts* of the metacarpals. This position was:

    a. rotated too steep

    b. rotated too shallow

    c. rotated correctly

    d. improperly flexed

57. A *lateral* view of a finger shows closing of the interphalangeal joints. This was caused by:

    a. flexion of the finger

    b. tilt of the finger

    c. rotation of the finger

58. Which view of the wrist is designed to desuperimpose the greater and lesser multangular bones:

    a. PA

    b. oblique

    c. lateral

59. A lateral view of the wrist demonstrates part of the head of the ulna posterior to the radius. The position was:

    a. correct

    b. rotated toward pronation

    c. rotated toward supination

    d. tilted

60. In order to perfectly superimpose the two bones of the forearm for a lateral wrist projection, the *hand* must be:

    a. in true lateral
    b. slightly supinated
    c. slightly pronated

61. A frontal view of the elbow demonstrates the head of the radius overlapping the capitellum of the humerus. The elbow was:
    a. improperly flexed
    b. improperly rotated
    c. improperly tilted
    d. correctly done

62. A lateral view of the forearm shows the two condyles of the humerus shifted off of each other vertically (superior-to-inferior). This indicates:
    a. the patient's wrist is not all the way down on the film
    b. the patient did not get his shoulder down level with the film
    c. the patient's humerus was rotated
    d. this appearance is correct for a lateral forearm

63. A *transthoracic* lateral view of the humerus shows the two humeral condyles shifted off of each other side-to-side. This indicates:
    1. the hand was not supinated properly
    2. the x-ray beam was not angled properly
    3. the humerus was rotated
    4. the humerus was tilted
    5. the patient was leaning sideways into the film
    a. 4 only
    b. 3 only
    c. 1 or 3
    d. 2, 4 or 5

64. With proper positioning, on the *transaxillary* view of the shoulder the head and neck of the humerus will appear just as it does on the:
    a. external rotation AP shoulder
    b. internal rotation AP shoulder
    c. transaxillary shoulder view with hand in "neutral" position

65. A lateral view of the scapula demonstrates the lateral border of the scapula and glenoid fossa superimposing the lateral ribs. The body position was:
    a. correct
    b. rotated too steep
    c. rotated too shallow
    d. flexed
    e. tilted

66. Use of a wedge filter is recommended for the:
    1. AP foot
    2. lateral foot
    3. PD calcaneus
    4. lateral calcaneus
    5. AP ankle
    a. 1 only

    b. 1 and 2

    c. 1 and 3

    d. 2 and 4

    e. all of these

67. A lateral view of the foot shows the thick first metatarsal bone projected inferior to the heads of the other metatarsals. To correct this position, the patient must:

    a. roll his knee down closer to the table

    b. roll his knee up farther away from the table

    c. rotate the lower leg more laterally

    d. do nothing — the position is correct

68. A view of the ankle shows the distal fibula completely desuperimposed from tibia, with the tibiofibular and talofibular joints both opened. This view is a(n):

    a. 45-degree external oblique

    b. 45-degree internal oblique

    c. 15-degree external oblique

    d. 15-degree internal oblique

69. A lateral view of the ankle shows part of the distal fibula extending posterior to the tibia. The patient's thigh was abducted:

    a. insufficiently, with the knee too far off the table

    b. too much, with the knee lying on the table

    c. correctly, with the knee resting on a sponge

70. A knee view shows the patella over the medial femoral condyle and the proximal tibiofibular joint fully opened. This position was:

    a. a straight AP view

    b. an AP view rotated 10 degrees

    c. a proper internal oblique view

    d. an internal oblique view over-rotated too laterally

71. A lateral knee view demonstrates the posterior surfaces of the two femoral condyles close to each other, yet one of the condyles superimposes both the knee joint and the subpatellar space. This was caused by:

    a. lateral knee rotation

    b. medial knee rotation

    c. failure to angle the x-ray beam cephalic

    d. failure to flex the knee 45 degrees

72. An axial view for the patella shows the rounded anterior edge of the tibial plateau closing off the subpatellar space and superimposing the undersurface of the patella. The view was taken with the patient sitting, holding the film over the distal femur. The error was that the:

    a. knee was overflexed too tight

    b. beam was angled upward too much

    c. beam was not angled upward enough

73. To obtain a clear view of the acetabulum and head of the femur for a groin (cross-table) lateral projection of the hip, it is essential to:

1. abduct the unaffected thigh
2. hyperflex the unaffected thigh
3. externally rotate the affected thigh
4. rest the unaffected foot on the table

   a. 2 and 4
   b. 2 and 3
   c. 1 and 2
   d. 1, 3 and 4

74. In order to place the femur in true lateral position for a unilateral projection, it is usually necessary to rotate the pelvis toward the affected side. This is the:
    a. Holmblad method
    b. Danellius-Miller method
    c. Lauenstein method
    d. Kuchendorf method

75. On an AP pelvis projection, the greater trochanters are seen to partially overlap the necks of the femurs. This is due to:
    a. rotation of the pelvis
    b. internal rotation of the legs
    c. failure to internally rotate the legs
    d. improper abduction of the legs

Chapter 9

76. A Caldwell view of the skull shows the petrous ridges at the middle of the orbits. Which of the following could have caused this appearance:
    1. insufficient caudal tube angle
    2. excessive caudal tube angle
    3. over-flexion of the head
    4. over-extension of the head
    5. head tilt

    a. 1 only
    b. 1 or 3
    c. 1 or 4
    d. 2 or 4
    e. 2, 4 or 5

77. A PA projection is taken with the orbitomeatal line perpendicular to the film. Which of the following x-ray beam angles would project the petrous ridges just below the *inferior* rims of the orbits:
    a. 12 degrees caudal
    b. 12 degrees cephalic
    c. 22 degrees caudal
    d. 22 degrees cephalic
    e. 30 degrees caudal

78. An open-mouth Waters view shows the lower teeth superimposing the sphenoid sinuses. To correct this error:
    a. angle the beam caudally

b. tilt the head slightly

c. close the mouth slightly more

d. extend the chin upward more

e. flex the chin downward more

79. On a Waters view the petrous ridges are seen in the middle of the maxillary sinuses. The patient cannot extend his chin any further. Which of the following would correct the view:

a. tilt the film 15 degrees away from the forehead

b. angle the beam 5–7 degrees cephalic

c. angle the beam 10–12 degrees caudal

d. angle the beam 15 degrees cephalic

e. angle the beam 20–22 degrees caudal

80. On a Townes (Grashey) view the petrous ridges are seen only one-half inch above the superior rims of the orbits and lie at a shallow angle about 15 degrees from horizontal. Which of the following caused this problem:

a. the patient did not get his chin flexed down enough

b. the patient flexed his chin down too much

c. too much caudal beam angle was used

d. the beam was centered too superior

e. the head was tilted

81. On a Townes (Grashey) view, the petrous pyramids appear assymetrical. The opisthion (mid-point of the foramen magnum) and the EOP are seen to the *right* of the junction of the petrous ridges and the bony nasal septum. The patient's face was:

a. tilted to the patient's right

b. tilted to the patient's left

c. rotated to the patient's right

d. rotated to the patient's left

82. A lateral view of the skull shows vertical (up and down) shifting of the orbital plates of the frontal bone as well as the posterior fossae of the occipital bone. This is due to:

a. rotation

b. flexion

c. extension

d. tilt

83. Superimposition of the lateral rims of the orbits is a *poor* criterion for determining head rotation on lateral views for:

a. sinus series

b. facial bone series

c. skull series

d. nasal bone series

84. A lateral skull view shows the posterior surfaces of the mandibular rami shifted off of each other side-to-side about one inch. How much was the head rotated:

a. 5 degrees

b. 10 degrees

c. 15 degrees

d. 20 degrees

85. On a submentovertex view of the skull, more cranial wall can be seen laterally to the *right* ramus of the mandible than can be seen on the left.

    a. the top of the patient's head was tilted to the right

    b. the top of the patient's head was tilted to the left

    c. the patient's head was rotated to the right

    d. the patient's head was rotated to the left

    e. the patient's head was too flexed

86. A submentovertical projection of the zygomatic arches can be obtained by:

    a. using reduced FFD in bilateral projection

    b. hyperextending the head in bilateral projection

    c. tilting the head 15 degrees to each side for unilateral projections

    d. all of these

    e. none of these

87. A Rheese view shows the optic foramen projected in the middle of lower half of the orbit. The patient's head was:

    a. too flexed

    b. too extended

    c. rotated too shallow (too lateral)

    d. rotated too steep (toward PA)

88. A lateral oblique view of the mandible shows the upside gonion projected about one inch above the downside gonion. To correct this position:

    a. Tilt the head an additional 10 degrees toward the film

    b. Tilt the head an additional 20 degrees toward the film

    c. Reduce the cephalic angle of the x-ray beam by 15 degrees

    d. Rotate the face 20 degrees toward the film

89. A lateral view for a mastoid series shows the upside EAM projected 1 and $\frac{1}{2}$ inches directly below the downside EAM. This view was taken with:

    a. 15 degrees caudal beam angle, no head rotation

    b. 15 degrees of head rotation, no beam angle

    c. 5 degrees caudal beam angle, top of head tilted 5 degrees downward from chin

    d. a double 15-degree beam angle

90. A Stenver or Arcelin view shows the petrous pyramid extending into the orbit. This position was:

    a. rotated too shallow (too lateral)

    b. rotated too steep (toward PA or AP)

    c. flexed too much

    d. extended too much

Chapter 10

91. The actual amount of metallic silver deposited in a given area of the film determines the _____ of that area:
    a. gray scale
    b. visibility
    c. contrast
    d. density
    e. noise

92. The amount of light which can pass through a given area on the film is called its:
    a. penumbra
    b. visibility
    c. tone value
    d. density
    e. contrast

93. A radiograph which is very dark overall but also shows a few bright white areas was most likely:
    a. overexposed
    b. underexposed
    c. correctly exposed
    d. fogged
    e. blurred

94. The mAs should be considered the primary control for image:
    a. density
    b. contrast
    c. sharpness
    d. magnification
    e. noise

95. If blue-sensitive film is used in a green-emitting screen, which of the following will occur:
    a. loss of contrast
    b. loss of density
    c. loss of sharpness
    d. mottling

96. With all other factors unchanged, OFD is increased, image density will:
    a. directly increase
    b. directly decrease
    c. not change at all
    d. may change slightly, but will NOT likely be a VISIBLE change
    e. may be affected INDIRECTLY, but it does not directly control it

Chapter 11

97. A radiograph with many different shades of density possesses:
    a. low contrast

    b. short gray scale

    c. high tone value

    d. fog

    e. high noise

98. A radiograph with only a few different shades of density possesses:

    a. high contrast

    b. long gray scale

    c. low density

    d. low tone value

    e. low noise

99. Which of the following should always be optimized at a medium level:

    a. sharpness

    b. magnification

    c. contrast

    d. shape distortion

    e. noise

100. Desirable gray scale in the image is lengthened by increasing:

    a. fog

    b. tissue atomic number

    c. mAs

    d. penetration

101. Which of the following is *most* essential to producing a radiographic image:

    a. adequate penetration

    b. adequate intensity

    c. adequate collimation

    d. adequate exposure length

    e. adequate distance

102. A radiograph made with proper mAs, but excessive kVp would appear:

    a. dark but with some contrasty, light areas

    b. dark but with foggy gray areas

    c. light but with washed-out gray areas

    d. pitch black with no visible detail at all

    e. medium density with high contrast

103. An x-ray beam with the ability to penetrate more different types of tissue will result in what change in image quality:

    a. higher contrast

    b. longer gray scale

    c. increased tone value

    d. increased mottle

    e. more sharpness of detail

104. With all other factors unchanged, if field size is reduced, image contrast will:

    a. directly increase

    b. directly decrease

    c. not change at all

    d. may change slightly, but will NOT likely be a VISIBLE change

    e. may be affected INDIRECTLY, but it does not directly control it

105. With all other factors unchanged, if OFD is increased, image fog will:
    a. directly increase
    b. directly decrease
    c. not change at all
    d. may change slightly, but will NOT likely be a VISIBLE change
    e. may be affected INDIRECTLY, but it does not directly control it

Chapter 12

106. Which of the following is NOT a cause of scatter radiation:
    a. increased mAs
    b. increased kVp
    c. increased field size
    d. increased patient thickness

107. Which of the following is NOT affected by fog in the image:
    a. contrast
    b. gray scale
    c. resolution
    d. sharpness of recorded detail

108. Fog is a form of:
    a. signal
    b. information
    c. noise
    d. blur

109. Production of scatter radiation is *most* dramatically affected by:
    a. x-ray beam energy
    b. x-ray beam intensity
    c. the amount of tissue exposed
    d. film size used

110. Fog increases:
    a. penumbra
    b. umbra
    c. gray scale
    d. density

111. *All* scatter radiation:
    a. can be eliminated with grids
    b. reaches the film
    c. is produced within the patient
    d. is secondary radiation

112. At the edges of an image, fog:
    a. reduces penumbra
    b. spreads penumbra
    c. has no effect on penumbra
    d. increases visibility

113. A radiograph whose lightest density is a medium gray has most likely been:

    a. overexposed
    b. underexposed
    c. correctly exposed
    d. fogged
    e. blurred

114. False images can be created by:
    a. misalignment of the x-ray beam
    b. artifacts
    c. tomographic motion
    d. angling of the film in relation to the part

115. Which of the following can reduce BOTH contrast and gray scale at the same time?
    a. high penetration
    b. high screen speeds
    c. high grid ratios
    d. high levels of scatter

116. Which of the following is NOT a form of image noise:
    a. false images
    b. mottle
    c. fog
    d. artifacts
    e. signal

117. Scatter radiation emitted from the patient is random in direction, but follows the:
    a. overall direction of the primary beam
    b. inverse square law
    c. shortest path to the film
    d. law of isometry

118. Fog can destroy image:
    a. contrast
    b. gray scale
    c. visibility
    d. all of these
    e. none of these

Chapter 13

119. Which of the following should always be *maximized:*
    a. density
    b. contrast
    c. magnification
    d. elongation
    e. sharpness

120. Which of the following is equivalent to low sharpness:
    a. high umbra
    b. low tone value

    c. good blur

    d. short gray scale

    e. high penumbra

121. Which of the following is equivalent to low penumbra:

    a. low sharpness

    b. high sharpness

    c. high blur

    d. low distortion

    e. low magnification

122. mA has no effect upon image sharpness *because* it does not relate to:

    a. scatter proportions

    b. geometry

    c. intensity

    d. exposure rate

    e. distribution of photons

123. Smaller focal spot sizes cause:

    a. less magnification

    b. less density

    c. less "off-focus" radiation

    d. more anode heel effect

    e. less blur

124. Which of the following would be reduced when changing from a par speed calcium tungstate screen to a high-plus speed calcium tungstate screen:

    a. density

    b. contrast

    c. sharpness of detail

    d. magnification

    e. shape distortion

125. With all other factors unchanged, if OFD is decreased, image sharpness of detail will:

    a. directly increase

    b. directly decrease

    c. not change at all

    d. may change slightly, but will NOT likely be a VISIBLE change

    e. may be affected INDIRECTLY, but it does not directly control it

Chapter 14

126. The ratio between focus-film distance and focus-object distance is the primary control for image:

    a. magnification

    b. shape distortion

    c. density

    d. contrast

127. Short FFD may intentionally be used on TMJ or SC Joint procedures to:

    a. achieve adequate density

    b. magnify the anatomy of interest

    c. blur and magnify obstructing anatomy

    d. enhance contrast

128. With all other factors unchanged, if FFD is decreased, image magnification will:
    a. directly increase
    b. directly decrease
    c. not change at all
    d. may change slightly, but will NOT likely be a VISIBLE change
    e. may be affected INDIRECTLY, but it does not directly control it

129. With all other factors unchanged, if OFD is reduced, image magnification will:
    a. directly increase
    b. directly decrease
    c. not change at all
    d. may change slightly, but will NOT likely be a VISIBLE change
    e. may be affected INDIRECTLY, but it does not directly control it

130. The formula for calculating magnification factors is:
    a. FFD/FOD
    b. FFD/OFD
    c. FFD/FFD–FOD
    d. OFD/FFD–OFD

131. The image of an object on the film measures 10 inches across. The FFD used was 25 inches and the object was set 15 inches above the film. How big is the object:
    a. 2″
    b. 4″
    c. 3″
    d. 5″
    e. 6″

Chapter 15

132. The projected image of a bone on a radiograph is twice as wide and three times as long as the real bone. The image is:
    a. magnified
    b. distorted
    c. unsharp
    d. both A and B
    e. both B and C

133. Foreshortening is a form of:
    a. magnification
    b. noise
    c. umbra
    d. distortion
    e. artifact

134. Beam-part-film alignment is the primary control for image:
     a. magnification
     b. shape distortion
     c. sharpness of recorded detail
     d. resolution
135. With all other factors unchanged, if the CR is angled to be perpendicular to an object which is tilted in relation to the film, image shape distortion will:
     a. directly increase
     b. directly decrease
     c. not change at all
     d. may change slightly, but will not likely be a visible change
     e. may be affected *indirectly,* but it does not directly control it
136. Which of the following does NOT directly affect the degree of shape distortion in an image:
     a. object thickness and shape
     b. angle of the object in relation to the film
     c. angle of the x-ray beam in relation to the object
     d. centering of the x-ray beam to the object
     e. focus-film distance
137. Which of the following types of objects, if any long axis they possess is kept parallel to the film, will show the most shape distortion when an x-ray beam is angled 25 degrees to them:
     a. a wedge-shaped object
     b. a thick, flat object
     c. a thin, tubular object
     d. a thick spherical object
     e. a small spherical object
138. Shape distortion is controlled by:
     a. screen speed
     b. tube movement
     c. focal spot size
     d. alignment
     e. distance

Chapter 16

139. Information can be lost if an image has:
     a. excessive contrast
     b. excessive gray scale
     c. excessive blur
     d. any of these
     e. none of these
140. The ability to distinguish two adjacent details as being separate and distinct from each other defines:
     a. contrast

     b. sharpness of detail

     c. resolution

     d. visibility

141. Image resolution depends on:

     a. sharpness of recorded detail

     b. contrast

     c. visibility

     d. geometrical integrity

     e. all of these

142. Which of the following is NOT a component of image penumbra:

     a. geometrical penumbra

     b. absorption penumbra

     c. fog penumbra

     d. all of these are components of penumbra

143. Density trace diagrams show how both sharpness and contrast in an image affect its:

     a. edge gradient

     b. acutance

     c. density

     d. gray scale

144. The total resolution for an imaging system is measured by physicists as:

     a. acutance

     b. modulation transfer function

     c. spatial frequency

     d. quantum mottle

145. Density trace diagrams show that the ability to distinguish adjacent details as being separate and distinct details depends upon:

     a. visibility factors

     b. geometrical integrity

     c. both of these

     d. neither of these

146. An image with a steep edge gradient, and therefore a high contrast/penumbra ratio, will present:

     a. high resolution

     b. low visibility

     c. low geometrical integrity

     d. low distortion

147. Resolution can be measured in:

     a. LLP/mm

     b. MTF

     c. S/C

     d. seconds

148. Which shape of object produces the worst absorption penumbra:

     a. trapezoid

     b. upright triangular

  c. cuboid
  d. spherical
149. Motion does NOT affect which of the following image qualities:
  a. overall contrast
  b. false images
  c. shape distortion
  d. sharpness of detail
150. Which of the following contribute to blur:
  a. geometrical penumbra
  b. absorption penumbra
  c. motion
  d. parallax
  e. all of these

APPENDIX 3

ANSWERS TO REVIEW QUESTIONS IN APPENDIX 2

1. C	31. C	61. A	91. D	121. B
2. D	32. D	62. B	92. C	122. B
3. B	33. C	63. C	93. A	123. E
4. D	34. C	64. B	94. A	124. C
5. C	35. A	65. B	95. B	125. A
6. A	36. A	66. C	96. B	126. A
7. C	37. C	67. A	97. A	127. C
8. B	38. B	68. D	98. A	128. A
9. D	39. A	69. B	99. C	129. B
10. A	40. C	70. C	100. D	130. A
11. C	41. A	71. C	101. A	131. B
12. A	42. A	72. B	102. B	132. D
13. C	43. C	73. C	103. B	133. D
14. B	44. D	74. C	104. A	134. B
15. B	45. D	75. C	105. B	135. A
16. D	46. A	76. B	106. A	136. E
17. C	47. B	77. C	107. D	137. D
18. B	48. C	78. E	108. C	138. D
19. A	49. D	79. C	109. C	139. D
20. A	50. A	80. A	110. D	140. C
21. A	51. C	81. D	111. D	141. E
22. C	52. D	82. D	112. C	142. C
23. C	53. C	83. C	113. D	143. A
24. C	54. D	84. B	114. C	144. B
25. B	55. B	85. A	115. D	145. C
26. A	56. C	86. D	116. E	146. A
27. B	57. B	87. D	117. B	147. A
28. C	58. B	88. B	118. D	148. D
29. D	59. B	89. A	119. E	149. C
30. A	60. B	90. B	120. E	150. E

INDEX